YOGA

for Business Executives and Professional People

By the same author

PHILOSOPHY, AN INTRODUCTION
PHILOSOPHY OF THE BUDDHA
TAO THE KING BY LAO TZU
WHAT MAKES ACTS RIGHT?
LOGIC FOR BEGINNERS
TYPES OF INTUITION
YOGA, UNION WITH THE ULTIMATE
DIRECTORY OF AMERICAN PHILOSOPHERS
THE WORLD'S LIVING RELIGIONS

YOGA

for business executives and professional people

by ARCHIE J. BAHM

THE CITADEL PRESS NEW YORK

FIRST EDITION

 Published by The Citadel Press, 222 Park Avenue South, New York, N. Y. 10003. Manufactured in the United States of America. Published simultaneously in Canada by George G. McLeod, Ltd.

Library of Congress Catalog Card No.: 65-15493

To ELAINE, my daughter

Contents

YOGA

for Business Executives and Professional People

CHAPTER I

What Is Yoga?

A man standing on his head, a woman giving food to a beggar, a monk sitting cross-legged hidden away in a silent cave, a man emptying his bowels in a river, a priest intermingling the flames of several fires in a Kali temple, a pupil listening to and learning from his teacher, and a business executive sitting at his desk stretching his fingers, straightening his spine and taking a few extra breaths—all these may be practicing yoga. The term "Yoga" properly applies to an amazingly wide range of interests and activities, though we cannot go into all of them here. The purpose of the present volume is to explore only a very restricted phase of yoga, namely, that which pertains directly to physical and mental health through breathing and posture exercises—which can also aid in reducing anxiety, temporarily and in the long run. The traditional name for this restricted phase of yoga is "hatha yoga."

Furthermore, we shall limit our pursuit to those aspects of hatha yoga which appear to be clearly in accord with Western medical knowledge and physical education theory. We will avoid anything which may be called "occult." We shall deal only with what each reader may try out for himself to see whether he can obtain the practical results achieved by others.

Hatha yoga, as we shall show, is largely a matter of common sense. Appreciation of it will require a little experimentation, some discovery of how the fruits of relaxation may follow from certain simple actions and the development of healthy habits—at least if one would retain continuing feelings of freedom from nervous strain and fatigue.

Before launching into our exposition of hatha yoga, we will mention briefly the other major varieties of yoga, not for the purpose of exploring them, but to sketch out a map of the immense, panoramic cultural background from which they have come and to make it clear that not every book with "Yoga" in its title deals with precisely the same thing.

The vast array of kinds of yoga has come to be classified customarily under four main headings. However, each of these four kinds contains a complex of subvarieties, and all four intermingle. Each, at times, seems to absorb all of the others. The four are called "karma yoga," "bhakti yoga," "gnana yoga" and "raja yoga." We shall devote a brief section to each. Other well-known types have been subsumed under these four; but these other types may also be considered independent varieties, as we shall show.

First, however, we should look at the general meaning of the term yoga. It is a word of many different meanings. Yet, despite all the differences that we shall indicate, it retains a common core of meaning throughout. The Sanskrit term *yoga,* like its English relative "yoke," refers to union, or reunion, and hence the return of the individual self to an original state in which its being and nature were perfect. Hindus typically conceive ultimate reality as quiescent, peaceful, undisturbed by anything. Different schools of thought do disagree about some characteristics of the self in its ultimate condition. The Jain and Samkhya-Yoga schools hold that each self exists as an individual independent of all other individual selves. The Advaita Vedanta school believes that a self loses all individuality by becoming aware of its mergence into a single world soul, atman, in which all difference, which is believed to be illusory anyway, disappears completely. Theravada Buddhism claims that a self exists as an impermanent, momentary self-awareness which mistakenly believes itself to be an enduring entity. Nevertheless, despite these differences, all schools idealize ultimate reality as a condition in which all disturbances, including all desires, distinctions, attachments, yearnings and anxiety about the future have ceased to exist. Since ultimate reality is perfectly pacific, any self which has become roused out of the original ultimate blissful peace has as its goal in life to return to, or to restore itself to, such beatific bliss. The term yoga refers not only to the final act of reunion, which is also called *moksha* or *mukti,* but to any step which brings one even the least bit closer to his ultimate goal.

Thus the word yoga is at once a term for the ultimate goal of religion and for every act or intention which is directed in the right way. Any endeavor which increases the peacefulness of one's state of mind, and correspondingly decreases its tension and anxiety, may properly be called *yoga.* The age-long experiences of Hindu rishis in searching for ways to remove mental disturbances have resulted in some very practical measures which can prove useful to whoever desires to employ them as a means to relaxation, even though he may not be at all interested in—and may disbelieve in—the more distant goal of perfect quiescence which motivated Hindu endeavors in the first place.

I. KARMA YOGA

Karma yoga presupposes a Law of Karma, a universal principle of reciprocity according to which each good you do will beget a good reward, whereas each evil you do will result in an evil return. This principle is presumed to operate universally, without exception, automatically and without favor to anyone. Since acts can be right or wrong only to the extent that they are voluntary or intentional, one's "doing good" or "doing evil" consists essentially in having good or evil intentions. Intentions naturally result in actions whenever conditions permit. But intentions which cannot be carried out only because the opportunity does not arise nevertheless count as actions, good or bad, so far as the Law of Karma is concerned. In fact, intentions to act in certain ways become established as habits of intending to act in those ways.

Thus, tendencies to act become latent in one's nature. They perpetuate the direction of one's desires either toward greater evil, zeal and anxiety or toward greater good, willingness and calmness. Ultimately, he who genuinely desires peace will intend and act in such a way that more peace will come to him. He will even intend a more peaceful desiring of peace.

On the other hand, a person whose disposition causes him to want excitement will desire, and do, what brings him aroused passions and frightening tensions, and eventually such troublesome desires (those bound to be frustrated) that he will become perplexed even regarding whether or not to desire more desiring.

Anything so universal as the Law of Karma applies everywhere: one finds it operating in every phase of life. In dealings with one's friends, neighbors, members of the family, employees, employers, customers, fellow citizens, or passersby, one wishes them well or ill and acts accordingly. If custom, codes or law enter into one's circumstances, his attitude toward them, involving willingness and good will regarding outcomes of acting relative to them, generates fitting rewards. When opportunities for social service present themselves, whether for easing the pain, hunger or fear in individuals or for promoting public welfare, one's intentions automatically come into play and spontaneously generate fitting fruits. Thus whatever one's duties appear to be, whether to husband, employer, country or God, one's intentions regarding them automatically beget results.

One may recognize that some good deeds reap good rewards immediately. When one pays a compliment or gives a gift to a friend, a similar compliment or gift may be returned immediately. But some results must be delayed. How long? We do not know. But if the Law of Karma is a principle of universal justice, we can expect justice to prevail in the long run. If one's karmas—or "good karmas" and "bad karmas," as the seeds which eventually bear fruit are called —do not yield obvious results in the present, then they will do so in the future. One argument for a future life, or for a series of reincarnations, is that when one's good and bad karmas do not balance in one life, then justice demands another life. A surplus of bad karmas will lead to rebirth in a more miserable (less calm) status, whereas a surplus of good karmas will bring about rebirth in a more lofty and peaceful (less anxious) body, stratum of society or social situation.

Without presuming anything regarding the reader's views on reincarnation or cosmic justice, we may nevertheless assert that a person's actions do have effects upon his future somewhat in accordance with his intentions. Whether or not principles of reciprocity function with precision, we believe that they work sufficiently well so that the more willingly one accepts the situation in which he finds himself as desirable, the more he tends to create for himself a present and future set of conditions conducive to greater satisfaction and freedom from disturbance. A person may rankle at his duties. Hindu theory holds that when a person does his duty for the sake of rewards rather than for duty's sake, he is less likely to receive rewards. "For duty's sake" here means doing willingly what he ought to do, however such duty is conceived, regardless of whether or not he will ever receive recompense. To will to do good even without reward is a better act than willing to do good only if good is to be returned. Hence whoever seeks what is best for himself will do good regardless of results.

Although orthodox Hinduism, like traditional Christianity, believes that full justice can be done only in "future life," anyone, regardless of his beliefs about life after death, may observe that a principle of reciprocity operates naturally, and more or less justly, in human nature. It does so in such a way that one who produces an attitude of confidence in others finds others coming to have confidence in him. We tend to distrust those who distrust us. So the amount and intensity of anxiety prevailing in our business and professional lives is due in part to our own unwillingness to do more than is required of us without promise of being fully rewarded.

II. BHAKTI YOGA

Bhakti yoga is the "way of devotion." A person may devote himself to his spouse, to his parents, to his children, to his country, to his God, to his studies, to his profession, to his corporation, or to his specialized responsibilities. The more one devotes himself to whatever he has committed himself to, the more he unites himself with it, the more he projects himself into it and the more he finds his own worth and value identified with it. Such identification is a kind of yoga. This is because the more a person feels at one with whatever he is dedicated to, the less he feels himself opposed to it. Feelings of opposition naturally generate tension and anxiety. These naturally subside as one's feeling of opposition transforms itself into a feeling of unity or identity.

Again, although orthodox Hinduism often channels its forms of devotion into service to local deities (much as we submit to our enjoyable Christmas duties, if not to Paul's wrathful and loving God), bhakti yoga encompasses devotions of all kinds. What is most important is the completeness and unselfishness with which one devotes himself, rather than the particular object or cause to which he is devoted. For bhakti yoga and karma yoga, although distinct in nature, remain inseparable. One's devotions (which obviously involve intentions) produce good karmas; unless, of course, one deliberately devotes himself to doing evil, or serves only because he expects rewards. And when, following the way of karma yoga, one dedicates himself to doing his duty, especially duty for duty's sake, he is already pursuing the path of devotion.

III. GNANA YOGA

Gnana yoga is the "way of knowledge." (The *gn* in "gnana" and the *kn* in "knowledge" have etymological connections, illustrating the surprisingly intimate relations between Sanskrit and English and, for that matter, among all of the Indo-European languages.) This way to, or toward, the goal of life involves a study of philosophy, or of the nature of knowledge and reality, so that achievement of insight into the truth will lead naturally to a commitment of the will to believe what is true, and consequently to acting in accordance with such truth.

Although different schools of Hindu philosophy disagree regarding details concerning the nature of knowledge and reality, all agree that, in its most ultimate state, being is quiescent, undisturbed by anxieties or cares for things of this world. All of them agree that, no matter how complex, prolonged or arduous the task, or how intricate the ethical precepts and problems encountered along the way, the ultimate goal of ethics, of religion and of life consists in achieving eventually such a state of quiescence. A person can pursue the way of knowledge under a teacher, by reading what others have said, whether in ancient scriptures or modern books, and by his own meditating upon the life he lives. The more he knows about and accepts the truth that ultimate reality is quiescent, the closer he approaches his goal. The way to know such quiescence is by progressively embodying it within himself or himself within it. Hence, the more fully he knowingly realizes his identity with what is ultimate, the more completely he feels himself united with it. Such feeling of unity with the ultimate is a kind of yoga.

Again, although the emphasis in gnana yoga seems distinct from those of karma and bhakti yoga, since it stresses learning, reading and thinking rather than concern for rewards or devoutness, nevertheless it too intermingles or merges with them. For one who is devoted to his studies, to learning, reading and thinking may, nay must, be fully devoted to them if he expects to achieve complete insight. Such devotion functions as bhakti just as much as any other kind. And, since knowing the ultimate and best in the way of knowledge, reality and value is obviously a good, when one seeks such knowing he is intending to do what is best. Such intending and acting begets rewards in accordance with the Law of Karma just as much as other kinds of intentions and actions. Here, too, paradoxically, when one studies for truth's sake rather than for the sake of rewards from such study, he builds up an ever greater store of good karmas. (Here we may observe the Hindu way of justifying that attitude required in all honest investigation–an attitude which, in Western science, is said to aim at "objectivity.")

IV. RAJA YOGA

Raja yoga is sometimes referred to in English as the "path of concentration." However, the term "concentration" must be explained before such reference can become clear. Concentration here has two different meanings, both of which are involved, but in different ways.

First, concentration pertains literally to "con-center-ation," a process of centering, centralizing or unifying all of one's diverse, and thus divergent, aspects together. Ultimate reality remains unitary and awareness of it can be achieved only by eliminating attention to diversity. The process of eliminating such attention is thus a process of concentrating attention. Anything which aids in reducing awareness of diversity and increasing awareness of unity is a yoga.

The second meaning of concentration in English has to do with "concentrated effort," though such effort, paradoxically, cannot succeed until it becomes "effortless." Since one can hardly eliminate attention to the various sensuous, intellectual and social attractions without some effort, effort is needed. And the more effort put forth to attain "single-mindedness," the quicker it will be attained. But so long as a person focuses upon such effort, rather than upon the goal in which effort will have been eliminated, he will be short of the goal. Hence, the concentrated effort, referred to in this secondary meaning of concentration, requires an act of will sufficiently strong to overcome its own willfulness to attain the end before it can be attained by concentration, union or yoga, in the first and primary sense.

The ultimate aim of raja yoga, as of all the traditional yogas being considered here, is attainment of complete quiescence. The means, which have become standardized under raja yoga, emphasize a fairly well-defined series of specific kinds of steps to control attention. Whereas karma yoga stressed good deeds and good intentions, especially doing duty for duty's sake, and bhakti yoga urged devotion, especially utter and complete devotion as a way to eliminate selfishness, and gnana yoga advised study, reflection, knowledge of the truth, especially such knowledge as brings one actually closer to the goal, raja yoga advocates deliberate control over all mental acts, including sensing, remembering, imagining, inferring, intending and even self-awareness.

Although the various emphases clearly differ, raja yoga also intermingles with, or rather incorporates into itself, all of the other yogas. Karma yoga is presupposed; for one can hardly expect himself to be able to practice raja yoga until he has earned enough good karmas to be rewarded with a sufficiently favorable condition in life where it becomes possible for him to practice it. (And each good intention motivating his practice of raja yoga increases his store of good karmas.) Bhakti yoga is presupposed, not merely because devotions are involved in karma and gnana yoga, but because one cannot make much progress in raja yoga without devoting himself completely to it. (And his devotion to the various steps in raja yoga is a kind of devotion, or bhakti yoga, just as much as any other kind.) Gnana yoga is presupposed since one can hardly progress very far through raja yoga toward a goal which he does not comprehend. One does not gain much genuine comprehension, or knowledge, of the nature of the goal until he has actually experienced some progress toward it through the ways which raja yoga emphasizes.) Thus, while raja yoga presupposes something of each of the other yogas, those who favor it hold that all the others are means to it for it alone can bring one actually to, or even close to, the ultimate goal.

Raja yoga, conceived as a way or path, has been organized traditionally into eight steps or stages. Perhaps the most famous formulation of these stages is that attributed to Patanjali whose yoga sutras include a systematic statement of the eightfold path or the eight "limbs" of yoga. For details of this formulation, see my recent volume, *Yoga: Union with the Ultimate,* A New Version of the Ancient Yoga Sutras of Patanjali (Frederick Ungar Publishing Co., New York, 1961).

This volume also includes an introduction not only to the many kinds of Hindu yoga but also to Buddhist, Taoist, Confucian, Moslem and Christian yogas. The eight steps may be summarized as follows:

1. "Abstention" *(yama)* refers to refraining from all kinds of evil intentions and, consequently, from all kinds of evil actions. Prominent among the results of this are unwillingness to harm life in any way *(ahimsa)*, unwillingness to lie, deceive or speak harshly or slanderously *(satya)*, unwillingness to steal or take anything at all which is not given *(asteya)*, unwillingness to be greedy, passionate or incontinent in any way *(brahmacharya)*, and unwillingness to own or to accept from other people more goods than are needed *(aparigraha)*. Willing acceptance of all moral taboos regarding evil intentions or actions reaches its culmination in the development of habits of automatic and spontaneous restraint of any tendency to follow a temptation to do evil. Abstention is not merely a preparation for social acceptance by others and a moral clearing of the ground for further advance. It involves a phase of yoga which might be called "negative peace." By restraining his desires to manage things his own way, a person achieves diminution of his own aggressiveness and thus becomes relieved of both outer conflict with others and the inner strains involved in pressing forth his own willfulness. Thus each abstention is itself already a yoga.

2. "Devotion" *(niyama)* refers to the positive side of intentions and actions. *Niyama* consists in having good intentions, just as *yama* consists in refraining from bad intentions. But, further, *yama* and *niyama* involve more than merely momentary or recurrent willingness to avoid evil intentions and embody good intentions. They function as enduring tendencies which come to embody themselves so completely in one's nature that he becomes unreservedly devoted to them. *Niyama* means giving oneself entirely over to having good intentions

for positive action. It exists in experience as complete willingness to do what is needed, just as *yama* occurs as complete unwillingness to do what is evil.

Niyama also applies to all needed positive actions. Five varieties have been distinguished: (a) "cleanliness" *(sauca)* or purification of the body by washing, seeking wholesome foods and cherishing good thoughts; (b) "serenity" *(santosa)* or a pervading feeling of contentment with things as they are; (c) "self-discipline" *(tapas)* or wanting to do all that is required to achieve the goal; (d) "self-study" *(svadhyaya)* or seeking to understand the true nature of self; (e) persistent endeavor to attain the ideal self *(isvara-pranidhana)* or supreme state of completely quiescent self.

3. "Posture" *(asana)* refers basically to a bodily position which is comfortable, effortless, and stable. Asana without further qualification commonly means Lotus Posture (see Plate 136) but, as we shall see, the term has been extended to include many other standardized postures and even series of positions. These postures, although all yogic in nature and purpose, may serve as exercises for conditioning the body in preparation for more advanced yogic effort, as well as being steady, comfortable and pacifying in themselves. Since most of the present volume will be allotted to consideration of asana, or of "the asanas," further discussion of its nature will be omitted here. Asana is yogic both because it promotes quietude of all bodily stirrings and because it prepares the way for the following stages.

4. "Breathing," or controlled, relaxed and energizing breathing *(pranayama),* pertains not only to inhaling and exhaling air but also to surrendering the whole self, bodily and mentally, to breathing. One must look beyond the detailed varieties of instruction, which include such directions as inhaling first through the right nostril, then through the left and then through both, to a more profound conception

of breathing. A person may breathe with his whole body rather than with just his nose. He may feel himself so fully identified with his breathing processes, deepened and slowed, regularized and steadied, that he experiences his whole self as a slowly, rhythmically pulsating being.

Such experience may be yogic in many senses. First, the regularizing of breathing induces a feeling of stability and thus of unity. Secondly, one's feeling himself identified with his breathing process constitutes another aspect of unity. Thirdly, his attending to his breathing, and to himself as a breathing being, draws his attention away from other distracting and disuniting attractions. Finally, his attaining an overwhelming soothingness which becomes habitual prepares the way for undisturbed attention to the next stages of yoga. An additional and important aspect of *pranayama* is the growth of energy and a sense of power, as well as euphoria, which is both needed for, and conducive to, the stages which follow it.

Again, since a whole chapter of the present volume will be assigned to exploring the nature, ways and values of breathing, further details will be omitted here. Perhaps, however, we should mention in passing certain additional developments related to raja yoga. Some of these are called, collectively, "laya yoga" and pertain to a deliberate effort to attain, control and direct, by specific acts of attention, the energy produced from deep, prolonged body breathing. However, consideration of the elaborate theory regarding the nature of *kundalini* ("coiled" or "serpent" power) and directions for developing and controlling it, remain beyond the scope of the present work.

5. "Retraction of the senses" *(pratyahara)* refers to cessation of sensation by withdrawing attention from all sensory stimuli, thereby eliminating awareness also of sensory objects. This process is yogic in several ways. First, a person may pro-

ceed to master attention to each one of the different senses —seeing, hearing, tasting, smelling, and touching. When successful, one is no longer disturbed by awareness of sensuous objects, their movements, any desire to own or change or destroy, or any stimulation by, or distraction by, them. Secondly, as one loses awareness of objects and sensations, he withdraws attention inwardly and thereby becomes more self-contained or self-unified. Thirdly, as external disturbances fail to arouse him, he achieves a more quiescent state of mind. Finally, this stage too is preparatory for those which follow.

6. "Fixation of attention" *(dharana)* pertains to "singlemindedness," or holding the mind steady by fixing it upon a single object. Before the senses have been completely withdrawn, one may practice dharana by focusing his gaze upon some immovable thing, such as a distant mountain peak, the tip of his nose or, as popularly depicted, his navel. But after attention to the senses has been withdrawn, one needs to focus upon some imaginary object. Focus he must, for otherwise his more or less vivid memories, his creative imagination, his intellectual inferences, his desires for more, for a better (hence different) future, all keep his mind stirred up in a variegated flux of activity. As everyone knows, dreams may turn into terrifying nightmares even when one no longer attends wakefully to sensuous objects. Yogic quietude becomes profound and pervasive only after one has mastered his thought processes as well as his senses.

7. "Fusive apprehension" *(dhyana)* names that process and state of mind in which the self as intuiter and any mental object which is intuited tend to merge into each other. Awareness of opposition between subject and object becomes insignificant, even when it does not completely disappear. The very object, which was selected for holding one's gaze steady or one's attention focused singlemindedly, grad-

ually ceases to be an object distinct from the subject. This fusion is the most yogic or unified stage thus far considered. But it too leads to another.

8. Finally, "fully integrated consciousness" *(samadhi)* consists in disappearance of awareness of self, even as merged with its object. Awareness then becomes pure or perfect. Its unity is so great that no distinctions whatsoever appear in it. Its quiescence is complete. It cannot be disturbed by anything since no distinctions between one thing and another, not even between self and object, past and present, or desire and satisfaction, exist to provide any tension or any act of attention within it. Whether or not this is the final stage or a stage just prior to stagelessness, and what other subtle veils preventing final insight into reality must be discriminated and overcome before entering fully into the most ultimate state *(kaivalya),* cannot be gone into here. These have been dealt with in some detail in my *Yoga: Union with the Ultimate.* But we should mention that Patanjali allocates almost one fourth of his sutras to *samyama,* a process in which the last three of the eight stages function together. The three operating yogically as one are more yogic, in the sense that they help one toward the goal more rapidly, than either of the three alone. However, as one approaches more closely to the goal, the last stage alone and by itself is more yogic than even the three functioning together.

Before discussing hatha yoga specifically, two more common terms naming types of yoga will be mentioned. The first is "mantra yoga." Mantras are forms of speech which have their effects upon the mind. Some ways of speaking, some kinds of expression, some words, some sounds have effects which others do not have. These effects may be good or bad. Regarding them we may have good or bad intentions, and thus involve ourselves more deeply in good or bad karmas. Hence mantra yoga may be thought of as a phase of karma yoga, though the emphasis here is upon sounds and their meanings. Some sounds have more power to arouse and others to quiet. Those which disturb, arouse, irritate or distract us produce evil whereas those which pacify, soothe, and relax us promote good. The omnisonal syllable *om,* or *aum,* traditionally has been deemed the most holy, most sacred, most satisfying and most pacifying of sounds. Pronunciation of it is most yogic when one enunciates it, not just with his vocal cords or his mouth, but, as in body breathing, with his whole body or, better, with his whole mind-and-body or his whole self. When one gives over his whole being to the embodiment of *om* within himself, he thereby enjoys bhakti yoga also.

Yet mantra yoga, in popular practice, often degenerates into magic, as when one recites a formula for the purpose of influencing some issue in which fulfillment of his own desires is at stake. Hindu theory embraces mantra yoga as a type of yoga because one who indulges in it does so with certain attitudes and intentions in mind, and thus automatically sows seeds which eventually ripen as fruit called "good karmas" and "bad karmas" that inexorably conduct one toward, or further away from, the ultimate goal.

The second is "tantra yoga." Tantra yoga seems, in some respects, the most complex, subtle and sophisticated variety of yoga since it, too, presupposes all of the other varieties and adds a further dimension involving sexual orgasm, conceived as experiencing a loss of self in a cosmic identity, and requiring years of preparatory training in karma (including mantra), bhakti, gnana and the various stages of raja yoga. Nirvana, the goal, is pictured as a mystical ecstasy in which all self-awareness disappears in a boundless sea of bliss. The goal is much the same as that described in raja yoga, but an emotional tone of bliss prevails in the final stage of extinguished self-awareness. Since tantra yoga involves additional difficulties of needing to resist the dangers of succumbing to temptations to become desirous and of overcoming awareness of maleness and femaleness and opposition and differentiation involved therein while making progress in the practice of *samyama,* it is doubtless the most difficult of all yogic endeavors to bring to a successful conclusion. Hence, it is perhaps the most rare variety, most occult in its management and most secret in its teaching and transmission of doctrine and techniques.

The purpose of this long summary of kinds of yoga is to help the reader to realize, first of all, that the term "yoga" has an immense range of proper meanings and that he should not expect to find hatha yoga, the subject of this volume, dealt with in every treatise where the term "yoga" is used. Secondly, hatha yoga has emerged out of a long-enduring, rich, profound and complex civilization. Although, in what follows, we shall single out and explore only those phases of yoga which may be used, with convenience, assurance and immediately observable results, for purposes of relaxing our everyday tensions, the reader should know that these results, and the particular directions for achieving them, are in effect products of centuries of experimentation by people who devoted themselves to relaxation on a much grander scale. They were seeking an ultimately complete and total quiescence, whereas we shall draw from their more extensive experiences only those techniques which can bring us such measures of relief from nervous restlessness as we may happen to want and be willing to work for. The reader does not need to know or believe any of the other doctrines surveyed in order to attain relaxing results from simple hatha yoga exercises. But he should appreciate their virtues more if he realizes that these practices have been distilled from the practical wisdom of a centuries-old civilization.

V. HATHA YOGA

We turn now directly to the question "What is yoga?" meaning now "What is hatha yoga?" The term "yoga" will be used throughout the remainder of this volume to refer to hatha yoga unless otherwise explicitly indicated. Although, on the one hand, hatha yoga may be thought of as a phase of raja yoga, that phase comprising the third and fourth stages mentioned above, on the other hand, many experts in hatha yoga consider it a relatively self-sufficient, independent area of living. To those who see the goal of life as beyond life, hatha yoga is merely a means to an end. But some hatha yogins believe that life as lived from day to day has its goal already within itself. Nirvana exists as a state of mind, as an aspect of living which can be enjoyed here and now. One may now avoid living in constant anxiety, tension, torment and terror. These nirvanic states are ends in themselves and a person practices yoga for the sake of living peacefully, if not continuously then recurrently, or as often as he can find opportunity for escaping from daily torment. As will be noted in the following discussion of values of yoga, enjoyable relaxation may be attained both immediately in some small degree and also enduringly by those who develop persistent habits of relieving themselves of accumulating tensions and reviving their energy.

Hatha yoga, for our purposes, pertains primarily to those traditional ways of controlling posture, breathing and attention and several additional aids, which can yield either, or both, temporary relief or relatively enduring composure. I shall add some suggestions of my own which may be helpful for beginners. But I shall not try to exhaust all of the more intricate and extreme suggestions which lifelong yogins recommend as variations for their advanced students.

Hatha yoga, then, has to do primarily with relaxation of

tension. Such relaxation may be partial or complete. It ranges all the way from a momentary pause in, or reversal of, growing anxiety to a resurging of mental energy and a feeling of complete restedness. The more momentary or less enduring one's relaxation, the less yogic, or less yogically successful, it must be judged to be. The more complete, pervasive and persisting one's feeling of repose, the more yogic it is.

Each of the different parts of yoga has its own kind of contribution to make in bringing about relief from tension. (1) Breathing, which will be discussed first, may alone, without additional attention to posture, be redirected in such a way as to yield relaxing results. (2) Posture, which will be considered in Chapter III, may also, without deliberate attention to breathing, bring relief. But combining it with certain breathing techniques and other aids enables it to render its consequences more quickly or more wholesomely. Each of the many standard varieties of posture can contribute somewhat uniquely to the total result; and, although a person may prefer, or be able, to use only one or a few of the standard postures, the use of more of them tends to contribute to a more complete feeling of at-homeness in his present circumstances. (3) Each of the aids which will be mentioned in Chapter V may reinforce the services of breathing and postures, and should be considered mainly as supplementary to them. Yet some of these aids may be employed independently, especially at times when use of breathing and posture techniques seem inconvenient. (4) Finally, and this may be considered a relatively unique feature of the present volume, many "little yogas," as we shall call them, can be practiced at almost any time or place, with at first surprising and later reassuring and reliable effects. Usefulness of these, as with the more standard kinds of yoga, will vary with personal abilities and willingness to try to exploit them.

In closing our introductory remarks on hatha yoga, we

should note, perhaps, that it consists in what hatha yogins teach and what hatha yogins practice. One need not go to India to find out. For, not only do many volumes exist in English, but also many hatha yoga gurus ("guru" means teacher) live in the United States. So far as hatha yoga in America is concerned, it consists, in part, in what these men and women do and teach others to do, and what those taught, or self-taught, think and practice regarding it. For our purposes, hatha yoga consists basically in what we shall treat in the remainder of the volume.

CHAPTER II

Values of Yoga

Since the values of yoga depend upon the nature of yoga, and since the present work is limited to hatha yoga as just described, the values to be discussed here must be limited to those of hatha yoga so conceived. The following survey of values, and the later discussions of values of particular techniques, have been selected for business executives and professional people, keeping in mind their typical array of daily activities, responsibilities and anxieties. People weighted with complexes of responsibility naturally experience multitudes of frustrations. Their general problems involve growing tension and their greatest need often involves reducing such tension without losing their alertness, resiliency or ability to tackle additional changes without fatigue or irritability. Thus the values of yoga here bear primarily on such questions as how, how effectively, in how many ways and how conveniently it can cope with this general problem of growing tension.

The values of yoga for business and professional persons include not only those which may be achieved at home, or after hours, but also those which may be realized on the job. It is a matter of common knowledge that one who succeeds in working relaxedly becomes less fatigued and thus handles his tasks with greater ease, efficiency, adaptability and intelligence. When a person's tasks become so taxing that they cannot be accomplished without intense nervous strain, then if he can succeed in relaxing, even only partially and temporarily, while at work, he should be much better off than when he waits until evening or nighttime to put forth all of his recuperative efforts. Consequently, although I shall seek to reveal the values of yogic practices generally, I will endeavor to put special emphasis upon those techniques which may be employed during the day, in an office or in transit. I will do this, I feel, more extensively than has been done thus far in any other book on yoga.

The following classification of values, organized basically around the distinction between "physical" and "mental," is somewhat arbitrary. It is arbitrary, first, because the human person is an organic whole and, no matter how different the physical and mental aspects of a self may seem, each intimately and constantly interacts with the other. It is arbitrary, also, because not all of the values of yoga fit neatly into this classification. We will designate a third large section as Conveniences and group therein numerous miscellaneous advantages. Finally, we will notice some incidental or secondary values of yoga, such as possible increase in wealth or improvement of beauty. Although quite irrelevant so far as the basic aims of yoga are concerned, they do at times constitute additional values and may become motives, even primary motives, of some people for engaging in yogic practice.

Before launching into our systematic classification of values, we should note two other sets of distinctions which are needed to give proper perspective.

The first of these differentiates between more specific values, such as relief from discomfort in particular parts of the self or particular organs of the body (eyes, neck or limbs), and more general values, such as relief from weariness, depression or overwhelming anxiety. Although yoga can be of some help in dealing with specific discomforts, such as headaches, stiff neck, tired feet, spinal soreness, abdominal distress and muscular pains, its primary emphasis is upon general well-being. By attending to practices for improving, regaining or retaining general good health, a person is likely to find that some of his more specific difficulties tend to disappear. If one's general store of energy increases, more of it becomes available for consumption by particular organs. Tensions or strains affecting specific organs may be relieved, in part at least, by attention to the welfare of the whole organism and by a more balanced exercise of the body as a whole.

The standard yogic postures and exercises were designed to improve health generally rather than to give relief to a local pain. Yet, in describing the values of each of such standard postures, we will point out that some of them do benefit particular organs more directly than others. A sluggish or overworked stomach, for example, receives a great deal of attention through inner massages in torso exercises. A fatigued brain gains refreshment from a headstand posture. A normal yogic attitude toward dealing with difficulties in specific organs is to attend to them directly. If your eyes are tired, roll them. If your fingers have become stiff, stretch them. If your ears begin to ache, wiggle them or jiggle a finger in them. But yogic manuals do not normally catalogue aids for dealing with each organ individually. They focus, rather, upon series of poses and movements which induce more general beneficial results. Attention focuses upon specific postures and exercises rather than specific ailments. Benefits which some of these postures and exercises can have for specific ailments will be indicated as we consider them.

The second set of distinctions has to do with immediate versus long-range benefits. Many persons will be more interested in immediate effects. These will be given some attention here both because the immediate effects are, indeed, worth-while in themselves and because awareness of these effects may convince the curious that further benefits await them if they pursue yoga further. But the long-range values will prove most worth-while for those persistent enough to attain them. The distinction should be obvious enough in itself. It is not a sharp one dividing immediate and future values into two totally different classes. Rather the values experienced immediately become enlarged, more enduring and more pervasive with longer practice. The long-range values will be experienced in the future as immediate enjoyments, in addition to serving as improvements in the physiological and psychological foundations of one's being.

I. PHYSICAL HEALTH

According to Swami Sivananda, whose *Yoga Asanas* went through ten editions between 1934 and 1955, the benefits of *pranayama* (yogic breathing practices) include the following: "The body becomes strong and healthy. Too much fat is reduced. There is luster in the face. Eyes sparkle like diamonds. The practitioner becomes very handsome. Voice becomes sweet and melodious" (page 180). Clara Spring, in *Yoga for Today,* includes "radiant health, abundant vitality, a beautiful well-functioning body" as "birthrights" which yogic practices help to maintain (page 12). Indra Devi, in *Forever Young, Forever Healthy,* page 25, predicts: "You will be able to enjoy better sleep, a happier disposition, a clearer and calmer mind. You will learn how to build up your health and protect yourself against colds, fevers, constipation, headaches, fatigue, and other troubles. You will know what to do in order to remain youthful, vital and alert, regardless of your calendar-age; how to lose or gain weight; how to get rid of premature wrinkles, and keep a smooth skin and clear complexion."

These sample statements are typical summaries of some of the benefits to be expected from yogic exercises. While cautioning the reader against overbelief, we shall examine in detail some of the types of benefits available. The attainability of each of the stated goals is a matter of degree, the degree of achievement possible varying greatly with different persons. The attitude advocated here is that of experimental belief. That is, try out and see for yourself whether or not you can obtain the suggested values. Caution may be needed also against overdoing, for here as elsewhere overdoing turns a prospective good into an actual evil. Yet, also, whoever begins to try but gives up too soon cannot expect to gain the desired results.

The experimental attitude involves openness to trial and error, and also a willingness to persist in trials until each experiment has been given a fair test. Many persons can profit from some yogic postures but others cannot. Each person will succeed partly, but not completely, with most of his experiments. If a person does not achieve a minimum of success in his early attempts, he is likely to give up all further efforts. Hence, the present volume has been designed to initiate beginners into yogic practices also by way of "little yogas" (see Chapter V) in which the goal is minor but results can be recognized immediately.

A. Immediate Values

Two interrelated general types of values, which may be enjoyed in some measure rather quickly from some exercises, will be called (1) "reduction of fatigue" and (2) "restoration of vitality."

1. Reduction of Fatigue

Fatigue results from many factors. Some fatigue comes from having used up available energy during prolonged work. Such fatigue can be removed only by sufficient sleep, rest and nourishment. But sometimes it is due to the way in which we go about our work. We succumb to the anxieties involved in our duties so much that we maintain tense postures even during periods when anxiety has ceased to be necessary.

In all persons—and all animals, for that matter—nervous tension characteristically tends to increase muscular tension and thereby consume energy. As muscles become tensed, they tend to contract. Although such tensions and contractions may not be uniform throughout the body, or the same in all persons at all times, we can observe that nervous fingers seem forced to close in the direction of a fist. Our arms embody a tendency to bend from a straight into a contracted position and, unless they remain otherwise occupied, they draw themselves close to the body. When one stands, he tends to become restless in his stance as he becomes more nervous. And when he sits, he moves toward doubling his legs farther under his chair, if room exists, and to cross them at the ankles. Or he may try to cross his legs at the knees, when convenient and proper.

As a person talks or reads, his head tends to move forward, often downward. Strain on muscles in the back of the neck increases. As this condition persists, tension, both nervous and muscular, grows. Instead of holding the head upright so it maintains a position close to a straight line above the spinal column, one usually bends his head forward as he becomes more anxious. Some people remain in such a tense position for so long that a drooping posture becomes a permanent feature of their bodily contour. They develop a stooped stature. Furthermore, as one focuses his attention, energies and body upon the object of his endeavor, he crouches his whole body forward just a bit. Such bending increases strain in his back muscles and reduces the size of his chest and active lung capacity.

We need a general but workable analogy to picture the over-all effect of these separately mentioned contractions. The body responds to omnistrain as if closing up like a clam under attack or like a spider which draws in all of its legs when afraid. We can experience this process intuitively when suddenly shocked with fear; but at work the process occurs much more slowly, imperceptibly, unknowingly. Yet if we stop to think about the matter, we find ourselves, after a prolonged period of concentration, subconsciously pulling the muscles of our body in such a way that we are drawing the body into a shape in which it occupies the least volume. Now such a condition, involving both nervous and muscular tension, naturally results in fatigue as it becomes prolonged.

The problem which one faces, when he becomes aware of his condition, is how to reverse all of these directions. That is, he should somehow release the tensions in his fingers, from clenched fist toward full spread of his fingers. He should unbend his arms held close to the body and extend them outward. He should retract his head from protruding forward and downward, and lift it up and back. He should retreat from his forward-bending position by straightening his spinal column, and enlarge his chest and lung capacity.

Altogether, the problem is one of withdrawing from a crouching posture and replacing it by an expanding one. Instead of drawing all appendages into the smallest possible space, as we do in fright, one should feel expansive, free and fearless and try to extend himself in the direction of occupying the largest possible space. But, since doing this all at once may be impossible or improper under many circumstances, attention to a few reversals—even to a single reversal—at a time may provide partial relief.

Most yogic postures and exercises have been designed to counteract these crouching tendencies. Their purpose is, first, to give relief from tension and then to bring reduction of fatigue due to such tension. Each of the many specific types of techniques—stretching of muscles, slowing of pace, control of breathing, and change of attitude from care about external objects and future effects to present being and inner self-sufficiency—has a bearing upon this general problem.

Since fatigue results from nervous and muscular tensions, reduction of such tensions helps to reduce fatigue. If we cannot approach the problem of reducing nervous tension directly, we may be able to attack it by way of diminishing muscular tensions—for the two are interconnected. So deliberate attention to the taut condition of muscles may result, through releasing muscular tension and inducing muscular relaxation, in diminution of nervous tensions.

However, the need for continuing to work under conditions of partial fatigue often brings us back rapidly to our previous state of tenseness. We need not only relief from fatigue, but also renewed energy with which to maintain both our attentive activities and such continuing muscular effort as may be needed in our work. Hence, in business and professional life, a lift is welcome and needed, but it is not always enough. So we should turn to the second general type of immediate benefit which may result from yogic practices.

2. Restoration of Vitality

We refer here to refreshment, revivification, reanimation or regeneration. When we become fatigued, we need more than relief from sluggishness and irritability. We want more vitality—enough to regain pliability, adaptability and initiative. This requires some replenishment of energy. How can such replenishment be achieved?

Yogic practices aim not merely at reducing fatigue but also at refilling both muscles and nerves with energy. Reduction of fatigue and restoration of energy function interdependently and both may be accomplished by the same exercises, if one carries them out in the right way. Unclenching a fist may yield a feeling of relief, but for a few moments only. If general tension remains, especially if finger muscles have been contracted so long that the fingers assume a bent shape normally, the momentary benefits quickly disappear. Neither continued relaxation nor restoration can be obtained so easily. First of all, a longer period of finger stretching is needed. How long? No standard rules exist, and people differ. One must experiment and see for himself.

But the following suggestion seems in order. Consider how long your fingers have been held in a contracted condition. If you expect that full relaxation can come only by a complete balancing of activity, then should not your fingers be held in an extended position for as long as they were held in a contracted position? Can you expect that anything less than an equal length of time in the one position can adequately balance the tendency toward extreme tenseness established by holding the other position for so long a time? Of course, no one will recommend such complete equality. One can obtain relief in a shorter time. But the point of this remark is to prepare the reader for expecting that reversing and restoring will require more than just a very short time.

Without detailing the similar problems involved in unbending legs, head, neck and torso, we will proceed to explain why and how restoration of vitality takes place. When muscles become constricted, the size of the blood vessels, veins and capillaries is reduced somewhat. At least increased and often persisting pressure is put upon them. Circulation becomes partially inhibited. Such inhibition may be so minute as to be insignificant much of the time, especially when constriction is replaced with occasional loosening of muscles as one moves about. But when one holds the same position for very long periods, as sedentary people who must concentrate and sustain their efforts often do, the constriction persists and infrequent loosening fails to allow sufficient replenishment of an adequate blood supply. Thus the muscles, and in a similar way the nerves, become fatigued. So part of the problem involved in restoration of vitality consists in how to relax the muscles sufficiently, with both enough relief from tension and for long enough time so that the blood can circulate freely to eliminate wastes and impurities and to provide fresh nourishment to muscle and nerve cells.

Another part of the problem has to do with supply of oxygen in the blood, for increased circulation of blood which lacks sufficient oxygen still will not do the job properly. By retreating from a crouched position and enlarging the chest capacity, one makes it possible to breathe more deeply. But such a possibility is not enough. Nor is taking a few deep breaths, even though one may feel somewhat refreshed immediately. One needs to breathe deeply long enough to supply the oxygen of which the blood has been deprived for the long period during which lung capacity was diminished and breathing minimized under stress of attention to the day's tasks. In trying to decide how long such a period needs to be, again one has no definite rule to guide him. If the period of general stress has been prolonged, a longer period may be required. If the subject of attention has required greater concentration and more intense constriction of muscles, a longer period should be expected. The matter can be decided by each individual only by personal investigation. The conditions in an office vary and the amount of time or opportunity available may be limited and uneven. But anyone who knows how to turn his attention deliberately to breathing exercises for even short periods may find himself rewarded with some increase in vitality.

Many of the standard yogic postures and breathing exercises, which may be exploited in some offices for short periods, involve much of the body rather than a single set of muscles such as those in the legs, hands or neck. These postures and exercises aim at increasing basal metabolism, even if for only a relatively short period. But when they succeed in this aim, they provide some increase in body functioning and an improved tonus. A few of these postures aid other specific organs, such as the eyes, fatigued from reading or looking, and the brain, fatigued from thinking or attending. Teachers of yoga commonly claim that certain postures especially benefit eyes and brain, resulting in improved eyesight, improved memory and improved thinking ability, and that some such improvement may be noted almost immediately. We shall indicate these benefits in conjunction with specific postures when we describe them later.

For the present, we can say that some such improvement may be observed. But since the results to be expected vary with different persons, depending upon the condition of eyes, circulation generally and multitudes of other factors, again the proof of results must come from personal testing.

So much, then, for immediate values. Before passing on, perhaps we should note that yogic exercises may also serve as a temporary cure for insomnia, but this immediate effect should occur after working hours, and this item will be dealt with later.

B. Long-range Values

Yogic practices have been designed much more for the purpose of reaping long-range benefits than for grabbing the immediate values just mentioned. I will group possible long-range benefits into two large, loose and somewhat overlapping classes. I call these (1) primary values and (2) secondary values. In the first are included those values pertaining basically to the maintenance of physical health. These will be divided, somewhat arbitrarily, into those relative to (a) restoring health, if lost, (b) maintaining health, against constant dangers and (c) longevity. In the second class are included benefits which, in my own estimation, are derivative from, and additional to, or incidental to, the main goal which is to achieve the primary benefits. These too will be divided, for convenience, into those relative to (a) suppleness, (b) reduced weight and (c) body tonus. Some individuals, for personal reasons, may happen to consider these as primary. The classification is my own and should not be regarded as traditional.

1. Primary Values

Although all of the values classified here as "primary" pertain to sustaining health, we distinguish for initial emphasis the uses which have been made of yoga for restoring health. Many of our readers will be very healthy and interested only in maintaining, not in restoring, health. But most of those already enjoying continuing well-being will hardly be interested in reading a book on yoga which aims at preserving such health. This volume is not intended for the merely curious, but for those in need of relaxation and restoration of vivacity and pliability. If the successes reported regarding recuperation of partly lost health are sufficiently impressive, one may become convinced about, and develop greater interest in, putting forth the effort required to obtain the primary values. Certainly, for one who has lost his health, few greater values can be imagined than regaining health.

a. *Restoring health.* Many of the books written about yogic practices came into existence because their writers felt so indebted to such practices for their own recoveries that they needed to pass on hope and help to others.

Indra Devi, for example, introduces her *Forever Young, Forever Healthy* with the following statement: "This book is written with only one purpose in mind: to share with you the remarkable experiences I have undergone—experiences which transformed me from a sick, nervous unhappy woman into a happy human being, healthy and relaxed both physically and mentally." Her story illustrates how a Western woman who happened to go to India discovered a way to a worth-while and healthy life after serious illness.

How a sickly Indian boy, plagued by "almost every major disease—scarlet fever, dysentery, typhus, cholera, and the other contagious diseases so common in the tropics," regained —or, perhaps I should say, gained for the first time—health and strength, and enough of it to travel to Europe and found a yoga school, is illustrated in *Yoga and Health* by Selvarajan Yesudian and Elisabeth Haich. The opening chapter, "True Story of a Sick Boy," excites sympathy. The book is a solid contribution to yogic literature and its illustrations depict achievement which anyone must admire.

Harvey Day, author of *The Study and Practice of Yoga* and *About Yoga—The Complete Philosophy,* an Englishman, "suffered badly from malaria, which early affected my eyes and teeth." "Fortunately," he remarks in the Introduction to the first of these volumes, "I managed to gain health." Many of the postures are beautifully illustrated by Hazel Cleaver, "once a sick, weak child," who "now teaches dancing and was recently judged to have the most perfect figure in the Midlands."

V. G. Rele, in *Yoga Asanas for Health and Vigor,* generalizing about life in general as well as reporting his own experiences, comments upon "the sequence of causes that deteriorate health, particularly in middle life" (page 7) and asserts that, "as a recuperative measure, when health has been shattered after a long continued illness, these exercises will brace up the body quicker than any other system of physical culture" (page 3).

Recuperation, maintenance of health and longevity do not require three different sets of techniques. They represent three distinguishable kinds of benefits. But all of them can be accomplished by the same sets of practices. We turn, now, for explanation of all three, to an examination of the problems and principles involved in yogic efforts to maintain health.

b. *Maintaining health.* Health is not a matter of momentary relief from fatigue or of temporary restoration of vitality. Health is itself a long-range affair and depends upon enduring conditions. Some of these, such as heredity, early conditioning, nutrition, early and continuing diseases (such as hay fever and asthma) and contagious diseases, yoga can do little or nothing to eliminate or change. Yogic benefits must be sought within the framework of "givens," of existing conditions established in a person's physique. Its values are to be sought only where physiological conditions can be influenced, modified, changed. But these conditions are many.

As in immediate values, yogic efforts are focused upon ways for reducing tensions and fatigue and restoring energy. But here the stress becomes one of giving attention to habits —to tendencies which not only occur on any particular day but also continue day in and day out. We not only use up our energies at work and when away from work; we also fail to recoup our full vitality during the night's sleep (or sleeplessness). We arise mornings and return to our duties without having completely recovered our full measure of plasticity, vigor and strength. We develop habits of exhausting ourselves more than we can recover. We acquire habits of beginning and pursuing our day's work without sufficient vitality. The aim of a developed program of yogic posturings is to assure a fuller restoration of vigor and vivacity. This can be accomplished only by developing habits conducive to such fuller restoration.

As in immediate values, yogic endeavors regarding long-range physical health pertain primarily to (1) circulation of the blood and increased (or decreased) metabolism and

(2) purification of the blood through increased oxygenation. But again the emphasis is placed upon developing habits—both habits which will be conducive to constant improved circulation and purification and to habits which will lead to recurrent improvement of circulation and purification at times when tensions and fatigue recur. The ideal yogic life is one which is freed from as many strains as possible—a rural or forest hermitage where sufficient simple foods can be provided with a minimum of effort and absence of anxiety. But since such a condition remains largely idyllic, we shall view yogic habit-making in the light of the realities facing typical business executives and professional people. Both the ideal and the practical methods have to do with stopping injurious and degenerative habits and the establishment of healthy and regenerative habits—all such habits involving breathing and posture, where posture includes both mild exercise and a regular program of posture variations.

The general value, maintenance of health, may be more fully comprehended if we cite some of the specific kinds of physiological values at stake. Better breathing habits develop the lungs and tend toward a reduction or elimination and prevention of diseases of the lungs, such as tuberculosis. Better posture, especially exercises which massage the internal organs—somewhat neglected by both those who fail to take regular physical exercise altogether and by those who stress muscle-building sports—stimulate these organs. Stomach stimulation may result in improved digestion. Massaging of the intestines and colon can speed digestion and prevent constipation. Kneading the liver, spleen and the various ductless glands tends to relieve sluggish secretion. Improved circulation tends to reduce the dangers relative to all diseases of the body, including those of the circulatory, nervous, digestive, muscular, glandular, respiratory and reproductive systems of the body. The heart itself may be improved by yogic practices, especially in persons of middle age or older; at least many will judge so when comparing the effects of the moderate and relatively restful yoga postures and exercises with those of more vigorous gymnastics or with more sedentary activities.

Again, the attainment of values by individuals depends upon factors peculiar to their circumstances. One must experiment to discover for himself whether he can obtain these primary values. The business executive and professional person will consider his yogic efforts as supplementary to, not as substitutes for, his other ways of maintaining his health. Modern medicine and medical services have provided ways and means not available when yogic practices were first developed. A person suffering from chronic illness should consult his physician before embarking upon a yogic routine with grim determination. Unfortunately, so much misunderstanding exists among physicians regarding the nature and values of yoga that one may receive merely derogatory disapproval. One physician, Franklyn Thorpe, M.D., in writing the Introduction to *Yoga for Today* by Clara Spring and Madeleine Goss, remarks: "In the more than ten years I have been practicing Hatha Yoga almost daily for forty minutes upon arising, I feel that I have had the opportunity to give it the acid test from the standpoint of theory and practice as well as from that of anatomy and physiology. . . . What began as a chore I didn't have time for soon became a necessity equal to bathing, care of the teeth, or any of the other cleansing functions of the body. . . . My morning starts with an inner feeling of tranquillity and even exhilaration which lasts throughout the day."

c. *Longevity.* Nothing miraculous is proposed by yogic teachers when noting that longer life may, and often does, result from following yogic ways of health maintenance. Life naturally continues to survive unless its healthy functioning is interrupted. When both external dangers and internal diseases and habits leading to degeneration have been removed, one naturally lives longer. If life has value, then longer life should have greater value.

Swami Nikhilananda, director of the Ramakrishna-Vivekananda Center in New York City, writes enthusiastically in his edition of *Vivekananda: The Yogas and Other Works,* page 587, as follows: "The result of hatha-yoga is simply to make men live long; health is the chief idea, the one goal of hatha-yoga. He is determined not to fall sick, and he never does. He lives long. A hundred years is nothing for him; but he is quite young and fresh when he is one hundred and fifty, without one hair turned grey." Not all of us can or would care to become full-time yogins. But the frequent mention of both "longevity" and "rejuvenation" in yogic textbooks and the obvious youthfulness of observable practicing yogins stand as evidence that here is a value worth investigating. Certainly some of the causes of old age may be retarded. The extent to which they can be checked or decelerated by yogic endeavors must be recognized as one of the long-range primary values of yoga.

2. Secondary Values

Although the values grouped here have been designated as "secondary," they obviously overlap and are interdependent with those just discussed as "primary." We can hardly have either without the other. Some persons may, in fact, value more highly and aim more directly at those which we are calling secondary. At any rate, the present section is devoted to examination of values which may be found in and through (a) increased suppleness, (b) reduced weight and (c) improved tonicity.

a. *Increased suppleness.* Although I know, as we all do, that a nimble and agile body signifies both a nimble and agile spirit and general well-being, and that flexible muscles can be produced by limbering exercises, I was still somewhat startled by a simple observation recently. When Swami Chidananda, of the Yoga-Vedanta Forest Academy, Rishikesh, Himalayas, on tour in the United States, stopped briefly in Albuquerque on February 22, 1961, on his way to Uruguay, I invited him to address a group during the noon hour in the faculty lounge of the University of New Mexico Union. After removing his sandals and drawing his legs onto the chair under him to "get comfortable," as he put it, he gave us both an interesting talk and an inspiring ceremonial mantra (prayer). During his talk, he began to enumerate some distinguishable points by counting each upon his fingers. What surprised me was the extreme pliability of his fingers, for each was bent backward to about a ninety-degree angle with obviously natural ease. My own stiff fingers bent backward hardly at all, and then only under some pressure.

This surprise caused me to look again at the relatively youthful appearance of this mature man. His smooth clear skin, his complaisant deportment, his quick but graceful gestures, his melodious voice, his confident and appreciative spirit, and his quick and obviously well-informed mind all impressed me with his wisdom. This Hindu saint's lithe movements and fearless confidence, in what was for him a foreign and unsympathetic environment, expressed a profound and persistently pliable spirit sustained by a vigorous supple body, despite, or perhaps because of, a very simple vegetarian diet to which he kept most scrupulously. Swami Chidananda's elastic, flowing, yet sure and lenient behavior contrasted markedly with the more stiffly channelized movements and thought patterns of the guests who heard him. Would that American visitors to foreign countries could leave so favorable an impression upon those who must judge a nation by its traveling representatives!

"Except ye become as a little child," who can flex his body in almost any direction, you cannot retain, or regain, facility of movement, adaptability of response or suppleness of activity. The older a person grows, the stiffer his bones and muscles become, unless he effectively exercises his whole system to retard or counteract this tendency. The longer one delays, the more difficult he should expect his task will be. A person who restricts the movements of his muscles to minimal distances should anticipate a gradual fixation, and limitation, of his powers of movement to those minimal distances. The more repetitious his fixed movements, the more mechanical he becomes. But his machine-like motions should be interpreted as signifying that the corpse-like stiffness, which completes or perfects itself in death, establishes itself in one's body gradually to the extent that he permits himself to move merely mechanically. Retardation of stiffness, or retention of suppleness, is surely a highly prized value. Although yogic techniques need not be the only ones available to this end, the success of those who have used them calls us to consider and try out the suggestions which yogic tradition proposes.

b. *Reduced weight.* Most everybody now, at least almost every business and professional person, has become calorie-conscious. How to reduce excess fat—which spoils our contours, produces sluggish metabolism, overworks our hearts, occasions unreasonable demands for new clothes and makes us somewhat ashamed in social situations—looms as a major problem in America and for many individual Americans. For overweight middle-aged people, reduction of weight continues to be a pestiferously plaguing problem.

Perhaps the best way to illustrate how weight may be reduced through yogic practice is to cite an article by Wambly Bald appearing in the San Francisco *Examiner* of October 13, 1959. It begins like this:

"New York, Oct. 12. Would you like to lose weight without resorting to the miseries of dieting? Well, try the miseries of Yoga exercises instead. One staunch advocate is Metropolitan Opera star Robert Merrill, who has been practicing these exercises for two years, and keeps trying to win converts. In those two years he has lost twenty pounds and now he's down to a trim, rhythmic-breathing one hundred and sixty, even though he continues to eat like a lumber jack. 'At one time I went on a lot of diets but just couldn't lose any weight,' he said. 'Then along came Yoga and look at me now.' He punched his hard flat stomach and started breathing through one nostril. And to further demonstrate what it's all about, he did a little flip and stood on his head. After that he showed the lotus position, legs scissored under the body. Was he still breathing through one nostril? Yes, the other one. 'If people weren't so lazy they wouldn't have to worry about diets,' he said."

Franklyn Thorpe, M.D., previously cited as writing the Introduction to Clara Spring's *Yoga for Today,* tells of losing about fourteen pounds and four inches around the waist in ten years, an achievement which he attributes "mostly to breathing exercises, for I have never been on a diet of any kind." Clara Spring, a long-time devotee and teacher of yogic postures, herself declares *(ibid.,* page 11): "Where ordinary routines for reducing often bring corresponding loss of vitality and lowered resistance to disease—sometimes with definite injury to health—Yogic practices develop energy as weight is controlled."

There is nothing magical about how yogic exercises lead to reduction of weight. Two well-known principles are involved. (1) Yogic practices which reduce anxiety thereby tend to reduce anxious eating. When under nervous strain we tend to gulp our food without attaining much genuine satisfaction. So we want more and, when more is handy, tasty, attractive, we easily yield to our impulses, because we still feel that desires should be satisfied and hope that reaching for more food will somehow produce such satisfaction. But, as we know from long experience, this satisfaction does not actually occur very often. If, on the other hand, we approach our meals with greater calmness of mood, whether produced by habits which have calmed our life or by a yogic "quickie" (like a pause for prayer before a meal), we tend to be less likely to overconsume in a frantic effort to quiet our midday anxieties.

(2) Yogic breathing increases oxidation, thus burning up some of the calories we have ingested. Yogic exercises, although they do not consume the quantities of energy required by more vigorous gymnastic exercises, do use some. But they induce more continuous and deeper breathing which gradually burns, sometimes forcefully, many of the calories already ingested.

Furthermore, having attention called to one's ugly excess fat, when trying to perform even the simplest postures, may remotivate efforts to do something about overweight. Since one can hardly attempt any of the standard postures without becoming conscious of his weight, size and shape, when such attempts make him aware of them, he naturally acquires further incentive to act upon the matter.

Also, yogic aids may be employed between meals whenever one becomes tempted to search for a snack. One may deliberately turn to yoga, rather than to the icebox or snackbar, when he feels the need for a lift or relief from restless nervousness. But whether the calming effects of yogas, either "little yogas" or "big yogas," can calm one's daytime hankerings is something each person must discover for himself.

Finally, we should mention that for those whose eating habits, whether at meals or between meals, are believed to be due to feelings of weakness rather than anxieties, most yogic postures and breathing exercises are designed to increase one's strength. Hence, they may relieve feelings of weakness more effectively than additional eating. The exercises themselves, although consuming some energy, also store up energy which, when combined with oxidizing breathing, provide energy that is ready for use rather than for storage.

Although limits exist relative to the amount of weight reduction that can be accomplished by yogic efforts alone, the examples of both traditional yogins and businessmen devotees indicate something of probabilities derivable from a fair trial. Yogic exercises might, in contrast with gymnastics, be called "slimnastics," but the name should apply not to those exercises which represent only halfhearted beginnings. Both moderation and persistence are required by those who achieve and maintain reduced weight by yogic methods.

c. *Improved tonicity.* What is "tonicity" or "tonus"? One must have experienced for himself what we are talking about or the term can have little meaning. It involves both (1) a condition of one's muscles and of the organs which supply them with energy and (2) a feeling of facility in their use.

The muscles respond with easy yet energetic tension. They are under full control of one's wishes and they respond automatically, quickly and smoothly to one's slightest whim. Tonicity refers here to spryness not just of a single muscle or a few muscles, those used over and over again each day, but of those throughout the body, including many not so commonly used. Tonicity is characterized by a steady, abundant flow of energy not easily exhausted under the pressures of intense work. It involves a harmonious functioning of all portions of the body needed for any particular kind of action.

The feeling of facility may be accompanied by a feeling of buoyancy, a feeling of freedom and power, as well as by muscle suppleness, celerity of thought, smoothness in executing motions and feelings of assurance that one can direct his body in any way he chooses. One's step becomes springy, yet firm and sure. One's movements are direct, free from feebleness or frailty, yet elastic and resilient. One meets physical obstacles with rebound and redirects his efforts with minimum feelings of frustration, disgust or dismay. He retains high spirits in the face of resistance to his efforts, and adapts himself easily because he feels his physical strength to be, if not unbounded, at least fully adequate to meet his needs.

Such tonicity comes from exercise of muscles combined with regenerative rest. It is true that heredity, diet, disease, age and the demands of work determine one's condition. But the moderate yet regularly recurrent movement of muscles of the whole body gives the body a balanced and systematic workout without requiring exhausting efforts. It emphasizes re-energizing rests and combinations of movement and rest, which naturally rebuild an abundance of energy. Yogic exercises place special emphasis on abdominal muscles which are central to the whole muscular system, rather than to the more external muscles of arms and legs. Once the trunk has been toned up, sprightliness in the extending limbs results almost automatically.

Before leaving our discussion of immediate and long-range values of yoga, perhaps we should mention what may be obvious already. Anyone who has achieved the long-range values is more likely to obtain the immediate values. In fact, he is likely to be enjoying them most of the time. On the other hand, one will be neither motivated to try, nor be inclined to continue, yogic techniques unless he can experience as benefits worthy of his efforts some of the immediate values outlined. Thus immediate and long-range values are interdependent. This is true, also, of immediate and long-range mental values. Interdependence of physical and mental health is so well known that it hardly needs stressing here.

C. Comparative Values

Although we have not yet examined yogic exercises, the present section on Physical Health seems to be a proper place for discussing values of yogic methods in comparison with other programs for maintaining physical health which emphasize gymnastics and sports. Physical education systems originating in India and in Europe have much in common. Both are interested in physical health and vitality, freedom from disease and longevity. Both are expressions of, and adaptations to, human physiology and its needs and limitations. Both have discovered and employed some of the same exercises, such as bending forward to touch the floor with fingers, or twisting the body and stretching muscles for purposes of limbering them. Both idealize physical fitness, self-control and deep breathing. So one might easily magnify the differences beyond their true proportions. Yet differences exist and these will be stressed in the following pages.

For convenience, these differences will be arranged under six headings: (1) less violent, (2) noncompetitive, (3) less exhaustive, (4) less specialized, (5) less expensive and (6) supplementary. For those who prefer to have these values stated in positive rather than negative phrases, the headings could read as follows: (1) more quiescent, (2) more individual, (3) more efficient, (4) more general, (5) more inexpensive and (6) supplementary. Regardless of whether conceived in positive or negative terms, some of the values in these groupings will be found to overlap with those in others because they are interdependent.

1. Less Violent

A review of the various kinds of gymnastic exercises, such as tumbling, chinning, jumping, weight-lifting, shot-putting, and of the numerous kinds of sports, such as basketball, football, baseball, handball, tennis, swimming, skiing, skating, hockey or even ping pong, reveals that in every one of them some violent action is required. One has to rush his body from one place to another or push some ball or puck through space. An exerciser expects to strain his muscles at times but, in sports at least, the furiousness of one's efforts becomes forgotten when attention centers upon a moving object and upon playing a combative role where some victory is at stake. For vigorous, successful competition, one has to "keep in shape," not just for the sake of health and relaxation but for the purpose of winning or at least making a respectable showing. When size and weight are advantageous in competition, they come to be admired and developed. Speed and strength become idealized. Muscle building, especially of the arms and legs when these are most needed in handling balls or equipment, becomes a necessary means—sometimes even an end-in-itself.

Yogic exercises, on the other hand, all occur within a small area of space and consist mainly in taking and holding a stable position. The only movement needed is that for going from one stable position to another. A rest period, of short or long duration as one chooses, between each such position permits, or assures, reduction of violence. The aim of the whole procedure is relaxation and recuperation, so all activity should be pervaded with a spirit of gentleness. The ideal of violent, jerky, strenuous movement remains entirely missing. And muscle relaxation rather than muscle building continues as the goal.

2. Noncompetitive

Yoga is completely noncompetitive in spirit. Each practitioner should proceed at his own pace, in private, and have no standard of achievement in terms of which to compete with others—or even with himself. The goal is health and relaxation for the individual, not a show of prowess or of any achievement in which one takes pride. Each person should aim only to work within his capacity. He should not try to exceed his capacity just to attain a favorable comparison relative to the achievements of others.

Competitive sports naturally breed anxiety, the very thing one seeks to avoid when needing relaxation. Competition appeals to pride, excites ambition, stimulates exertion. It results, normally, in much frustration, since wherever there are winners there must be losers. When several contestants compete for a single prize, there must be many losers for one winner. Apart from the dangers of injury due to collision, competitive sports promote the arousing of antagonism, ill will and injury to pride. Appeals to sportsmanship may smooth ruffled tempers, but feelings of partial unfairness so often result that the energy required to survive under strained social relations in addition to straining muscles may be tremendous. Although competitive sports do provide some healthful and relaxing benefits, the danger of overdoing and of becoming involved in additional anxieties continues to be ever-present. Sports do get one's mind off his work. But when, to the nervous anxieties imposed upon us by our work, transportation and family, community and political affairs, we add anxieties of sports competition, strain piles upon strain until our capacities give out. Then we often develop headaches, fatigue, exhaustion and ripen our bodies for diseases. When "recreation" includes thrilling movies, exciting television programs and shocking news reports, there is no escape from strain. We develop "omnistrain." Competitive sports hardly provide the best remedy for omnistrain.

Yoga requires quietude, privacy and freedom from interference by others. It has quietude, personal rest and recuperation as its goal. It employs quiet methods and pacifying techniques. Thus it is quiet in its origin, quiet in its goal and quiet in its ways. The moment a competitive spirit attracts one's attention, his quietude is gone. Even the attempts of two persons, each trying to be quieter than the other, are suffused with suppressed turmoil.

3. Less Exhaustive

Competitive sports and gymnastics usually continue to be pursued until one is "pooped out." A person hardly expects to achieve maximum benefit until he has exerted himself to the utmost. But the aim of yoga is to attain a maximum amount of renewed strength in a minimum amount of time. "In active sports," says S. Yesudian in *Yoga and Health,* page 68, "we expend our strength and then have to lie down to rest. In the passivity of Yoga exercises, however, we collect a gigantic amount of energy which we store up within us. It is like building a dam across a river. The force is stored up, and this gives us an immense reserve of power. . . . Thus, no matter how tired we are when we come home from work, we can easily do passive Hatha Yoga exercises, as they cause no further fatigue. Anyone who has ever tried knows!" "If you practice relaxation," remarks Swami Sivananda in *Yogic Home Exercises,* page 77, "no energy will be wasted."

4. Less Specialized

Whereas some types of sports require strong leg muscles, for example, a standard yogic routine aims at calling all muscles of the body into play. It may be unsafe to generalize here, since some sports differ from others in degree of all-around muscular development. But yoga does not aim at muscle development in the sense of attaining stronger muscles. Rather it tries to bring them all into use in relaxing, limbering exercises. Its goal is not to develop bunches of muscles such as those admired in weight lifters, wrestlers or boxers. Instead it aims at maintaining a sensitive, supple, well-poised, healthy body which is ready to respond to every normal need.

Swami Sivananda, in *Yoga Asanas,* page 22, expresses this point in a typically Hindu way. "Ordinary physical exercises develop the superficial muscles of the body only. One can become . . . a beautiful physique. But Asanas (postures) are intended for the thorough exercise of the internal organs, viz., liver, spleen, pancreas, intestines, heart, lungs, brain and the important ductless glands of the body . . . which play an important part in the economy of nature in maintaining health in metabolism and in structure, growth and nutrition of different kinds of cells and tissues of the body."

5. Less Expensive

Gymnastics usually involve a gymnasium and all that goes into the cost of building, managing, repairing and maintaining it. They normally demand equipment, such as parallel bars, rings, horses, jumping poles and rods, dumbbells, punching bags, smooth floors and floor pads. They usually require special clothing, gym suits, gym shoes, sweatshirts, and locker rooms, bathing facilities and varieties of supervision. Competitive sports make use of balls and other instruments such as bats, racquets, hockey sticks, pucks. Specially constructed basketball courts, tennis courts, handball courts, squash courts, baseball diamonds, football stadia, swimming pools, polo grounds, ice arenas, golf courses are needed, as are supervisors or referees, rules and regulations, and sometimes judges. First-aid medicines and services seem to be standard requirements. Costs mount upon costs. Both public and private recreation programs and service fees in private athletic clubs add up to a staggering national total, to say nothing of the percentage of personal budgets spent upon "recreation."

But yoga is, or should be, completely inexpensive. No appliances are needed, if one has a carpeted floor or a not-too-soft mat. Though a person may wear such clothes as he pleases, nudity, which is possible in privacy, often proves the best condition. And nudity is costless. One does not even have to wash as many clothes. No shoes are required. There need be no costs of wear and tear on equipment, buildings or transportation, for one can practice yoga at home, in his bedroom or, for that matter, wherever he can find privacy and a few square feet of floor space. He is not exposed to the diseases of others in gymnasium shower and dressing rooms. He is exposed to less danger from injury. And he has no need for taking time off from work or other activities, since he can sandwich some yogic exercises in between them.

6. Supplementary

The more passive and static, quiet and private, health-maintaining techniques of yoga not only differ somewhat from the more active, moving, exciting and social activities of sports; they may be viewed also as supplementary. The differences need not be regarded as so antagonistic that anyone who devotes himself to the one cannot be a devotee of the other also. Together they give a variety which neither alone can provide. Yoga may be used when other systems are not available. Some persons may treat it as a substitute, especially older persons who cannot stand vigorous exercises, or poorer persons who cannot afford to join in expensive activities, or shut-ins or those isolated for whatever reason.

But others treat it as supplemental, in two ways: (a) It may provide additional variety and thus give relief from boredom resulting from usual patterns of behavior; (b) It adds a genuinely new dimension to one's physical health program.

Still others treat yoga as a self-sufficient system, for apparently yogins have maintained their health by means of it for centuries. We suggest that younger executives may find it supplementary to their more vigorous and social interests. But older persons should find it to be increasingly suited to their otherwise declining vigor. The comparative values of yoga and other systems may well change with changing circumstances, such as age, sex, degree of isolation, physiological development or degeneration. So, although we have pointed out many types of difference which are easy to observe, the full extent of values of yoga for individuals can be known only by personal re-experimentation from time to time.

II. MENTAL HEALTH

Since the present work has been restricted largely to hatha yoga techniques relative to breathing and posture and, in a minor way, to control of attention, the values of yoga for mental health discussed here are intended to be limited to those which flow from use of these techniques. We have no intention of exploring either the other varieties of yoga or values which may result from following them. Of course, since the breathing and posture practices of hatha yoga were conceived and nurtured in a psychological, philosophical or religious perspective which idealizes quiescence as the ultimate goal, we can expect some overlapping of values. Here, however, our aim is merely to attain relief from disquietude rather than to become totally absorbed into perfect quietude.

Just as the values of yoga for physical health tend to vary with age and other circumstances, so the values of yoga for mental health may be expected to differ likewise. Younger people, naturally more active and virile, with more of a future ahead of them, should be more ambitious, more attentive to, and more anxious about their future. Older people, on the other hand—especially the very old—are not only less active and vigorous, but with most of their life already lived, should expect to be less ambitious, less concerned about, less anxious about their future. Unless they have already succeeded in accepting their age as desirable and enjoyable, "the last of life for which the first was made," their main anxiety, if such it should be called, may be that of how to reduce their anxieties. Whoever has already fully eliminated his fears and willingly acts his age may have nothing more to gain from yoga. But those who remain worrisome about or in old age, despite all their other efforts to quiet their mental disturbances, may profit mentally from yogic endeavors.

The following mental health values have been arranged primarily into two groups, immediate values and long-range values, with a concluding section on comparative values. The classification is my own, and the differences between immediate and long-range values must be regarded partly as a matter of degree. To the extent that they also differ in kind, we should note that those of each kind not only supplement but support those of the other.

A. Immediate Values

Two opposing but interdependent types of values which may be experienced without much waiting are (1) reduction of tension and (2) restoration of pliability.

1. Reduction of Tension

Since the amount of benefit obtainable should be expected to fluctuate with the extent to which one devotes himself to a full fifteen-to-thirty-minute round of exercises, we should distinguish between the immediate effects of such a full round and those of "quickies" which we will call "little yogas." The effects of the former should be considerable whereas those of the latter will probably be minimal and transient.

Quickies bring only a bit of relief, a surface subsidence, a letdown of tension. They may be likened to a sigh of relief, a cool drink of water, a "seventh-inning stretch," or a few puffs from a pipe or cigarette. They cannot save us from sinking back soon into the same rutted routine with its fatiguing pressures. One danger with quickies is that, when the effect also wears off immediately, we either give up in disgust or seek to repeat and repeat, like a chain smoker, with only minimal relief. If a person then develops a mania for such reliefs, he thereby adds another dimension of anxiety to his suffering with omnistrain. From the view of those advocating a full round of exercises, development of a mania for quickies is certainly a mistaken use of yoga. Yet, even so, a little may be better than none, may be just enough to get one through some extremely trying situations, and may assure him that the little values experienced can lead him to greater values if he is willing to try.

Those who approach a full round of exercises—something not available to most beginners—reduction of nervousness, irritability and confusion, depression and mental fatigue may also be experienced. These different kinds or aspects of tension may be indistinguishable in one's experience as such. More traditional accounts of these benefits speak of "freeing the mind from mental disturbances," "calming the spirit," or "steadying the mind." One experiences a relief from the pressure of his "compulsions." His nervousness, especially any jitteriness, should subside or disappear. He should experience laxation, or "unlaxing," or, as we more commonly speak of it, "re-laxing." The extent to which these benefits may be expected will depend in part upon whether or not one can approach and participate in them willingly and wholeheartedly; for one who tries to practice postures with anxiety cripples his chances for very much benefit.

2. Restoration of Pliability

Reduction of tension and restoration of pliability serve as "two sides of the same coin." The former is negative, or a negation of something negative, whereas the latter is positive in emphasis. Tension, here referred to as "negative," is not an evil in itself, but it becomes evil when carried too far—so far that the strain endured in maintaining it becomes debilitating. But pliability, not so much of muscles as of mind, is clearly a positive value to anyone who has felt his mind entangled in torpor or slugged into inactivity despite his most willful exertion to keep it lively.

The positive side of the benefits from a full round of yogic exercises may be described as renewal of mental agility. Both mood and capacity for alertness, attentiveness and willingness to tackle problems revive. One may not be able to rekindle boundless enthusiasm late in a working day; early morning, or even noonday, efforts to recharge mental energies can revive a full measure of willingness. Traditional phrases, such as restored "spiritual vitality," intend to convey the complex idea of mental spryness, agreeableness, resiliency, and feelings of confidence and self-sufficiency. Some even testify to attaining feelings of buoyancy and euphoria; these then provide a background or mood of well-being and assurance such that one naturally more fully enjoys both his ability and the worthiness of being more tolerant and generous.

Little yogas, on the other hand, can be expected to yield little more than a lift or a "pause that refreshes." But the more standard postures and breathing procedures, those which engage the whole body and rehabilitate the circulatory system, replenish the brain as well as the muscular system and thereby regenerate mental powers. The same reinvigorating blood supply which refreshes the brain may also "improve eyesight" by replenishing energy exhausted in tired eyes and "increase the power of memory" (Sivananda, *Yogic Home Exercises,* page xvii). Déchanet, reporting on his own experiences in *Christian Yoga,* page 13, observes that yoga "frees certain intuitive and affective powers." Yet these more immediate values must be judged as minor in comparison with the long-range values also obtainable.

B. Long-range Values

The more enduring values relative to mental health appear to fall somewhat naturally into two large groups. These will be called (1) "personal" and (2) "social." The values constituting each of these groups may also be observed to have their "negative" and "positive" sides or aspects.

1. Personal Values

a. The negative side of long-range personal mental values has to do with reduction of mental ills. These may range all the way from vague feelings of frustration, persecution, insecurity, on the one hand, to acute and specific types of insanity, on the other. It is a mistake to interpret hatha yoga as a miraculous cure-all. But its attack upon, and diminution of, some basic mental ills may indeed be just enough to pay dividends that grow in magnitude. If, through use of yogic techniques, we can merely halt and reverse some mental cancer, some compulsive complex that keeps us chained to unrelenting, omnipresent and gradually increasing anxiety, we may reset a course which will bring us around to a healthier adjustment. We are all at times insane. We are all, in some degree, insane. Overwhelming waves of omnitension and omnistrain, which may catch us in periods of physical and mental exhaustion, can produce a spiritual explosion which leaves us so helpless that we are at a loss to know how it all came about. By recurrent, regular efforts to reduce tension through yogic exercises, we may stay and finally reverse our tendencies toward insanity.

Although one may picture the long-range values resulting from steady, habitual practice as merely extensions of the immediate values, he must, sooner or later, also recognize some values which differ in quality and kind rather than merely in degree. For the long-range effect should be removal, not just of temporary anxieties which recur when caused by a particular day's problems, but of lifelong tensions, caused by life's problems. That is, the task here is removal not merely of momentary, daily, weekly or monthly fears, which require their own specific efforts at removal, but also of built-in, basic, tendential fears, or fears constituting deep-lying and profound anxieties that pervade our outlook no matter what particular fears may momentarily provoke us. For example, as one gets older, he begins to fear that his life has not been sufficiently worth while, that he has fallen short of his goals, that he has failed to attain his proper ambition, that he has lost out in the race to keep up with the Joneses or in his attempt to measure up "in the sight of God"—however he happens to conceive his shortcoming. These more profound, more enduring, more pervasive fears regarding the larger values of life cannot be helped much by quickies.

Thus, when Ramacharaka, in his *Hindu-Yogi Science of Breath,* page 10, says one may, by controlled breathing, "practically do away with fear and worry and the baser emotions," he refers to the growing ability of a devoted practitioner to diminish the power which both momentary and permanent fears have over us. One seeks to develop habits of resistance to the disturbing effects of excitement, ambition, antagonism and frustration. The long-range goal of yoga is not just momentary relaxation, but the living of a relaxed life.

b. Turning from the negative to the positive side, we shift from avoidance of fear to acceptance of faith in life. The goal of yoga (as of all sound psychology, profound philosophy and mature religion) is confident living. Its aim is to replace pessimism and its varieties such as cynicism with a "yea-saying" appreciation of life, not only on any given day, but as a gracious, wonderful whole. When you achieve the yogic spirit, then you can say with the Stoics, "I accept the universe." If you cannot accept all of it, because some problems remain unavoidably troublesome, then you will accept the troubles which you have as (1) yours and (2) enough for you, without wishing you had still more troubles (either greater ambition or other people's troubles).

Poise, serenity, contentedness, patience, assurance—all of these are positive mental values attainable by anyone who has achieved a willingness to be at peace with himself and the world. The confidence desired is not just enough to do the day's work but enough to live one's whole life—and one can do his day's work more confidently if he has already predisposed himself to living his life with trustful serenity. Thus a person seeks through yoga not merely momentary mental agility, but an agile life; not just momentary pliability, but a continuingly pliable existence; not just momentary relief from disturbance, but a permanently peaceful perspective.

Although not everyone who undertakes to experiment with yoga can expect to achieve or maintain the goal described by Shri Yogendra, *Yoga: Personal Hygiene,* Volume I, page 29, as "exuberant and exultant health," he should notice the sun more often when it shines. Swami Sivananda idealizes the goal as "ecstatic joy" (*Yoga Asanas,* page 180). Déchanet, a Roman Catholic monk who was led into yoga by his Catholic predecessors, gives a vivid account of how he uses yogic techniques as aids to worship. He describes a "euphoria that pervades the story of my experiment. I wish to make it clear that this euphoria is real and lasting and spreads through the various levels of my daily life, physical, psychical and spiritual" (*Christian Yoga,* page 25). Even though few of us will achieve anything like perpetual exuberance, ecstatic joy or euphoria, attainment of a more trusting outlook on life provides a spiritual soil from which spiritual roses have a better chance to grow. The pragmatic experimentalist will say: "Try it and see."

2. Social Values

a. If we first look at the negative side of possible social values of mental health from yoga, we can observe a twofold opportunity: It may reduce your annoyance with others and others' annoyance with you. If you become less irritable, you tend to irritate others less and tend to be less irritated by what others do when they present themselves as problems to you. Your obdurate, demanding, insistent, morose attitudes can make you hard to get along with. Diminution of these should make you less difficult to deal with. The social effects —upon your colleagues and clients, superiors and inferiors, to say nothing of family, public officers and service specialists —could be overwhelming.

b. On the "positive" side, a twofold consequence may be noticed: You tend to be easier to get along with and you tend to find others easier to get along with. Or, if your personal improvement grows beyond mere contentment to exuberant appreciation, you may find both more people liking you and you liking more people. You become more adaptable, reliable, steady, alert, responsive, ever-ready, patient, gentle and humane. When this happens, you become recognized as a more desirable person to deal with. If you develop a buoyant spirit, you will find that buoyancy is catching. Others, seeing you as cheery, tend to respond in kind, reacting more cheerily to you. Your rewards increase. These rather obvious platitudes regarding possibilities should not be taken as guarantees regardless of circumstances; sometimes a cheery suggestion begets wrath from another suffering under an ugly mood. But tendencies nevertheless exist and you may profit from them.

We need not dwell upon the long-range costs of social irritability in business and professional activities, especially at the managerial levels. Loss of job or client or employee or spouse may bring on a crisis. A sharp, insistent temperament exudes irritants which may so pervade the atmosphere as to affect whole offices, companies, colleges, communities, families and even entire professions. The morale of an office is a most important aspect of business and professional life. The prevailing temperament of leaders or spokesmen tends to determine the quality of the company, its "corporate image," and the kind of confidence with which its clients can trust it. Although it is too much to expect that one can, by yogic techniques, generate some social euphoria, yet we all know that some companies, some offices, some committee meetings, some college classrooms, have an air of relaxation, trust and assurance about them which pay off in dividends, as well as being enjoyable in themselves.

Although any executive must try out for himself the benefits possible from yoga, he may then want to introduce yogic efforts and ideals to his associates or employees. Although the full benefits can be obtained only from daily devotions of several minutes, preferably mornings and evenings, one may adopt "yoga breaks" in place of "coffee breaks," or use a few minutes for a private headstand in place of a trip to a smoking room. Even though yogic exercises are personal and private, a cooperative approach to problems of how to enable a company to benefit from them may result in original ways of obtaining such benefits in unique professional situations.

I cannot refrain from closing this section on social values without quoting at length from the effects of yoga upon character as noted by Déchanet in *Christian Yoga*. "Yoga also produces a more active, willing and generous disposition. It quickens the life of faith, of love of God and our neighbor. It quickens our sense of duty and responsibility as men and, above all, as Christians" (page 26). "It follows that Hatha Yoga influences character to the good. One man, after some weeks of practice, admits he no longer knows himself, and everyone notices a change in his bearing and reaction. He is gentler, more understanding. He faces experience calmly. He is content; the pinpricks of life affect him less or not at all. He is in command of his own will and goes about his studies without fear and anxiety. His whole personality has been altered and he himself feels it steadying and opening out; from this there arises an almost permanent condition of euphoria, of 'contentedness' " (pages 41, 42). "You will feel that gentleness and sympathy come more readily. You will not feel like venting your spleen on others as frequently as before, and if it should occur, you will regret it all the more. You will make a kind of pact of non-violence with yourself. You will still have fits of impatience often enough, and even of anger. But something will be telling you that this is not only bad but even useless, and that it really is not worth the trouble to fly out and get beside yourself for nothing. A great need for sincerity will bring you to detest, more than others do, not only lying but all forms of duplicity and dissimulation. You will sense the more keenly whatever is not genuine, and even what is merely conventional in speeches and words, and also in attitudes that men think they can take up in order to edify, but more often they take up lest they should lose face" (page 105).

C. Comparative Values

We will now compare the mental health values of yoga with three groups of alternatives. The first group consists of other psychological traditions or other systems of mental health maintenance. The second group consists of other kinds of physiological activities which aim at yielding healthy mental rewards. The third group consists of different kinds of drugs or medicines—including tobacco, tea, liquors and sedatives—which have been used quite commonly to relieve tension. These three groups, and a needed notation about supplementariness, will be classified as follows: (1) psychological, (2) physiological, (3) pharmaceutical, (4) supplementary.

1. Psychological

Although hatha yoga, at least so far as breathing and posture are concerned, is not primarily a psychology but a physiology, the mental health results may nevertheless be compared with the goals of certain psychological systems. We have not, in this volume, gone into *kundalini* or other psychological theories and practices sometimes associated with hatha yoga. Our occasional references to attitude and attention do pertain to psychological aids and natural accompaniments of yogic breathing and posture exercises. But the mental health values of yoga referred to here are limited to those already discussed in Sections A and B.

The vast array of psychological schools must be dealt with by means of a brief sketch that is suggestive rather than exhaustive. These schools will be lumped together under three classifications: (a) hedonistic, (b) voluntaristic, (c) quietistic.

(a) Hedonistic schools insist that good consists in pleasant feeling, evil in pain or unpleasant feeling. If too much nervous tension is experienced as unpleasant, then a person should turn to more pleasant alternatives, when possible. He may divert himself with sweets, for example; and the omnipresence of candy stands wherever people meet may be interpreted as some evidence of uses made of this mode for quieting desires and relieving tensions. But how well does this method work? Those with mounting anxieties must eat increasing amounts of candy. Observation of persons who use this method indicates that it results in increased avoirdupois without lasting results so far as permanent reduction of tension is concerned. Yet, on the other hand, fat people often seem more jovial than thin ones; their movements are slower because they cannot manipulate their great weight easily. Thus sweets-eating techniques of calming nerves may have some virtues. But most business executives and professional people will be unwilling, knowingly, to follow this method because of other handicaps involved.

(b) Voluntaristic schools are many. Only four varieties will be mentioned here: romanticism, Freudianism, existentialism and traditional theism.

Romanticism idealizes exuberant self-expression, obedience to impulse, abandonment of self wholeheartedly to desirous self-indulgence. Inhibition, by law, other people, conscience or "reason," is evil because it thwarts desires and builds up tensions. Freedom from tension should be sought by throwing off inhibitions and pursuing one's own spontaneous impulses. Such people never know when to stop, for to stop doing what you want to do is evil. Violent and erratic temperaments, however, make such people unfit for business or professional positions, except as actors, artists, operatic stars or possibly as "fast-buck" salesmen. They enjoy the thrill of telling off the boss or customers too much to hold a position of responsibility for very long.

Freudianism, although it has made profound, permanent contributions to psychological theory and practice, appeals primarily to sexual interests in ways which are distracting in most kinds of business and professional work. However much nightclub expense accounts testify to deliberate employment of sexual stimulants in business, such techniques are used not so much to relieve tension as to stimulate passion and to obtain irrational solutions by emotional involvements which may take their toll later in worries about exposure to bribery or blackmail—even if on a petty scale.

Existentialism idealizes anxiety as an end-in-itself, positing the belief that only in those moments when one faces momentous decisions is one "authentic." But the cost in energy to maintain one's self in a constant state of authenticity, in persisting anxiety, is too great for most people to bear. It appeals primarily to the young, who have energy to waste, or those who, because they can find no escape from self-imposed torment, rationalize such self-torture as somehow central to the very meaning of life itself. Even if existentialism is not a wholly perverted perspective of life, its ideals involve increase of, not relief from, tension. Thus it can hardly be much of an asset in most businesses or professions.

Traditional theism (and neo-orthodoxy) conceive "sin" as willing to go against the "will of God" and "salvation" as becoming willing to submit one's will completely to the will of God. Apart from difficulties in knowing the will of God, and the impossibility of an imperfect person's achievement of this willingness completely except by an act of Grace by God, the availability of this kind of appeal for relaxation appears in doubt to many. However, this method has worked for centuries, and it works for some today. It has been supported by the idea that God rewards hard workers, those who use their "talents" in accordance with God's will. Those who accept their daily lot of troubles as the will of God can, so long as they willingly accept such will, find comfort and relief in the feeling that things will come out right. Periods of prayer, if needed to reassure or reassess one's willingness, provide more of that "peace which passeth all understanding." Many businesses have prospered because they had confidence that their operating policies were in accordance with the will of God.

But all of these voluntaristic psychologies join in emphasizing the importance of will and in solving the problem of tension and anxiety by increased willing. The romantic, who is tensed by inhibiting frustration, frees himself by willing more violently. The Freudian, whose tension is interpreted as due to suppression of his libidinous Id, seeks relief through libidinous expression. The existentialist, who idealizes authenticity as best when one is aware that his whole being is at stake in his wholly unmotivated willful deciding of his own fate, concernfully urges himself into more and more willful appreciation of life by constant magnification of his fear of total extinction. The traditional theist, willfully trusting in "the Everlasting Arms," feels he must willfully reassure himself that his willingness to do God's will is complete; whenever doubt arises, as it so often does in the face of business injustices, he must reassert his will to believe; for any time when such will becomes weakened, it must be strengthened by more emphatic resolve.

All of these varieties of voluntarism see the solution to life's problems in terms of stronger or more active willing. Yoga, on the other hand, considers will as the primary source of our tensions, anxieties and physical and mental exhaustion. It seeks not a more active but a less active will. The way to relieve tension is to seek quietude. If willfulness, ambition or a sense of urgency increases our nervous tensions, then use of methods which decrease these must be sought. Breathing and posture exercises can reduce our anxieties partly because, in the process, our willfulness is distracted, retarded, softened; the peacefulness of feeling that we have had enough undercuts the sense of urgency out of which so much of our willfulness grows.

(c) Quietistic schools, prevailing mainly in the Orient, compete with yoga in stilling our wills. Jainism, Buddhism and Hinduism, and most of their multitudinous subschools, join in believing that more peaceful living can come from deliberate, habitual diminution of the ardor of our wills. Taoism and Confucianism, the predominant Chinese schools, also idealize a more harmonious life to be gained by restraint of meddlesome willing. Zen, which has roots in both Buddhism and Taoism, is the chief rival of yoga for attention in America today. Our discussion of quietistic schools will be limited to Zen as a prime example.

Zen and yoga overlap regarding ideals of alert, supple, patient and efficient dealings with affairs in everyday life. Although having some common sources in ancient Hindu philosophy, they differ in two main ways.

(1) The goal of raja yoga, which remains the goal of hatha yoga for orthodox yogins, is attainment of an ultimate state of reality, consciousness and value *(satchitananda)* in which quiescence is perfect. Most can attain it only beyond this present life, which is full of disturbances. The goal of Zen is attainment and maintenance of an attitude such that one experiences each present and passing moment as itself the ultimate in the way of reality, consciousness and value. For Zen, the world as presently experienced is the best of all actual worlds, and whoever fails to appreciate it as such loses and wastes his present ultimate reward. Hatha yoga and its breathing and posture exercises must be regarded as means to a more ultimate end; Zen experiences are ends-in-themselves.

(2) Hatha yoga, at least as we have presented it here, emphasizes physiological techniques and seeks mental health and its values primarily by way of improving physical health. Zen attends mainly, if not exclusively, to psychological techniques and lets physical nature marvelously take care of itself. One may "use" Zen for practical purposes, in business as in war (Samurai swordsmen and Kamikaze pilots), but physical agility flows more from mental spontaneity than mental from physical as in hatha yoga. Unfortunately, Zen is usually presented in unnecessarily enigmatic ways. Business and professional life may profit even more from Zen than from yoga; still, the definitely utilitarian, problematic business and professional life—which demands a worrisome attitude generating the tensions which the present volume is designed to

relieve—may find the unworrying spirit of Zen somewhat incompatible with its main efforts. But this is another story.

2. PHYSIOLOGICAL

Physical exercises pursued under the guidance of other systems of physical health, whether those devoted to gymnastics or sports, or to any of the specialized techniques about to be mentioned, also have consequences for mental health. We cannot take time to explore the relative merits of, or even survey all of, the various schemes for attaining mental health by physical means. Some advocate walking "on all fours" like our presumed four-footed ancestors did. Some advise prolonged fasts. Some believe you can diet your way to mental health—by fruit juices, or buttermilk and cheese, or yogurt, or chili, or curry, or vegetarian or raw-meat diets. Some suggest self-flagellation, some walking several miles each day, some continence, some copious sexual indulgence, some enduring a cold silence, some sunbathing and nudist exposure, some Turkish, Swedish or other hot baths, some massages and colonic irrigation, some specially mechanized body rolling chairs or beds, and some rowing machines. Singing and dancing also have physiological values for mental health. It is unsafe to generalize upon the comparative values of yoga relative to all of this vast array of possibilities. Since people differ in abilities, tastes, needs and opportunities, each individual must discover for himself the relative merits of different systems. The two millennia of successful use of yogic methods, together with the immediately observable benefits previously noted, may combine to give an inquirer motive to explore further for himself.

3. PHARMACEUTICAL

Although we can only guess, today probably the most commonly used ways to obtain relief from mental tensions are neither "psychological" nor "physiological" but "pharmaceutical." By pharmaceutical we mean all those ways in which we intentionally employ chemicals of one sort or another as the primary agent for achieving our goal. These include not only "drugs" or "medicines," which range from prescription concoctions designed for individual needs to standard over-the-counter pills, but herbs and their liquids—some of ancient origin, such as teas, tobacco and spiritous liquors; some of more recent discovery, such as carbonated beverages and colas. For convenience we classify these agents under four headings: (a) tobacco, (b) soft drinks, (c) liquors and (d) pills.

(a) The term "tobacco" covers all that is chewed and snuffed as well as smoked, whether smoked in a pipe or as cigars or cigarettes—each kind available in multitudes of varieties and competing brands. The profitableness of manufacturing tobacco products has been so great that commercial enterprises have helped promote cigarette smoking as an integral part of our contemporary way of life. One may, indeed, get a momentary lift from a drag on a cigarette. If it were not so, sales would not continue. But it is a mere quickie, and its merits and demerits should be compared with those of yogic quickies. The believer in tobacco claims that when one puffs to light or smoke tobacco, he almost automatically takes some extra, healthful breaths. Also, some relief from tension may come when a person turns his attention from business worries to manipulating and drawing upon a cigarette. And smoked tobacco may stimulate the organism, whether through aroma, flavor, heat or nicotine. But, on the other hand, in the long day's work too many stimulants may be precisely what is *not* needed. Yogins will claim that the quieting benefits from the breathing needed for puffing and the temporary distraction from business anxieties can be attained better through yogic quickies.

Furthermore, quite apart from possibilities regarding cancer or other respiratory ailments, the smoke inhaled with air breathed may bring into the system additional impurities which the circulatory system must eliminate. Aftertaste in the mouth, odor on one's breath, annoyance to others who dislike smoke, ashes scattered accidentally, and the nuisance of ashtrays which have to be emptied and cleaned, must count as ills of tobacco smoking—to say nothing of the costs of tobacco, of damage by fire, of higher insurance rates. Petty annoyances resulting from running out of cigarettes and having to borrow some, and from the tendency which increasing nervousness has in leading to chain-smoking and to publicly observable (hence publicly confessed) nervousness, may become part of the picture. By contrast, a yogic quickie —such as sitting straight or deliberate, deep, lengthened breathing or finger stretching costs nothing, injures nothing and may be executed quite unobtrusively. Since no one stands to profit from advertising a yoga slogan—such as that appearing in the battle between tobacco and candy manufacturers recently, REACH FOR A LUCKY INSTEAD OF A SWEET—we can hardly expect popularization of some slogan such as REACH LIKE A YOGIN AND NOT FOR A WEED.

(b) Arbitrarily meaning by "soft" drinks, teas, coffees, cocoas, colas and carbonated beverages, we shall take but a quick look at a vast subject.

"Tea began as a medicine and grew into a beverage." Then it "entered the realm of poetry," grew "into a religion" (symbolized by "The Tea Ceremony"), and a philosophy or a "whole point of view about man and nature," according to Okakura Kakuzo, whose *Book of Tea* is a classic which no cultured tea drinker should admit he has not read. Ignoring the claims of those who regard tea as a cure-all, skimming over the varieties of teas (such as the more exotic jasmine or sassafras, and the plainer green, black or blended), the differing ways of preparing (steaming or boiling, slow or fast, in metal or china pots, with tea leaves afloat or bagged), and "barbaric" ways of "fixing" (with lemon, milk and sugar or ice), we note merely that long and widespread usage testifies to genuine refreshment.

But the yogin may claim that the tea drinker's sigh of pleasure is accompanied by moments of relaxation because with the sipping of tea one automatically takes some extra breaths, slows the pace and deepens the stroke of his inhalations—something the yogin does deliberately and from which he benefits intentionally, not just accidentally, and without all the bother of cooking—making a fire, washing teacups, disposing of soggy tea leaves, or of paying anything for tea, teacups, fire or service.

Coffee drinking is too well known for profitable comment here. But coffee drinkers may be divided into two main types. The first consists of those who drink coffee as often as they can get it and use it not only for eye-openers in the morning but for pacifiers repeatedly during the day and for nightcaps at bedtime. They drink such great quantities that it ceases to be much of a stimulant when they do drink it. The second consists of those who drink coffee mainly because they want to enliven their brains and thus must give it a rest whenever the desired stimulating effect is not forthcoming. But, in any case, coffee is a stimulant. Constant drinkers may so saturate their physiological systems that they can no longer be goaded by increased dosage. If and when coffee stimulates one's body and brain, it may indeed provide some temporary refreshment. And, as in tea drinking and smoking, one may turn his attention away from his day's worries, take a few extra breaths and stretch his legs a bit, especially if he walks a few steps during his "coffee break."

But again, the yogin can claim that some of the effects obtained from coffee drinking can be obtained more directly and surely from yogic efforts, and with less cost and fewer aftereffects. For one can hardly become "drugged" by yogic exercises whereas he may easily become groggy from drinking too much coffee. Coffee stimulates; yoga relaxes. The body must eventually rest from such stimulation so it can recuperate its unirritated energy; when coffee prevents one from sleeping, it prevents recuperation. But yoga is itself recuperative; so if one can somehow replace his "coffee break" with a "yoga break," he should both have more unirritated energy for use during the day and be in less danger of sleeplessness at night.

Cola drinks also stimulate and may be regarded, like coffee and tea, as tension promoters, despite their temporary, sometimes obvious, refreshing effects. Cocoa, or hot chocolate, and carbonated beverages may also provide momentary lifts. But all, if they do not provide food, or if they add more calories than are needed, burden the body with chemicals which must somehow be eliminated. Yogic breathing and posture exercises do not overload the body with extra waste but aid in hastening excretion, both through the lungs and by means of intestinal massage and increased blood circulation.

(c) Liquors, or alcoholic drinks of all kinds, including wines and beers, have been used for purposes of relaxation for centuries and few who have experienced the effects of liquors upon body and mind will deny that relaxation may be achieved. However, when comparing the relative merits of yogic methods with use of liquors for purposes of relief from tension, certain other consequences need to be noted. These may be divided into those affecting the executive or professional person himself and those affecting clients or guests, when liquor is served as part of the way of transacting business.

If the executive drinks his liquor in private (as he should practice his yoga in private), he may be able to gauge the amount required for achieving needed results. However, even so, disadvantages may be noted. Liquor not only relaxes but often dulls the intellect and reduces critical faculties, alertness and conscientiousness which need to be retained while at work. Yogic exercises tend to refresh and revive in these areas, rather than dull them. Liquor in small quantities must be absorbed by, and disposed of by, the circulatory system. When consumed in large enough quantities, it may result in a hangover with its attendant difficulties.

In addition, the problem of dealing with alcoholic odors in an office can hardly be avoided. Many corporations, public and private, have rules prohibiting use of liquor on the job. If executives use liquor, problems of fairness sometimes arise: "What's good for executives should be good for employees." Even disregarding the costs of liquor, problems of storage, washing glasses, the tendency to increase consumption as one grows more nervous leads naturally to excess. Results here—ranging from decreased ability to handle office problems to drunkenness, drunken driving, unintentional betraying of trade secrets, losing one's position of trust and prospects of becoming an "alcoholic"—all appear as demerits compared with yogic practices, which can hardly result in any of these.

Turning to consequences of liquor usage where clients are concerned, first of all, office odors again present a problem. Those antagonistic to liquor usage tend to be annoyed with, and to distrust, persons who drink liquor. Some clients don't drink and may be insulted. The problem of trying to decide when to and when not to offer a drink introduces additional anxiety into the day's work. Then, when the executive has several clients and joins each in a drink, he may soon imbibe too much. Such a policy leads to problems of providing options to cater to different preferences, of keeping a variegated stock, of mixing drinks, of storing liquors and accouterments, of providing service and washing glasses, to say nothing of costs, tax-deduction problems, thefts, breakage and the like. Although these days one can hardly expect to invite his clients to a yogic session in his office, one who refreshes himself yogically in private may be able to meet his clients with such a buoyant spirit that the conviviality which others seek to obtain through drinking liquor can be achieved more naturally.

(d) We use the popular term "pills" here to refer to sedatives in whatever form, from aspirin to whatever the latest brand of tranquilizer happens to be. Nowadays these may be effective; they are simpler to keep, in pocket or purse, and to take unobtrusively, than tobacco, coffee or liquor. Yet they must be purchased, whereas yogic benefits are free. They may leave one groggy or dopey, whereas yogic exercises tend to clarify the mind. To recover quickly from their depressing effects, one often requires a stimulant, such as coffee, whereas yogic exercise elevates. Those who become dependent upon a sedative-stimulant cycle may find themselves demanding both more sedatives and more stimulants to achieve desired effects, until they saturate their system with drugs and caffeine in such quantities as to overtax their circulatory systems. Furthermore, most pills merely reduce tension and do not, in themselves, refresh, revitalize and restore energy as yogic exercises tend to do.

4. Supplementary

One may become as zealous an advocate of yoga as of anything else, urging yoga as a cure-all to replace all other methods of achieving relaxation and mental health. But the view advocated here is that business executives and professional people consider yoga as supplementary to other methods. Many will find themselves unable to succeed in their attempts to adopt yogic methods. Many will find it impossible to give up other methods to which they have become accustomed. Many will find yogic ways impractical in their occupational and other circumstances. In any case, the view presented here commends an experimental attitude and effort. Some will succeed where others fail to attain the possible benefits. Those most likely to put forth sufficient effort to succeed will be those who have found other methods unsatisfactory or unavailable in their situation. Advancing age may often be conducive to yogic experiment. Those, even though young, who are interested in adventure and novelty or in adding another tool to their fund of techniques, may explore yogic challenges.

One who has acquired yogic skills, but not yogic habits, may still employ them as intermittent supplements to other ways of relaxing. A confirmed smoker or drinker may turn to yoga when his supply of drinks or smokes runs out, when he is tired of smoking or drinking or when he needs more restoration of pliability than these can give. Some may habitually try coffee in the morning and yoga in the afternoon. All of our suggestions about yoga have been emphasizing use of yogic methods on the job. But many will find their greatest applicability after hours, at home, or even during the night. One who adopts a morning-and-evening pattern of yogic exercises may still pursue all of his other methods during the day. So, although some will seek to use yoga exclusively, as yogins have done for centuries, most readers of this volume will find yoga of value mainly as a supplementary method. Those who do should find some improvement in their immediate and long-range mental health.

III. CONVENIENCE

One of the most striking features of hatha yoga is its amazing flexibility and adaptability to varying conditions. Some other methods of seeking health and relaxation seem suited primarily for the young, not the old; for men, not for woman; for those with money, not for the poor; for those with periods of free time, not for the busy; for those with large areas, not for shut-ins; or for the already healthy, not for the ill or feeble. The purpose of the present section is to survey some of the ways in which yoga is adaptable.

These ways seem to bunch themselves into three sections: variations in physiological conditions, such as those of age, sex, strength and size; variations in opportunities due to conditions of space, time and mode of living; and variations in beliefs, such as religious or moral, and in attitudes, such as willingness or reluctance to try something new.

A. Physiological Conditions

That yogic practices rival or surpass in variability most other methods for maintaining health and relaxation may be illustrated by noticing ranges relative to age, sex, strength and size.

1. Yoga may be practiced by children, youth, the middle-aged, the old and the aged. Although systematic, detailed treatment of yoga for children is beyond the scope of this book, we may note some advantages specifically relevant to children. The young child's bones, tendons and muscles often are more flexible and he can attain some of the standard postures with greater ease than an adult.

Parents who want to help their children attain a sense of personal achievement, especially a feeling of superiority over adults in some area—something very much needed by them in order to acquire a measure of self-respect in competition with others where they are normally frustrated—may find a unique opportunity here. Yogic exercises may be used for kindergarten breaks when weather conditions do not permit going out-of-doors. A distraught mother may quiet, even if only temporarily, her wildly excited brood, or enliven her bored only child, with yogic games. Many South Asian schools give mass instruction in yogic postures to classes out-of-doors, just as American schools sometimes conduct group calisthenic exercises in the open air. Early establishment of yogic aptitudes may ease readoption later in life when genuine needs develop. Pictures of two youngsters, one a three-and-a-half-year-old seated in the Lotus Posture, may be seen in the January-February, 1955, number of the *Self-Realization Magazine,* page 34.

Youth can be expected to be too vigorous and preoccupied with other things to develop much interest in yoga, although anyone prevented from engaging in more vigorous activities may profit from such interest. The middle-aged may be able to enter most fully into the patterns of standardized postures. Swami Sivananda remarks that "People of twenty or thirty years of age perform all Asanas nicely. Practice for a month or two will render all rigid tendons, muscles and bones very plastic" (*Yoga Asanas,* page 24).

But performance of *all* of the asanas or postures is not the goal of yoga. The goal is health and relaxation. So those whose lives continue to be pervaded with anxieties and threatened with degenerative illnesses have most to gain from yoga. Again, thorough pursuit of the special values of yoga for the aged is beyond the scope of the present volume. But we cannot help remarking that the older one gets, the more he is likely to profit from yogic measures, provided he can accept with equanimity the principle that he should merely stretch himself as far as he can with comfort rather than create in himself anxieties from futile aiming at extreme goals.

2. Yoga is suited to both men and women. Although traditionally yoga has been pursued, and written about, more by men than by women, as is true with many other occupations in patriarchal societies, yoga may be even more suited to the needs and abilities of women than to those of most

men. Especially those women who stay at home much of the time, and who either cannot or will not use public gymnasia and sports facilities, may find yoga a most convenient way to improved health and mental quietness. Compared with their working husbands, they are likely to have more privacy, softer floors or more convenient pads and places, more periods when they are off duty, while the baby is asleep. This book is written for business and professional people, not for housewives. Perhaps another volume devoted to surveying the peculiar advantages of yoga for women should be written. But professional women—those too exhausted from the day's work to refresh themselves through sports—may find yogic breathing and modest posture exercises ideally suited to their needs.

Pictures of women performing various postures may be seen in such books as Alain's *Yoga for Perfect Health,* Day's *The Study and Practice of Yoga,* Devi's *Yoga for Americans,* Sitadevi Yogendra's *Yoga: Physical Education* and Spring's *Yoga for Today.*

3. The benefits of yoga are available to both the strong and the weak. Those bursting with strength may extend the number of times they perform each posture, increase the vigor and rapidity with which they act, pursue the more difficult postures and their variations to further extremes, and rest less during such processes. But also the weak, feeble and ill may benefit from the simpler procedures and from breathing efforts even more effectively than the strong. Pictures of postures usually depict pinnacles of achievement rather than ordinary practices of beginners, amateurs, the weak and the aged. Although we cannot assert that yogic benefits will be obtained in inverse proportion to one's strength, we can affirm that no matter how weak or strong a person is, he can derive some benefit from yoga.

4. Size, regardless of whether one is tall or short, fat or

thin, is not a handicap in benefiting from yoga. Although thinner people may more easily attain the standard postures, fatter people have more to gain from breathing and posture exercise. Human bodies come in a wide range of sizes: some people have long arms and short legs, or vice versa; some have long torsos and short limbs, or vice versa. Having short arms and long legs may appear as a handicap, but only to those who misinterpret the goal of yoga to be imitating some pictured posture rather than feeling relaxed, supple, agile and in a state of euphoria.

B. Opportunities

Yoga is advantageous because of its adaptability to so many differing conditions of living and working. These may be illustrated by surveying some variations relative to place, time and occupation.

1. Even for standard postures only a small space is needed. So, unless a room is extremely small or particularly crowded with furniture, almost any room will serve where privacy is possible. No huge gymnasium or playing field is required. A private office, or even an office with only noon-hour privacy, may be sufficient. At home, a bedroom and, when traveling, a hotel room, may be all that is needed.

2. Yoga is adaptable to both amounts of time available (since practices range from long and leisurely series to momentary quickies) and time of day or night. Although morning and evening practice periods may be most common and convenient, some persons have less privacy at home than in the office and may be in greater need of relaxation at noon, midafternoon or at quitting time than at home. Many will find their chief opportunity, and need, at night. We have made little mention of insomnia thus far, but business and professional people seem particularly addicted to carrying tensions to bed with them and to remaining disturbed through-

out the night. Some yogic exercises may be performed in bed, and some on the floor in the dark, in such a way as not to disturb a sleeping spouse.

Furthermore, some devotees report that when they practice yoga regularly they need less sleep. Others refer to *yoganidra* or "yoga sleep" which is "better than sleep"; especially for one who dreams fitfully and awakens fatigued from his nightful of dream battles, yoga sleep, which involves remaining sufficiently conscious to control the focus of attention to prevent it from wavering and wandering off into uncontrolled nightmares, may yield a much more relaxing and refreshing night than ordinary sleep. Sleepers easily disturbed by nightmares, especially in the morning hours, may profit from deliberately setting their alarms for a 3:00 A.M. exercise session and reap a "second night's sleep" afterward.

3. "Occupation" refers here to however one's time is occupied—to differing conditions of work or lack of work. Even in committee meetings one may, if not a speaker, sit up, unobtrusively stretch some muscles and breath slowly and regularly. Or, in business and professional conversations, one may deliberately reduce his speaking speed. If one can become aware that his rapid speaking is itself conducive to nervousness, both in himself and in his clients, he may intentionally reverse his tendency to increase speed and intensity. A definite slowdown, noticeable to his fellow conversers, may induce a spirit of leisure in them also and yield an additional increment of relaxation during business transactions.

Or, at mealtime, a diner may exert a bit of effort to diminish the speed of his biting, chewing and swallowing, with noticeable results. One of the functions of a pause for prayer before meals, a yogic prayer if no other, may be to reduce tenseness and "anxiety eating." Also, time required for transportation to and from the office, to say nothing of traveling occupations, may be used for relaxing, if one can plan and develop habits for this purpose.

But also those prevented from working, such as shut-ins—whether from illness, crippling conditions, contagious diseases or hay fever—may utilize yoga. Occupational restrictions which confine one to a hospital room, at home, or in prison may constitute opportunities for seeking health through yoga.

C. Beliefs and Attitudes

Too many people mistakenly think of hatha yoga as a mysterious, occult Hindu religious sect, deducing that its beliefs and practices must therefore be inconsistent with their own. It is true that hatha yoga has been pursued for Hindu religious purposes, but it may be employed by anyone else as well. Even in India, hatha yoga is practiced not merely by the followers of the Samkhya-Yoga school but also by Vedantists, Jains and Buddhists. "One may continue to be a Hindu, a Christian, a Mohommedan, a Russian or an American, a Socialist or a Fascist, a Theosophist or a Freemason or whatever one happens to be or styles himself and he can still follow Yoga and receive the fullest benefit. It does not require one to disown his beliefs, creed, religion or heritage," says Shri Yogendra in *Yoga: Physical Education,* Seventh Edition, page 26.

A Roman Catholic monk, J. M. Déchanet, O.S.B., has written a fascinating book entitled *Christian Yoga* in which he describes in detail both something of the history of references to yogic practices within the Catholic tradition and his own experiences in using yogic methods to further his own orthodox aims and methods. "It is certainly true," he says, "that the practice of Yoga makes for increased suppleness and receptivity, and thus for openness to those personal exchanges between God and the soul that mark the way of the mystical life, without becoming confused with the latter.

But Yoga also produces a more active, willing and generous disposition. It quickens the life of faith, the love of God and our neighbor. It sharpens our sense of duty and responsibility as men and, above all, as Christians" (*Christian Yoga,* page 26). This English edition, with its *nihil obstat,* published by Harper and Brothers, New York, and Burnes and Oats, Ltd., London, 1960, is a translation of a third French edition of *La Voie du Silence* (Desclée de Brouwer, Paris).

Déchanet explains various ways in which yoga aids religious practice, giving details as to how particular postures have specific effects of use in worship. For example: "I know very well how much can be derived from ten minutes of the Pole posture, followed by another ten in the Full Backwards Bend or Reintegration posture, when breathing has become so slow and deep that it may seem as if the breath reaches the base of the intestines or the perineum. Then there is no difficulty in attaching yourself wholly to the subject of prayer. . . . The activity of the various vital currents really enters into play in prayer. An extraordinary sense of calm sinks into the mind, while from the depths of the soul there rises up towards God a silent concert, as it were, of praise and adoration" (*ibid.,* page 17).

Turning from beliefs, religious or cultural, to attitudes, or conditions of doubt concerning the practicability of yoga, we should reiterate again that the experimental attitude is needed. One does not need a professional *guru* or teacher to introduce him to initial experiences of benefit. Nor is yoga something exclusively for professional yogins. Results are experimentally verifiable. Expert yogins are available as teachers, however, for those interested in technical perfection.

IV. OTHER VALUES

Five kinds of values, which do not fit conveniently into the foregoing classifications, remain to be considered. They must be regarded as secondary or derivative for present purposes. Usually they remain unmentioned in traditional treatises on yoga; even here they should appear as incidental. Yet what appears as insignificant to one person may appeal as magnificent to another. These five kinds of value pertain to beauty, sex, knowledge, pride and wealth.

A. Beauty

Beauty of figure, graceful carriage, melodious voice, glowing face and charming smile have all been mentioned as possible rewards of yogic practice. Swami Sivananda says that "By practicing the Asanas regularly, men and women will acquire a figure which will enhance their beauty and that suppleness which gives them charm and elegance in every movement," and "be endowed with a peculiar glow in his face and eyes and a peculiar charm in his smile" (*Yogic Home Exercises,* pages xix, xxii). Clara Spring, expressing an American woman's point of view, reminds us that "A number of world-famous beauty courses contain certain exercises based on Yoga" (*Yoga for Today,* page 12).

B. Sex

Although most traditional treatises on yoga favor abstinence, yogic endeavors may be adapted in various ways to sexual needs. Those who are physiologically weak and partially or wholly impotent may restore potency as they regain their physical health. Steadier practice of milder yogic exercises may yield results when more vigorous bodybuilding workouts end in undue exhaustion. Those who approach sexual matters nervously rather than relaxedly may profit from previous relaxing yogic exercises. Indra Devi remarks that "The wives of several of my students have often told me that since their husbands had taken up Yoga exercises, their marital relationships had undergone remarkable changes.

Dr. Rudolf von Urban in his very informative work *Sex Perfection and Marital Happiness* tells that a relaxed condition is one of the essentials for a harmonious sex relationship because when hurried and strained it leaves the couple (the woman especially) dissatisfied and irritated, adversely affecting her entire well being" (*Forever Young, Forever Healthy*, page 113).

C. Pride

Pride, and especially anxiety about pride, is something which hatha yoga seeks to diminish or eliminate. We are not advocating pride, but some will choose to consider pride a value anyway. To one who has been dejected because he cannot do his work properly when he becomes tired, irritable, crochety or haggard, any degree of refreshment may be accompanied by additional degrees of self-respect. Furthermore, one who has benefited from yoga may be moved to help his friends who are obviously in need; he may instruct others and be rewarded with appreciation due a gracious teacher. However, warning is needed. Although we can no longer appreciate the fact that yoga was regarded as a "secret doctrine" for ages, indiscriminate broadcasting still seems unwise. Instruction should be given, not to the merely curious, but to those only who ask for it and seek it earnestly. One may take private pride in his private achievement of the asanas; but when one shows off his yogic prowess as a parlor trick, he puts himself in the role of a circus clown and may expect ridicule or humiliation rather than pride. If one seeks to be proud because he is better than other people, his pride is that kind which "goeth before the fall." But if he succeeds in achieving skill which provides him with health and self-confidence, he may justly raise his self-esteem simply by observing himself living the improved results as an achieved fact.

D. Knowledge

Readers of treatises on yoga soon become familiar with a recurrent refrain. Yogic theory and practice lead to increased self-knowledge. Although many of these treatises extend the meaning of yoga beyond hatha yoga, as interpreted here, the values of self-knowledge indicated are intended to include those derivable from using breathing and posture exercises for attaining and maintaining health, physical and mental, and relaxation. The knowledge is not merely that of the practical kind relating to techniques, but especially of a spiritual sort pertaining to grasping something about the nature of the self at rest.

This knowledge of self may be contrasted, not only with knowledge of the world of objects, things and other persons, but also with knowledge of the way the self behaves when it asserts itself and projects itself aggressively, and of the way a self reacts to stimuli, responds with fear and anxiety and interacts with other persons and things. Knowing the self at rest, at peace, as a *being* rather than merely as an agent or *doer,* is a genuine kind of knowledge which usually gets lost in the rush of activities and push of desires. Ideals for realizing your self, as a being or be-er rather than merely as doing or do-er, continue to be largely missing from Western philosophy, psychology, religion and education. The value of discovering one's self and of enjoying one's self as it *is,* rather than as it is going to be, is indeed a value as well as a kind of knowledge. Again, the attainment of this kind of knowledge may be beyond some people; the only way to know that there is such knowledge and such a value is to try and see.

E. Wealth

About the last thing one should expect from yoga is wealth. Yet, when certain facts are pointed out, it becomes obvious that here is a value not to be overlooked. First of all, as Swami Sivananda argues, "Health is wealth. . . . If you do not possess good health you cannot prosper in any walk of life" (*Yogic Home Exercises*, page xiv). We need but review any of the factors listed under Physical Health and Mental Health to see that they have a bearing upon our ability to deal with the problems in our businesses and professions. Many factors affecting our day-to-day and long-range capacities for achieving business and professional goals may be influenced by yogic endeavors. One can hardly calculate results, but still can easily sense the significance of improved health for business success.

Not only may one acquire more financially from good health, but he need spend less upon measures to alleviate illness. The costs of physicians, medicines and hospitals, and of psychiatrists and mental hospitals, are so astronomical as to need no further comment. But another aspect of yoga reduces expenses: in reducing anxiety and desirousness, yoga tends to diminish our desires and the expenditures we make trying to satisfy those desires. A person who achieves peace with himself, even if only part of the time, has less motive for spending money to win the battle for satisfaction of his cravings. The previous detailed lists of ways in which yoga is less expensive than most other methods of attaining and maintaining health and relaxation may be recalled here as contributing to one's capital. Although attainment of wealth is not a primary aim of yoga, few who know the value of health for attaining wealth—especially as one experiences declining health under loads of high responsibility—can doubt that improvement of health through yoga may have a high financial value.

CHAPTER III

Breathing

I. IMPORTANCE OF BREATHING

We must distinguish between (1) the importance, indeed, the necessity, of breathing for life, (2) the importance of healthy (sometimes called "proper" or "correct") breathing, and (3) the importance of controlling or deliberately modifying our breathing habits for purposes of "correcting" them.

A. Necessity for Life

You know—even though you may have forgotten—that you are essentially a breathing being. Breathing remains so constant a feature of your existence that you naturally cease to be aware of the fact. Only when shortness of breath or need for more air demands some readjustment does breathing attract your attention. But how absolutely, how continuously and how marvelously you depend upon breathing for your existence, nature and welfare is usually not sufficiently appreciated.

Yogic treatises on breathing customarily recite some obvious facts: (1) For human beings, without breath there is no life. Other animals also must breathe to live, and oxygen intake in some form is necessary for plant life down to its lowest forms. (2) From birth to death one must breathe. The independent life of a newborn child begins with his first gasp; it is unsafe to sever his umbilical cord and detach him from the oxygen supplied by his mother's blood until he can breathe for himself. Life is "an uninterrupted series of breaths" (Alain, *Yoga for Perfect Health,* page 57). And, after his last gasp, a man soon dies. (3) "Man may go without food for a few months and without water for a few days, but without air he cannot exist for a few minutes" (N. V. Gunaji, *Scientific and Efficient Breathing,* page 1). (4) All other functions of the body and mind depend upon breathing.

Enthusiasm for proper appreciation, however, often leads to overstatements. Worshipful praise, re-echoed throughout the centuries, appears in words attributed to Shivagama: "A more useful science than the science of respiration, a more beneficial science than the science of respiration, a greater friend than the science of respiration has never been seen nor heard." Although it is true, in a sense, that "breath is life" and "life is breath," such poetic summaries do not warrant saying that "life is *nothing but* a series of breaths." When Ramacharaka (*Hindu-Yogi Science of Breath,* page 8) says that "breathing may be considered the most important of all the functions of the body, for, indeed, all the other functions depend upon it," one must caution against mistaking a necessary for a sufficient condition. *All* of the necessary conditions of the body are "most important" for, indeed, all other functions depend upon each of them.

B. Importance of Healthy Breathing

Everyone knows how to breathe. Breathing takes place automatically, spontaneously, naturally. So it seems foolish to think that one can be told how to breathe. Yet, one's breathing naturally becomes modified and restricted in various ways, not just momentarily, but habitually. We develop unhealthy habits unawares. Not only do we drift into slouched positions with diminished lung capacities and shortened breaths as individuals, but we live in social conditions (in school, factory, home, office and movies) which normally induce sluggish tendencies in our systems.

Yogic enthusiasts sound the cry: "Civilized man does not know how to breathe" (Yesudian, *Yoga and Health,* page 49, and Alain, *Yoga for Perfect Health,* page 57). Alain continues: "Anxiety has taken him by the throat so that he hardly *dares* breathe deeply any more" (*ibid.,* page 58). What is the reason for "forgetting" how to breathe?

Not only is it true that "a connection always exists between respiration and mental states" (Eliade, *Yoga: Immortality and Freedom,* page 56), but also this connection is a two-way relation. Improper breathing produces diminished mental ability and mental tensions result in restricted breathing. Although most of the present chapter will be devoted to improving breathing habits so as to refresh and sustain vigorous mental activity, the problem of the section is to see how prolonged mental concentration and anxiety tend to cripple our breathing capacities. The best way to become convinced of the powerful effects which attention to work has upon breathing is to observe the phenomenon in others or in yourself.

The more fully a sedentary person devotes his attention to a perplexing problem, the more he tends to lean forward, draw his arms together, bend his head down; all of these movements make for reduced lung capacity. The more intense his concentration, the more tense his muscles become. Those of his arms, neck and chest contract; such muscular tenseness clamps down upon or constricts the muscles which move the thorax and control inhalation and exhalation. His breaths become shorter and shorter. After an extended period of intense focusing, one may notice that his whole system seems to be frozen in a position of adjustment for dealing with his problem intensely. He may deliberately take a breath and then notice that his system sinks back again into its tensed adjustment so that he immediately stops breathing again.

We become fatigued not only from decreased circulation of the blood, but from decreased availability of oxygen for the blood because we have almost stopped breathing. We have forgotten to breathe; as our duties, responsibilities and their attendant problems become more demanding, we develop habits of forgetting to breathe. In this way, we "forget how to breathe."

Try an experiment suggested by Swami Vishnudevananda. He directs us to focus attention upon the ticks of a clock placed at a distance of about twelve feet. If other matters distract our attention, we should put forth still more effort to experience the ticking with undivided attention. If we fail at first, we should try again and again until we succeed in keeping the ticking clearly in mind for at least a few seconds. "Now let us see what happened. . . . The majority must have completely suspended the breath; the others, who have less concentration, must have had very slow breathing. Thus it proves that where there is concentration of the mind, the breathing becomes very slow or even suspension may take place temporarily" (*The Complete Illustrated Book of Yoga*, page 221).

If no clock is available, you may devise your own experiment. Or, you may deliberately observe the breathing patterns of others as they clamp themselves to their duties or submit themselves to the demands of their ambition. But you will realize the full significance of the problem only as you become aware of how your own anxieties first constrict your breathing and then debilitate your mind.

C. Need for Controlled Breathing

Thus a need develops for doing something to reverse not only the tendencies toward restricted breathing which occur during each day but also the habits which develop from hardening these tendencies as they recur day after day, month after month, year after year. Conviction of need can come only after the significance of the problem has been realized. But also conviction that something can be done about the problem may be possible only after one has observed beneficial results from attempts at reversal in oneself or others.

Before trying yogic methods, many readers may find it more convenient to observe how some of their own usual techniques of relaxing work relative to increasing oxygen supply to the brain by reversing tendencies to constricted breathing. A smoke, a coffee break, a trip to the restroom or, for those who can manage it, a belly-shaking laugh, requires some readjustment of constricted breathing patterns. The effects of these little reversals, like "little yogas," may be noticed; and more smokes, breaks, trips or jokes may be sought deliberately. But for those whose occupations continue to be tedious or intense, something more will be needed. Deep breathing exercises and stretching of muscles, especially those primarily concerned with controlling inhaling and exhaling, should be sought. More violent sports can prove valuable here for those who have energy, time and opportunity. Going for a walk is a common technique in oldsters. Setting-up exercises in the morning should be beneficial, especially for those whose dreams intensify concentration and restrict breathing during the night.

The purpose of this chapter is to provide opportunity and initial incentive for experimenting with some of the traditional yogic methods for modifying breathing patterns.

Hopefully, efforts will continue until one has produced permanent changes in his habits. But many may not be able to make such permanent changes. They can, nevertheless, develop habits of inducing temporary reversals by daily efforts at deeper breathing. Those who try and succeed, but forget again, may then discover the importance of deliberately scheduling breath-control exercises.

Before exploring traditional advice, we will take a glance at the nature of breathing. Awareness of the intricacies involved in what takes place so constantly should deepen our appreciation of the importance of breathing and of how suggestions for improvement must take physiological foundations into consideration.

II. WHAT IS BREATHING?

Even if you know the importance of breathing, you may still have little idea about what breathing is. Our survey of a few of the complex and intricately interdependent conditions of breathing will deal with (1) stages in breathing, (2) kinds of breathing, (3) organs of breathing, (4) processes in breathing and (5) ways of controlling breathing.

A. Stages in Breathing

Begin analysis of the nature of breathing by noting first what is obvious: breathing consists of two stages, "breathing in" or inhaling and "breathing out" or exhaling. But we are unprepared for the varieties of methods of control until we recognize two other stages which usually go unnoticed. The first consists in the pause, which may be short or long, between inhalation and exhalation. The second consists in the pause, long or short, between exhalation and inhalation. These two "resting" stages may or may not be very restful since the whole respiratory system, including its muscular and nervous mechanisms, undergoes a reversal of direction and multitudes of minute adaptations take place whenever each such reversal occurs. Thus each single act of normal, unmodified breathing entails four distinguishable stages: (1) inspiration, (2) retentive pause and readjustment phase, (3) expiration and (4) extensive pause and its readjustment phase. All four are entailed in a complete act of respiration. Technical names will be assigned to these stages later.

B. Kinds of Breathing

A quick preliminary sketch of different kinds of breathing may give us a panoramic view of some more obvious distinctions before we become involved in the detailed, technical elaboration of kinds in Section III. Some of these distinctions appear rather superficial whereas others seem more profound. I cannot accept as wholly successful the following attempt I've made to arrange them in an order of increasing significance.

1. Although yogic treatises do not normally do so, Déchanet rather boldly distinguishes two ways of breathing: "One for men, the other for women" (*Christian Yoga,* page 110). He says that a woman's breathing rhythm is more rapid than a man's and that her upper chest expands first, whereas a man's breathing rhythm is slower and his abdominal expansion comes first. Although, doubtless, physiological differences in men and women do affect their breathing, I suspect that, the world over, women breathe more placidly than men and that the differences which Déchanet notices may be related partly to size of body rather than sex. Smaller bodies may be expected to have a shorter, and perhaps more rapid, rhythm stroke than larger bodies. The fact that women live longer than men, on the average, may be due to many factors; but a study of breathing habits in men and women, especially in the older ages, may prove enlightening. However, distinctions of sex do not normally play a significant role in discussions of breathing.

2. Noisy versus quiet breathing is a distinction which has its significance in other conditions. Snoring may indicate deep slumber; wheezing, asthma and panting, shortness of breath; and other noises, clogging of nasal passages. But traditional yogic exercises do deliberately seek to control the loudness or softness of breathing and, in addition to giving directions for increasing loudness and softness, often combine both increases and decreases in subtle ways, synthesizing them in larger, more encompassing experiences, as in mantric chanting of the sacred symbol *om*.

3–9. Fast and slow, regular and irregular, jerky and smooth, deep and shallow, forced and effortless, voluntary and involuntary, and mouth and nose breathing may be noted. Each of these ways of differing is recognized and exploited in yogic exercises, though these exercises aim at attaining control over breathing habits and they should end in development of habits of slow, smooth, regular, effortless breathing.

10. The distinction between "high," "middle," and "low" breathing, where most of the expansion is in the top, middle or bottom parts of the chest and lungs, and the joining of all three in "complete yogic breathing," will be dealt with in detail in Section III.

11. The distinction between the mere passage of air in and out of lungs (with related physiological and mental effects) and experiencing breathing as an affair of the whole body, the whole self, even of the whole universe (which becomes more significant as one penetrates into traditional yogic theory and goals) will be explored in Section IV, on *pranayama*.

12. The distinction between nervous and relaxed, or anxious and peaceful, breathing—which is a main focus of concern in the present volume—will be elaborated upon in Section V.

The purpose of this quick, incomplete survey has been to provide an initial glimpse into the complexity of problems involved in any attempt to obtain a thorough grasp of the nature of breathing.

C. Organs of Breathing

You know, as does anyone who has received an elementary introduction to physiology or to health and hygiene, that your body consists of several systems (digestive, circulatory, nervous, muscular, skeletal and reproductive), including the respiratory system. You can hardly forget for long that you have a nose, throat and lungs. But you may not always keep in mind the more technical names for the multitudes of parts of your breathing apparatus. Some of these parts will be recalled, as follows: nose and mouth, pharynx and larynx, trachea and bronchi, lungs and thorax.

1. Nose and Mouth

Your nose, which is a good place to begin our summary of a few of your principal parts, is not a simple affair. It consists not only of an outer shape and skin (which often receives more attention than your inner nose), but also of two air passages (nostrils or nares).

Your nostrils not only differ in size and shape from those of other people (somewhat in proportion to your differing from them in total size, shape and facial features) but may also differ from each other (because, as with right-handedness and left-handedness, you may have come to breathe through one nostril more than another). Whether relatively long or short, large or small, straight or crooked, they vary in circumference and contour throughout their length. The bottom or floor surfaces of the nostrils tend to be more horizontal and the top or roof surfaces have been shaped more like an arch.

Your nostrils depend for their size and shape partly upon the structure of your skull. The floors of your nostrils rest upon two upper jawbones in the front and two hard palate bones in the rear. The bone which serves as part of the floor of the brain cavity also functions as a roof for the nostrils, as do the nasal bones of the protruding part of the nose which form what is called the "bridge." A bony and cartilaginous septum separates your two nostrils. Irregularities exist also because the bones serving as the outer sides have scroll-like bulges in them and because the body structure is modified by and adapted to various openings, such as those of the tear ducts, which serve as drainage tubes for liquid secreted to wash dust from the eyeballs, the sinuses and finally the pharynx.

The several nasal sinuses, including the better-known frontal sinuses in the forehead above the eyes and the maxillary sinuses on each side of the nose, play various roles in breathing, thinking, illness and yogic exercises. Most of us realize their existence when they become infected, as with colds, hay fever, or noxious gases or dusts, resulting in headaches. Some sinuses appear to perform an important function in cooling the brain. Nervous activity uses energy which seems to generate heat that needs to be conducted away. Thus, somewhat like the radiator of an automobile, the sinuses may serve as a cooling system for the brain, which supplements the circulatory system wherein the blood serves as a coolant. What role, if any, the backward and forward movement of air against the membranes of the nostrils and sinuses has in generating or discharging static electricity, and what relation such static electricity has to nervous currents in the brain, needs further study. Nevertheless, we all know that we seem to be able to think better when we have a "clearer head" resulting from well-ventilated sinuses. Yogic breathing and posture exercises not only increase oxygenation through the lungs and circulation of the blood within the brain, but also tend to enlarge and clear the sinus cavities for freer air circulation.

The skin lining the nostrils consists primarily of membranes which do not dry out easily in the presence of moving air. They are kept moist by secretions called mucus which sometimes dries and hardens into a cake which must be expelled. Hairs embedded in such membranes, especially near the outer opening, often grow into sieve-like mats which catch and repel small objects, insects and dust. Olfactory end-organs are embedded in these membranes and some areas have a thick, spongy tissue which expands, so much sometimes—especially when irritated by infections or allergies—that it closes the nostril completely. Although yogic exercises may be insufficient by themselves to relieve clogged nasal conditions, they may help considerably.

The mouth, too, is an important air passage—especially when we need more air than can be forced through the nostrils, as when we gasp for air or pant or puff, and when the nostrils are closed by swollen membranes or mucous discharge. Membranes lining the mouth and tongue seem to dry up from air movements more rapidly than nasal membranes though saliva, secreted by the salivary glands in the mouth, aids in maintaining moistness. The oral passage may be closed by the lips, by the tongue pressed against the teeth or roof of the month, and sometimes with the aid of the soft palate. Directions for opening and closure, partial or complete, of the mouth constitute parts of some directions for traditional yogic exercises.

2. Pharynx and Larynx

The pharynx is that opening behind the nasal cavities and mouth which is bounded by the root of the tongue and is lined with tissues called tonsils which may become enlarged, as adenoids, partially obstructing the passage of food and air. Two Eustachian tubes, which permit adjustment of atmospheric pressure in your middle ears, open from the sides of the pharynx. The pharynx ends in the esophagus or tube leading to the stomach and the larynx or "voice box," which contains the vocal cords and glottis and muscles needed for producing sounds. A cartilaginous epiglottis at the top of the larynx aids in closing it tightly so that solid and liquid foods will not be permitted to enter it during swallowing. Respiration is interrupted during swallowing. Yogins sometimes deliberately hold the epiglottis aperture closed to force holding air in or out of the lungs in certain exercises.

3. Trachea and Bronchi

The trachea or "windpipe" is a tube kept open against pressures because its walls consist in part of cartilaginous rings, or semirings. It is lined with a mucous membrane containing ciliated or hair-like cells which beat upward toward the nose and mouth and move mucus and the entangled dust particles in that direction. It ends by dividing into two other tubes called bronchi which in turn branch again and again until they terminate in bronchioles, thin-walled tubes which lead to tiny air sacs with their small dilations called alveoli where most of the gas exchange takes place. The mucosa of the trachea and bronchi contain ciliated epithelium; the cilia beat upward forcing both excess mucus and entangled dust, pollen and germs toward the throat.

4. Lungs and Thorax

Each of the two lungs consists of bunches of bronchioles and alveoli, blood vessels and capillaries, and elastic tissue, arranged in lobes and surrounded by a pleural membrane which secretes a lubricating fluid. The lungs, together with the heart, occupy most of the thoracic or chest cavity, bounded on the sides by the ribs and on the bottom by the diaphragm which separates the chest cavity from the abdomen containing most of the digestive system.

Since the pleural sacs are airtight, as is the inner lining of the thorax, and since the only opening from the outside is the trachea, air may be forced in or out of the lungs by enlarging or compressing the thoracic area. Three sets of muscles—those acting on the ribs, those acting between the ribs and those acting on the diaphragm—are primarily responsible for changing the size of the thorax, although other muscles of the body, such as those in the arms, legs and back, may twist the body so as to distort its usual shape and exert pressures which squeeze or expand the chest cavity. A blow on the abdomen, tight clothes, a full stomach or intestinal gas may also provide temporary pressures.

D. Processes in Breathing

1. Respiration

An average adult at rest inhales and exhales about sixteen times per minute. Each time, half a liter (about a pint) of air is drawn in and expelled. At the end of a normal expiration, one may force out an additional liter and a half of air, leaving, it is estimated, an additional liter in the lungs which cannot be forced out. Also, after normal inspiration, one may inspire an additional one and a half liters. So, with effort, it is possible to increase the amount of air inspired and expired during each breath from half a liter to three and a half liters.

Not all of the air breathed can be used by the body because some must remain to fill the nose or mouth, sinuses, larynx, trachea, bronchi and their larger branches. This is called "dead air" in contrast with "alveolar air" which participates in gas exchange. The shallower the breathing, the larger becomes the percentage of dead air in each breath. But also, in shallow breathing, less of the alveolar air is expelled and more impurities are retained.

Most yogic breathing exercises have the effect of increasing both the amount and percentage of air which enters actively into the purifying gaseous exchange processes described below.

The air inhaled normally consists of about 79% nitrogen, about 20% to 21% oxygen, about 0.04% carbon dioxide, with traces of other gases and varying amounts of water vapor. Exhaled air often consists of about 79% nitrogen, about 16% oxygen, about 4% carbon dioxide, with traces of other gases inhaled and volatile substances absorbed from the alimentary canal, and varying amounts of water vapor approaching saturation. Since the nitrogenous content remains approximately the same, the major, most significant change is an exchange of about 4% oxygen for about 4% carbon dioxide.

2. Oxygenation

When the percentage of oxygen exchanged for carbon dioxide remains the same, the total amount of oxygen and carbon dioxide exchanged per minute tends to increase as a greater air volume is breathed—other things being equal. "Other things" are not always equal, however, since one eventually reaches a limit relative to the amount of blood circulated by the heart through the capillaries in the alveoli. One may, by strenuous exercise, increase the volume of ventilation to ten times the resting level. Or one may deliberately force increased ventilation without exercise. When muscular exercise increases, more oxygen is needed by the body. When ventilation is forced intentionally, some increase in oxygen content and decrease in carbon dioxide content of the alveoli and blood may be expected, though limits exist here also. Part of the aim of both yogic breathing exercises and posture movements and rests is to "purify" (increase the ratio of oxygen to carbon dioxide) the blood and the various parts of the body to which blood circulates.

The interchange of oxygen and carbon dioxide is possible

because of the structure of the cells joining the alveoli and the capillaries and the laws and processes of gas exchange. The cells are not only flat and extremely thin but are so constituted that they permit, or facilitate, gaseous diffusion. The laws of chemical processes involved in gaseous exchange, and transportation in the blood, are much too complex to discuss here. But since the movement of carbon dioxide from the blood to the alveoli takes place by diffusion, rather than by secretion, the reverse process may take place also. That is, when the concentration of carbon dioxide in the alveoli is too great, some of it will move back into the blood. The significance of this fact for both involuntary breathing habits and voluntary efforts to increase oxygenation should not be overlooked.

3. Regulation

In addition to the processes involved in the gross changes in volume and composition of air inhaled and exhaled, and in gaseous exchange between respiratory and circulatory systems, the processes entailed in regulating our breathing patterns may be noted. When we begin to take a breath, why do we continue? How long do we continue? When do we stop? What causes us to stop when we do? What causes us to begin to exhale? Why does exhaling continue? How long does it continue? When does it stop? What causes it to stop? Even if we can answer these questions regarding a single inspiration and a single expiration, constituting a single cycle of breathing, can we answer questions concerning the pattern of such cycles? Will a second cycle be exactly like a first? May it also be different? Why? What causes our pattern of cycles to be regular? Or irregular? Why do we sometimes have fast regular rhythms, sometimes slow regular rhythms, and at other times fast irregular rhythms or slow irregular rhythms?

Although the answers to these questions are much too complex to go into here, we may note briefly certain relevant facts. A group of nerve cells in the medulla, the respiratory center of the brain, controls the contractions of muscles used in breathing. Inspiration takes place when the nerve cells of this group send impulses through motor nerves to respiratory muscles. When something, we do not know what, prevents these cells from sending impulses, inspiration ceases and expiration occurs. Apparently we do not use muscular energy and force to expel air but merely stop inhaling; then exhaling takes place automatically, without muscular effort. Since all respiratory muscles contract in an harmonious way, some organizing process in the brain marvelously coordinates their movements. Apparently the respiratory center cells function much like the pacemaker tissue of the heart, since they seem to induce rhythmical patterns of respiration without outside help, even though they are sensitive also to various influences which modify their action.

In addition to the involuntary regulation and regularization of breathing patterns, many involuntary reflexes also exist, such as those noticeable in choking, sneezing, coughing, hiccoughing and swallowing. It is almost impossible to breathe while swallowing food. Other reflexes may be noted, such as sudden holding of breath when you sniff ammonia and similar chemicals. Or if cut or pained anywhere in your body, you hold your breath. If your air supply has been cut off, you automatically gasp for breath. Emotional excitement, fear, anger, enthusiasm all stimulate breathing, as may sudden increase in either heat or cold.

Contrasted with involuntary mechanisms is voluntary control of breathing. You know that you can deliberately take a deeper breath or stop breathing momentarily. Such direct intentional control may be supplemented by indirect intentional control, as when we dance or kiss or drink or smoke or sing. We may deliberately run for such a distance that we get our "second wind," after which we breathe more easily even though exercising strenuously.

Part of the significance of distinguishing between voluntary and involuntary control of breathing is that yogic exercises aim first at changing unhealthy involuntary patterns voluntarily and then at an establishment of more healthy patterns. Whereas nervous tension produces some inhibiting influence upon deep, regular breathing patterns, deliberate effort to counteract these influences in such a way that our more completely spontaneous and uninhibited rhythmic patterns become restored is needed. Let us now investigate how traditional yogic techniques seek to accomplish this goal.

But we should notice that our question, What is breathing? has been only partly answered. The remainder of the present chapter will be concerned not only with traditional techniques but also with how these reveal more about the nature of breathing; not only with *pranayama,* but with how our conceptions and feelings regarding the nature of breathing may be expanded beyond our ordinary tendencies; and not only with breathing for relaxation, but also with how certain experiments may give us more insight into how "natural" and "nervous" breathing overcome each other.

III. TRADITIONAL TECHNIQUES

In expounding yogic ideals of breathing, I am duty-bound to reveal, illustrate and explain some of the methods that have become traditional. The problem of adapting such methods for use by contemporary business and professional people involves personal experimentation which may lead to discarding any method that does not prove to be of personal value. Knowledge of the reasons for these methods may be more important to the reader than the explicit directions themselves, for the methods are subject to some variations anyway. Once a person establishes habits of practicing healthful rhythms, the significance of specific directions relative to different types of techniques may be forgotten. But since some methods have survived—doubtless because their value has been proved again and again by generations of yogins—and have become standardized, a chapter on yogic breathing exercises would be inadequate without them. Even apart from their traditional values, the reader not only may find additional insights into the nature of his own breathing processes, and how to attain additional relaxation through them, but may also discover areas of physiological activity in which to pursue new kinds of experiments.

A. The Complete Breath

We may be surprised when reminded of an immediately obvious distinction between three or four kinds of breathing which we all use. These may be called "high," "low" and "middle" breathing and "complete breathing."

1. "High breathing" refers to what takes place primarily in the upper part of the chest and lungs. This has been called "clavicular breathing" or "collarbone breathing" and involves raising the ribs, collarbone and shoulders. Persons with asthma, a corset, a tight belt, a full stomach or who otherwise become short of breath tend to resort to high breathing. One may deliberately draw in his abdomen and force its contents upward against the diaphragm and into the chest cavity in order to cause high breathing. But he will soon discover that this is a very inefficient way of breathing. Not only does he breathe with only a small part of his lungs, but he exerts a great deal of muscular energy both in pressing against the diaphragm and in keeping his ribs and shoulders raised abnormally high. High breathing is naturally shallow and a larger percentage of it fails to reach the alveoli and enter into useable gaseous exchange.

2. "Low breathing" refers to what takes place primarily in the lower part of the chest and lungs. Since it consists mainly in moving the abdomen in and out and in changing the position of the diaphragm through such movements, it has been called "abdominal breathing" and "diaphragmic breathing." Sedentary persons who habitually bend forward while they read or write tend to slump into low breathing. Whenever one slouches or slackens his shoulder and chest muscles, he normally adopts low breathing. Try the experiment yourself —after taking a deep breath—of dropping your body forward into an effortless position often assumed when you feel utterly fatigued. Then observe how your abdomen continues to move in and out with a minimum movement of your ribs and chest muscles. Again, you may tend to take only short breaths and breathe inefficiently, though the body may ask for and take more without disturbing the upper chest muscles very much. We often use low breathing when sleeping. But whenever we become physically active, as in walking, running or lifting, we are likely to find abdominal breathing inadequate for our needs.

3. "Middle breathing" is a little harder to describe since the limits of variability are more indefinite. Yet it is breathing in which mainly the middle parts of the lungs are filled with air. It exhibits some of the characteristics of both high breathing, since the ribs rise and the chest expands somewhat, and low breathing, since the diaphragm moves up and down and the abdomen in and out a little. It has been called "thoracic" or "intercostal" breathing. But too often it also remains a shallow type of breathing.

4. The yogic ideal of a "complete breath" involves the entire respiratory system and not only includes the portions of the lungs used in high, low and middle breathing, but expands the lungs so as to take in more air than the amounts inhaled by all of these three kinds of breathing together

when they are employed in shallow breathing. The complete breath is not just deep breathing; it is the deepest possible breathing. Not only does one raise his shoulders, collarbone and ribs, as in high breathing, and also extend his abdomen and lower his diaphragm, as in low breathing, but he does both as much as is needed to expand his lungs to their fullest capacity.

Now one should not, in attempting a complete breath, strain himself in any way or put pressure upon any of his organs or muscles so as to produce discomfort. By practicing complete breathing, one may be able to enlarge his lung capacity so that, after practice, he can inhale more air than formerly. But this increased capacity should come gradually rather than by force. By repeating such a complete breathing too often or too rapidly in succession, he may absorb too much oxygen and become dizzy. One may continue to employ all of the muscles and all portions of the lungs in breathing without expanding his lungs to their maximum extent each time he inhales.

Proper yogic breathing employs all of these muscles and all or most of the lungs, but the extent of expansion and, especially, the rate of breathing may be progressively reduced to suit the body's needs for oxygen consumption under the conditions of exercise or rest which prevail. As one's cycle of breathing involves an increasingly larger lung area, his respiration may be decreased correspondingly while the amount of oxygen available for use remains the same—or even increases. Slower, deeper breathing not only stimulates the lungs into healthier action, and brings more of the body muscles into play, but it has the effect of calming the nerves, as anyone can observe for himself when experimenting by enlarging his breathstroke and decreasing his rhythm rate. Although other factors must be taken into consideration also, other things being equal, the slower one's respiration rate the calmer he feels. One may deliberately reduce this rate for beneficial effect, but he can continue this reduced rate for a length of time only if he also breathes more deeply.

Since the values of yoga for long life, health and continued relaxation can be attained most effectively only if one develops habits conducive to these ends, he will want to establish regular rhythms of breathing deeply and slowly. If he wishes these habits to become as deeply ingrained in his nature as his already developed traits of low, middle or high but shallow breathing, he will have to do something deliberately in order to effect the change. One may be able to devise his own program for revising his natural inclinations. He may need no further advice from yogins. But many will wish to consider as suggestions the traditional directions offered to beginners.

It is customary to give advice regarding the best postures for breathing practice. Hence many instructors advise practicing postures before experimenting with breathing. But, since deliberate use of complete breathing is normally requested in conjunction with many of the posture exercises, it can be experimented with in almost any posture in which one has free control over his chest and abdominal muscles. And, since the kind and degree of relief from anxiety which can come from breathing exercises is somewhat dramatic and intuitively obvious, one may be more immediately and fully convinced of the value of experimenting further with postures if he tries—and fails, as he is likely to do—to benefit from posturing first. Thus one may try his initial experiments right where he is, regardless of whether he happens to be sitting, standing or lying down.

Nevertheless, some advice may prove helpful. If you are sitting, sit upright with feet placed squarely on the floor, with your hands spread out upon your knees. If you are standing, stand erect with chin up, with arms hanging loosely at your sides, with fingers straightened, and with feet solidly planted on the floor and slightly apart. If you are lying on your back, use no pillow, stretch your body to its full length, and keep your arms and fingers straight, whether at your sides, spread out sideways or on the floor above your head. In any case, do not contort yourself into an uncomfortable position. Remove anything which will distract your attention from concentrating fully upon the breathing experience itself. Later, after you have mastered some of the postures and adopted one which is most comfortable and rewarding for you, you will automatically seek to sit, stand or lie when you become ready for your daily breathing exercises.

Gunaji (*Scientific and Efficient Breathing,* pages 45, 46) recommends some general principles to keep in mind while practicing. These include: (1) Breathing exercises should never be pushed to the point of weariness or exhaustion. (2) Exercises should not be repeated too often. (3) They should not be merely mechanical. (4) There should be no hurry or haste. (5) Attention should be concentrated on the exercise while it is being performed. (6) There should always be variety and change in the exercises. (7) Exercise should always be gentle and nonviolent. And, we may add, breathing should not be jerky or irregular, but smooth, steady and continuous.

A complete breath involves first inhaling slowly until your lungs are filled to capacity. Some recommend that you begin with abdominal breathing, gradually move into middle breathing, and finish filling the lungs with high breathing. Second, a pause, short or long, should occur at the end of inhalation. This, too, should not be forced at first, though, as we shall see, deliberate experiments with extending this pause play an important part in successful yogic practice. Third, exhale, also slowly, smoothly and completely. Again, some recommend beginning exhalation with high breathing, proceeding gradually to middle breathing, and ending with abdominal breathing and use of abdominal muscles to expel all air from the lungs. Fourth, another pause, short or long, should occur at the end of exhalation. This too should not be forced at first, though this pause may prove to be even more significant than the first as a stage in which to seek and find a kind of spiritual quiescence that can be most powerful in its relaxing effects. Each of these four phases of a complete breath needs more detailed examination.

B. The Four Stages of Breathing

Each cycle of breathing, usually thought of as merely a single inhaling followed by a single exhaling, may be analyzed into four phases or stages, each with its distinct nature and its traditional Sanskrit name. The transitions from inhaling to exhaling and from exhaling to inhaling involve at least reversals in direction of the movements of muscles and of expansive or contractive movements of lungs, thorax and abdomen. The time necessary for such reversals can be very short, as may be observed if one deliberately pants as shortly and rapidly as he can. Yet they can be long, as one may notice if he intentionally stops breathing when he has finished inbreathing or outbreathing. The effects of these pauses—especially when they become lengthened, at first deliberately and then spontaneously—seem remarkable. Thus in our analysis of the four stages of breathing we shall pay special attention to these pauses, how to lengthen them and how to profit from them.

The first stage, inhalation, is called *puraka,* and we have come to speak of a single inhalation as a *puraka.* A *puraka* is a process of drawing in air; it is expected to be smooth and continuous. If a person should pause one or more times during the process of a single inhaling, the process might be spoken of as a broken *puraka* rather than as a series of *purakas,* though the expectation of continuity is so thoroughly presupposed in traditional literature that concern about this possibility is largely missing.

The second stage, the pause after inhaling, is called *kumbhaka,* and consists, at first, of deliberate stoppage of flow of air and retention of the air in the lungs, without any movement of lungs or muscles or any part of the body and without any incipient movements. A beginner may experiment by using some force to keep such pause motionless. Quite elaborate instructions and techniques have been worked out for this purpose.

The third stage, exhalation, is called *rechaka.* It too should be smooth and continuous, though often the speed of exhaling is different from that of inhaling, as we shall see. Normally, muscular energy is used for inhaling whereas exhaling consists merely in relaxing the tensed muscles. Such relaxing forces air from the lungs as they return to an untensed condition. However, a person can force air out with muscular effort; so when he sits or stands erect and has his abdominal muscles under constant control, muscular effort may be used for both inhaling and exhaling. Especially if one deliberately smooths the course of his breathing and holds the cycles in regular or definitely irregular patterns, he is likely to use muscular energy at each stage, including the pauses. However, in a condition of complete relaxation, one should expect effort to be needed only for inhaling.

The fourth stage, the pause after exhaling, is also called *kumbhaka,* especially when the stoppage is deliberate or prolonged. Since the same name, *kumbhaka* is used for both pauses, some means of differentiating between them becomes needed. They are called *bahya kumbhaka* and *abhyantara kumbhaka,* but we shall name them the "empty pause" and the "full pause," respectively. One may stop and stop his breathing without having his lungs completely full or completely empty. But lack of a more convenient alternative leads us to adopt the terms full pause and empty pause as designative rather than as completely accurate descriptions. The fourth stage, the empty pause, completes the cycle which terminates as the pause ends and a new inhalation begins.

C. Arrested and Resting Breath

Since the two pauses have great significance, we must examine them further. Four aspects of the problem, and the significance of arresting breathing, and of resting during a pause in breathing, will be explored briefly. They pertain to (1) length of time during a pause, (2) techniques for holding breathing, (3) suggestions concerning practice and (4) the nature and benefits of *kevala kumbhaka* or "perfectly peaceful pause."

First, let us consider how long a pause may last. That it may be very short, even only a fraction of a second, should be obvious from a trial of quick puffs. But that it can be very long is not at all obvious until one attempts some serious experimentation. Try holding your lungs full of air and see how long you can do so. Immediately you can retain it for several seconds and even, perhaps, for minutes. If you happen to be fatigued and if your body needs constant replenishment of oxygen, you may be unable to hold your breath very long. But when you have become rested and relaxed and when your body is already well supplied with oxygen, you may hold your breath much longer. Yogins, seeking to extend the duration of a full pause, first breathe regularly, in one of the standard ways outlined below, for some time until the body becomes oversupplied with oxygen. Then they can extend a pause still longer without discomfort. The rule for avoiding discomfort should be followed always, except, perhaps, when experimenting to see how much discomfort results, or how soon discomfort is experienced, from deliberate extension of such pauses.

Apparently advanced yogins can stop breathing for an hour or more without discomfort. Some of them eventually can remain almost completely motionless for days, even having themselves buried for such periods in order to demonstrate ability to survive without food, water or very much air. When buried, such yogins do not stop breathing entirely, but their inhalations and exhalations become so long and slow and their pauses so prolonged that almost no energy is consumed and very little oxygen is needed. Even their heartbeats become so retarded that only a minimum of oxygen is needed by the heart muscles. Their cerebral activity almost ceases, so very little energy is needed to support the voracious capacity of the nervous system.

It is not the purpose of this volume to suggest that business executives and professional people bury themselves for days. Nor need they prolong breathing pauses for an hour or more. But, as we shall point out, there are some significant ways of attaining relatively complete relaxation by use of these pauses. One cannot retain his breathing for an extended duration as long as he is nervous, anxious or fatigued. So, in pursuit of extended pauses, he will have to do what is required to attain a state of rest; the state of rest, when attained, will have countereffects which reduce his nervousness. When one discovers how effective these techniques can be, he may then deliberately seek to exploit them for relaxation.

Secondly, let us acquaint ourselves with some traditional ways of prolonging pauses. Although a practitioner aims, ultimately, at inducing these pauses at will, without aids, he may also wish to experiment with the standard techniques—especially when he feels a need for them in prolonging pauses. These aids all involve deliberate attempts to block breathing passages in such a way that air does not escape of its own accord when chest and abdominal muscles become relaxed. Again, although one may find himself acting somewhat awkwardly and feel some strain when trying new, unusual types of muscular control, he will be able to use these ways only if he can do so comfortably.

These aids are called *bandha*. *Bandha* is a Sanskrit word related to our English words "band," "bind," "bond" and "bound." Each of the *bandha* employed for prolonging breathing pauses binds air in our lungs or closes and locks the air channels so that no air can escape or enter. Although more such *bandha* have been developed, we shall limit our consideration to four. The parts of the body mainly involved are the (a) lips and palate, (b) glottis, (c) chin and (d) diaphragm. The first two seem more important in prolonging full pauses and the last two more necessary for retaining empty pauses.

a. You could stop air from escaping from your lungs simply by closing your lips tightly if it were not for the fact that air can then escape through your nose (except when nostrils are clogged, as by hay fever or a severe cold). Pressing lips against the teeth may aid in tightening them. When your nostrils are clear, you may simply lift your soft palate against the roof of your pharynx and close the passage into the nostrils. You may do this deliberately or you may learn to allow this to happen automatically after some training. A little air pressure from your lungs may aid in holding the palate in such a closed position. (You may have learned to use—or may have spontaneously used—this method as a swimmer.)

b. You may prevent air from leaving your lungs by closing your glottis. Your glottis closes automatically when you swallow. All you need to do is to stop your swallowing movements at that point where your trachea is closed. This may be difficult to do at first, since an automatic reflex pattern has been built into your autonomic nervous mechanisms. But a little effort at trying to attain voluntary control over your involuntary processes should give you mastery of this technique. Of course, you may combine both the lips and the palate closure with the glottis closure to produce a still tighter lock.

c. A third aid or *bandha* is called the *jalandhara bandha* or "chin lock." This consists in pressing the chin close to the chest and dropping the head to help in maintaining immobility of muscle and air movements. This position proves more useful in holding an empty pause, for the pressure of the chin against the chest pushes the base of the tongue and the larynx up into the pharynx and against the palate, thus providing aid in resisting the pressure caused by the vacuum in the lungs.

d. A fourth *bandha, uddiyana bandha,* involves raising the diaphragm and keeping it immobile during an empty pause. Here the abdomen must be drawn in and up as far as possible; all air should be expelled before using this *bandha.* In order to attain complete control and more comfort, one may put forth some effort in one or more mock inhalations, without admitting any air, before assuming fullest relaxation possible during this pause. Of course, one may combine both chin lock and raised diaphragm techniques in retaining an empty pause. Both of these techniques can be employed in either a standing or sitting position and they are commonly employed together during sitting postures. We should note, also, that these two *bandha* appear to serve as strenuous and circulation-stimulating exercises rather than muscle- and will-quieting attitudes, though they do aid a person in attaining thorough mastery over his respiration cycle.

Thirdly, the problem of prolonging the duration of a pause, whether full or empty, should be approached with caution, patience and practice. One may, for example, gradually lengthen the duration of a pause by counting—perhaps by moving his fingers consecutively—some short units of duration and adding one unit to each successive pause. In this way, he can proceed gradually and gainfully, whereas if he tries to attain a prolonged pause on the first attempt, he is likely to overstrain himself, suffer some discomfort and feel no beneficial or restful effects. Whenever a series of increasingly extended pauses reaches the point where one feels he has to exert effort in order to hold the pause longer, he should stop. But by repeating such a series once a day for several days—or even several times a day for several days—he can observe a gradual increase in the length of the pauses which may be held with comfort. This problem, and success in dealing with it, is an individual matter; one should expect to attain considerable mastery over it before he is ready for the supreme feeling of repose which can come from suspended animation (*anima* is a Latin term for "breath").

Fourthly, let us attempt to describe the experience sought. No description can substitute for the experience itself. Yet some descriptive ideas may help the reader to know what to look for and whether the effort needed for experimentation will be worth his while. *Kevala kumbhaka* (perfectly peaceful pause) involves not only complete cessation of movement of air and muscles and also of all tendencies or urges toward such movements, but also complete cessation of all awareness of such movement and tendencies. The state experienced appears as one of complete rest. Urgency, interest, motive, will, desire—all disappear momentarily. Such general cessation of urgency involves disappearance of specific interests and anxieties, such as those of hatred, fear, ambition, love, hunger, thirst—including those tendencies to hate specific tasks, to fear particular persons, to demand specific rights or to zealously force oneself or others to attain indicated goals. During such a peaceful pause, quiescence is experienced as perfect. We do not need to cite the eulogies of yogins who depict it as so like the imagined goal of life, Nirvana, that they describe it as a "sip of eternity" or as drinking "the nectar of immortality" (Sivananda, *Yoga Asanas,* page 163). But we can say that anyone writhing under the pressures of multiple anxieties, who can experience for himself the utter peacefulness of *kevala kumbhaka* even for a moment, needs no one to tell him how restful such an experience can be.

Inexperienced critics will argue that we do not want to lose our ambition, our desires, our will, our fear of failure and our thirst for results. If we did, we would lose our business, fail to do our professional jobs, become victims of others' aggression and drift into lethargic slovenliness. But one should remember that he cannot stop breathing for long, even if he succeeds in prolonging the periods of pause. One has to devote almost full time to yogic practices before he can begin to lose his sense of direction and his basic, inherent, almost ineradicable sense of urgency to live and act and strive. The purpose of recommending consideration of experiences of *kevala kumbhaka* to business and professional people is to aid in retarding progressive overanxiety which can be as crippling in its way as excessive indifference (laziness) may be in its way. Suicides and suicidal tendencies, which result from the development of unbearable anxieties, may be retarded and prevented by sufficiently assiduous practice of yoga. The automatic mechanisms which spontaneously induce inhaling and exhaling, as well as heartbeats and hunger and thirst, can be modified and inhibited—but for only very short periods, so far as most people are concerned. Thus the effects of *kevala kumbhaka* can be expected to be but momentary or at best temporary, unless one deliberately seeks to pursue the rest available with more than ordinary determination.

Part of the value which may be expected from trying to achieve momentary (and prolonged) *kevala kumbhaka* is more than merely momentary. For (a) the effort required to achieve it will involve some reversal of one's normal direction of neurotic efforts and some distraction from specific business or professional worries, which may bring its own small or great measure of relief. And (b) the introduction of a moment of complete rest into a continuingly and increasingly cumulative process of developing omnistrain may be enough to reverse a devastating trend. Just as a single desire, like the camel's head in the proverbial tent, can grow into an overwhelming devotion to desirousness, so a single moment of complete rest may also serve as a camel's head to begin reversal of a trend which drags us inevitably into a condition of utter fatigue. The instinct for survival is so great in man and the substantiality of driving purpose is so strong in business and professional people, that they need not fear total loss or even much diminution of ambition from experiencing moments of perfect quiescence. Rather, attainment of awareness that they can arrive at such moments by deliberate use of self-controllable techniques should provide an additional source of confidence that they can push themselves into more ambitious ventures without fear that they will become "crack-up" victims of their own insatiable zeal. But a person is warranted in having such confidence only if he has already become master of techniques for attaining and profiting from the restful effects of peaceful pause.

Anyone who has tried to experiment with *kevala kumbhaka* will know that, in spite of successful efforts to achieve prolongation, the experience is self-terminating and, in spite of some slight reversal of anxious tendencies, one is soon again immersed in his more usual anxieties. The pull of tendencies, both innate, acquired and situational, to provoke attention and action, with their necessary tensions, is so powerful that a few moments of perfect rest are not sufficient to endow one with a peaceful personality. The experience must be repeated again and again, and even then, although it may aid in temporary reversal, it cannot be expected to overcome or counteract the much more powerful drives which nature, culture and individual ambitions have established so deeply within us. Yet, its pacifying effects should not be overlooked by anyone who has become overambitious and overanxious.

Even though one may experience moments of rest merely through breathing experiments, he is likely to find that he needs to combine them with other physical exercises and postures in order to attain a more lasting, more pervasive restful mood. Some will seek to obtain yogic benefits solely through use of postures and others may proceed no farther than breathing experiments; but both together can induce greater relaxation than either alone. We shall, in the following, refer to employment of complete breathing as part of yogic routines; whether one follows a traditional pattern or works out a procedure for himself, deliberate and habitual profiting by the relaxing benefits of *kevala kumbhaka* is a rest resource within the reach of most people—regardless of occupation, age, sex, religion or kind of ambition. Although one may more conveniently work it into morning or evening setting-up or relaxing exercises, this kind of rest-inducing technique is available as an on-the-job resource. One may be able to experience the lift from a moment or two of *kevala kumbhaka* that remains more beneficial than smoking a cigarette, a trip to the water cooler or another cup of coffee, while consuming less time for pausing from the task at hand.

D. Patterns of Arrest

In addition to those cycles of breathing in which (1) no voluntary pausing occurs after either inhaling or exhaling, (2) cessation of movement is caused by deliberate effort after a full inhalation, and (3) stoppage is produced by special exertion after a thorough exhalation, we will examine some other varieties of cycles. A practitioner can (4) voluntarily arrest inhalation at any time and (5) intentionally halt exhalation at any time. He may be able to achieve a more peaceful pause if he does not push inhalation or exhalation to extremes, especially when holding a pause at such an extreme requires some effort or strain. Since any volitional and muscular action needed to hold a pause may both distract attention from enjoyment of quiescence and require its toll in energy expended, the least strenuous conditions for pausing should be sought; although one may need to practice achieving the extremes in order to obtain complete self-mastery, he will have to discover for himself, through such practice, how induced pause can be enjoyed most beneficially.

Furthermore, as one becomes more expert in self-control, he may manage to induce pauses without effort, even though he can hardly do so without some minimum of willingness. Each of the foregoing five patterns of cycles may be so experienced. (1) We quite naturally breathe without appreciable pausing after either inhaling or exhaling. (2) We may develop habits of drifting spontaneously into a heady coma at the end of a slowly rising inhalation. (3) We can let ourselves go during subsiding feelings experienceable during a slowly declining exhalation and sink into utter stupor. One who recalls how, when exhausted from fatigue, he has suddenly slumped into a lifeless slouch, completely abandoning all further struggle may anticipate something of both the completeness and the spontaneity with which an effortless pause after exhalation can be felt. But we may also let go at any time in the breathing cycle, whether (4) inhaling or (5) exhaling. One can drift suddenly into a pause whenever he is willing, provided his other bodily, mental and environmental conditions permit. The degree of willingness is itself a factor both in the ease and spontaneity with which one enters a pause and in the length of time during which the pause may be enjoyed without discomfort.

Although one may effortfully induce or effortlessly sink into a peaceful pause at any time, he is likely to find that he can do either more conveniently and hold such a pause much longer if he prepares for it by several forced inhalings and exhalings in advance. Since the length of time during which a pause may be prolonged without discomfort depends mainly upon the supply of oxygen available in the circulatory system, any process of breathing which develops an oversupply of oxygen in the blood reduces the demands which our automatic inhalation starters make upon our respiratory muscles. Although one should, in general, never overdo anything, he may wish to experiment with oversupplying the oxygen content of his blood until he knows from experience how much forced breathing is desired to obtain a maximum or an optimum period of prolongation.

When one has prepared himself both with easy breathing habits and with firm and comfortable posture skills, he will be ready to enjoy the fruits of peaceful pauses. The amount and effectiveness of the relaxation experienced during the pauses of even skillful practitioners will vary, however, with the fatigue and nervous factors which at any time must be overcome. The powerful hold that overwhelming omnistrain has upon a person's system can be relaxed completely only by sufficiently great countereffort. No fixed rules can be given regarding how much devotion to breathing exercises is needed to vanquish the anxiety produced during any day's work struggle. Only through repeated experimentation can one develop the kind of self-knowledge and self-mastery needed in order to plan and execute his own program for relaxation.

E. Eight Standard Exercises

Although no one should be limited by, or even expect himself to be interested in, all of the following kinds of breath control, a tradition, which attributes its origin to Svatmarama Suri's *Hatha Pradipika,* continues to be respected by tradition-minded yogins. Each kind has its Sanskrit name, indicated below, though debate continues regarding the precise translation of some of them. We shall adopt an English descriptive term which most closely approximates the nature, function or most striking feature of each. These are, respectively, (1) right-nostril breathing, (2) loud breathing, (3) teeth hissing, (4) tongue hissing, (5) bellows, (6) nasal snoring, (7) swooning and (8) floating.

(1) "Right-nostril breathing" *(surya-bhedana)* refers to an exercise in which one inhales though his right nostril and exhales through his left, holding the inhaled breath as long as possible before exhaling. Although one may eventually develop an ability to do this without using his fingers to close either nostril, beginners, at least, should expect to use their fingers. One may close his nostrils in any way he chooses; but the traditional technique has become standardized as follows. After pressing the index and middle fingers of the right hand against the palm of that hand, use the thumb to close the right nostril and the ring and little fingers to close the left nostril. Left-handed persons may reverse this procedure. When both nostrils are open, the fingers rest on the bridge of the nose.

Properly performed, both inhalation and exhalation should be complete, and the process repeated ten to twenty times without pausing between cycles (with a prolonged full pause but no empty pause), and with continuous voluntary control over one's muscles to assure smooth, soundless breathing at all times. One should employ both the "chin lock" *(jalandhara bandha)* and diaphragm raising *(uddiyana bandha)*; he may use the lips and palate and glottis closures also if he chooses. Although one should never hold his breath to produce undue strain, still he is expected to feel, sooner or later, a pressure all over his body, from head to toes, or from the roots of his hair to the tips of his toenails, with perspiration oozing from his pores. Climatic conditions and amount of surplus water in one's body may have some bearing upon the result. But repetition of this exercise may enable one to continue it, after much practice, to as many as eighty repetitions in a series without discomfort.

The Sanskrit term *surya-bhedana* is a compound word. *Surya,* originally meaning "sun," has come to mean "right," and *bhedana,* literally meaning "blooming" or "opening out," has come to refer to the opening from which breathed air comes out, or nostril. Since both nostrils are used, the original description may have been much more complex, but with the emergence of a standardized series of exercises to be passed on from teacher to pupil through oral transfer, the phrase "right nostril" became sufficient to designate the type.

2. The "loud breathing" *(ujjayi)* exercise consists in drawing air in through both nostrils with the glottis held partially closed. This partial closure of the glottis produces a sound like that heard in sobbing, except that it is continuous and unbroken. The sound should have a low but uniform pitch and be pleasant to hear. Friction of air in the nose should be avoided; consequently no nasal sounds will be heard. A prolonged full pause should begin, without any jerking, as soon as inhalation has been completed. Closure of glottis, use of chin lock and closure of both nostrils are standard. Although one should prolong his pause as long as possible, it should be terminated and pass into an exhalation smoothly and slowly. However, when properly performed, exhalation proceeds slowly and steadily through the left nostril with the glottis partially closed as in inhalation. One may begin to

exhale with release of air pressure by lifting the finger from his left nostril, loosening his chin lock and then partially opening his glottis. Exhalation should be complete.

Although the total length of time required for a single cycle of breathing will vary with different persons, certain ratios of the periods needed for inhaling, pausing and exhaling are recommended. The period occupied by exhaling should be about twice as long as that occupied by inhaling. One may, and perhaps should, first practice inhaling and exhaling without a full pause. Then, when he feels himself ready, he should hold his breathing for a pause which is comfortable. With continued practice, this pause can be extended to a duration which is double that of the inhalation or equal to that of the exhalation. Some more advanced yogins, however, hold their pauses to four times the duration of inhalation and double the duration of exhalation.

Although it should be obvious that persons with lung, chest or heart ailments ought to indulge in breathing experiments only if they have been assured they can do so with safety, perhaps an additional word of caution may be wise. Kuvalayananda, in his *Pranayama, Part I,* page 47, cites an article, "Ujjayi Pranayama Explained," in the magazine *Yoga-Mimamsa,* Volume IV, and remarks that inhalation and full pause, "if developed beyond the right proportion, are likely to damage the lungs more than the heart; whereas an unduly deep exhalation is likely to affect the heart more than the lungs." Hence, as always, moderation in the performance of exercises should be sought.

3. "Teeth hissing" *(sitkari)* pertains to the sound made by drawing air in through the front teeth—either tightly closed or slightly opened—with the tongue tip playing an important role in regulating the air pressure and sound. This technique pertains only to inhaling, except that exhaling normally takes place through both nostrils, after a usual full pause.

One will find the sides of his tongue pressed against the teeth lining the sides of his mouth, if they are closed tightly, or expanding between the upper and lower sets, if the jaw is opened slightly. The sound, a kind of reversed hissing, like that made when one suddenly touches ice or a hot object or feels a draft of hot or frigid air, should be regulated so as to be smooth and to sound pleasant. The experience has been described as "sipping air." This technique usually cools the mouth and may have both a cooling and a relaxing effect upon the whole body. Lips should close at the end of inhalation, preparatory to holding the full pause with chin lock. Closure of the lips ends the hissing sound, *si*, with a "sip."

4. "Tongue hissing" *(sitali)* refers to the sound caused when air is drawn in through the protruding tongue folded into a tube. The tongue, pushed about three-quarters of an inch beyond the lips, is folded as much as possible like a tube, with such pressure on the tongue from the lips as may be needed to retain the tube-like position with a suitable opening held for the duration of the inhalation. The resulting tongue position may appear more like the lower portion of a bird's beak than a tube, but variable opening or closing of the tube-like passage in the folded tongue, in cooperation with faster or slower inhalation, makes possible variations in loudness and softness and smoothness of the reversed hissing sound. Again, a cooling effect may be noted and, indeed, sought through this and the foregoing technique whenever needed. The tongue is drawn back into the mouth and the lips are closed at the end of inhalation. Exhalation is through both nostrils.

I had a curious experience when observing and participating in a yogic devotional ceremony by Swami Chidananda in the University of New Mexico Union faculty lounge on February 22, 1961. The beautiful, enchanting sounds he made during a tongue-folded portion of the chant seemed to me to be coming through an imaginary tube extending far into and far out of his mouth. Breathing techniques may be combined not only with physical postures but also with sound and meaning (mantra) exercises to produce many varieties of psychophysical results which are both restful and amazing. Here is an area open for exploration which has remained almost entirely unexploited in Western cultures.

5. "Bellows" *(bhastrika)* consists primarily in forced rapid deep breathing which serves as a basis for many varieties of exercises, all of which may be described by the same name. Although air is forced both in and out, emphasis is placed upon expulsion or explosion of air. A series of such explosions, each following the other in quick succession without pause, either full or empty, may be called "a round." Beginners should limit a round to about five explosions, though the number may be increased to ten, or to any number needed to obtain the desired effect. The desired effects range from increased ventilation, increased blood circulation, increased clearing of nasal passages and increased thinking capacity to overwhelming pacification of all mental disturbances. Caution may be needed against such powerful explosions that the lung tissues will be injured and against extending a series so long as to become dizzy. As always comfort, not reckless excess, should guide our motives and manner.

Although one may begin his bellows experiments by breathing through his mouth or both mouth and nose, standard types limit breathing to either both nostrils or one nostril. The breathstroke in the rapid succession of breaths may or may not be very deep, but it is customary to finish or follow a round by the deepest possible inhalation and exhalation. A series of normal breaths should occur before undertaking a second round. A deepest possible inhalation and exhalation may, and perhaps should, introduce each round. Some nasal hissing can be expected, though unpleasant sound and fluttering of nasal skin surfaces should be avoided. Although one may stand if he wishes, proper performance of this technique can be done in a seated position allowing maximum relaxation of abdominal muscles and easy diaphragmatic breathing. Variations include using a full pause after each round, partial glottis closures and alternation of nostrils. Kuvalayananda, in his *Pranayama, Part I*, Chapters V and VI, explains details of four varieties and relates *bhastrika* to other types of exercises.

Since the temptation to go to excess in initial bellows experiments exists, I must suggest caution. If one is determined to push himself to the limit, he should lie down if there is any danger of his losing consciousness and falling to the floor. Forced breathing does produce relaxation and revitalization. One may observe approaching dizziness, drowsiness and diminution of consciousness. One may employ *bhastrika* as a means of inducing sleep. No harm can come, surely, from hyperventilation so long as one lies in bed; for when one loses consciousness his breathing pattern tends to rectify itself and return to normalcy. Excessive ventilation results in lightheadedness, giddiness or a feeling of floating in the air.

My own experience with hyperventilation came unexpectedly during a period of physical weakness when I was led to breathe slowly and deeply over a long period to regain strength. Then, while walking to keep an appointment, my kinesthetic sensory mechanisms seemed to remain "asleep" and I had the distinct feeling of walking on air. I could control my muscles but walked unsteadily since my almost insensitive feet seemed disconnected from my knees. Since I was undergoing treatment for heart arrhythmia, I feared a heart attack. But, despite my fear and feeling disconcerted at not being able to keep my appointment, I enjoyed a surprising sense of euphoria. Theravada Buddhists deliberately seek such euphoria during yogic exercises and believe that one has made little serious progress until he has experienced *piti,* or the floating feeling of "walking on air" that comes from hyperventilation. After having had such experiences oneself, one can realize how naturally miraculous fantasies appear to the naïve and credulous as genuine occurrences.

6. "Nasal snoring" *(bhramari)* differs from the usual mouth snoring in that the lips are closed and vibrations of the soft palate are caused entirely by nasal airflow. One may practice mouth snoring first in order to develop some voluntary control over the palate vibration process. But nasal snoring is more difficult. One should approach control attempts gradually. The soft palate must be lifted toward the top of the pharynx sufficiently to produce a flutter which may, at first, be very hard to control. The sound produced is commonly described as being like the buzzing of a bee. Although, in *bhramari,* one breathes both in and out through both nostrils and produces a snoring, buzzing or humming sound in both directions, he should expect somewhat different sounds from inhaling, which has a higher pitch, than from exhaling, which has a lower pitch. Although I, and probably most of my readers, cannot distinguish between the buzzing sounds made by male and female bees, it is interesting to note that *bhramari* is customarily described as involving rapid inhalation producing a high humming sound like that of a male bee and slow exhalation producing a low humming sound like that of a female bee.

Although one must see for himself what benefit comes from nasal snoring, I cannot refrain from passing on a description given by Kuvalayananda (*Pranayama, Part II,* pages 18, 16). "A beautiful sound produced by a combination of gentle vibrations of the soft palate and nasal friction will be heard. In the beginning this is rather rough and irregular but by practice it can be made so sweet and sonorous that the listener may feel as if a stringed instrument is being played upon by some dexterous musician." "By a continuous practice of this type there easily supervenes a condition of bliss in the minds of eminent yogins that defies all description." The enthusiast may explore still other versions of *bhramari* techniques and combine them with the varieties of gestures, postures, pauses and mantras with interesting effect.

7. "Swooning" *(murcha)* is recommended only for those already well advanced in the use of other breathing techniques. Its maximum benefit comes from repeated practice under controlled conditions wherein the practitioner knows what to expect. It involves a prolonged "full pause," held with a chin lock, until you experience the approach of fainting. Beginners may, indeed, faint. But experts remain seated upright, normally in the Lotus Posture, and attain a restful, pleasant suspension of consciousness. One breathes through both nostrils and may require several rounds and full pauses to attain his goal. If the approaching fainting appears to be leading to a collapse of posture, one may resist it until he regains physical self-control. When successful, one enjoys a prolonged, relaxed, euphorious, semiconscious swoon.

8. "Floating" *(plavini)* is not so much a breathing technique for getting air into the lungs as an air-swallowing technique for getting air into the belly. By both swallowing air until the stomach is bloated, when it sounds something like a drum if tapped, and keeping the lungs almost fully inflated, one can float in water for an indefinite time if otherwise undisturbed. By retaining a prolonged full pause and exhaling and inhaling very slowly, one is able, with the aid of an air-filled stomach, to remain afloat with comfort. This method may be combined with mineral baths, hot baths or other bathing techniques designed for relaxing, and with various postures, such as the Fish Posture, which can be performed

easily in water. However, *plavini,* like other breathing exercises, may also be practiced in a normal seated position. Whether the relaxation which comes from this exercise seems worth while is something one must judge for himself. Those suffering from stomach gas pains should avoid this method, unless they also master ways for expelling air through the esophagus (by belching or eructation) or anus (after learning from posture exercises which most effectively achieve this end), as needed.

The many aspects of breathing exercises, such as *kevala kumbhaka* or absolute suspension of breathing sought by raja yogins, need not detain us here. The beginner already has more suggestions than he can manage, and those dissatisfied with their own progress may consult a guru. No one or many of these exercises is necessary for achieving relaxation, but each has its own contribution to make. One may experiment with each to discover for himself the comfort and repose it can give before selecting one or more for inclusion in a daily routine. Since the maximum effects of breathing exercises normally come when combined with posture exercises, one should not expect perfect satisfaction from an impatient trying out of a few breaths. Some breathing exercises combine better with certain postures than with others, so one should not settle finally upon developing habits relative to such exercises until he has also made some progress with posture techniques. However, not only can he practice these exercises prior to and independently of postures—he can also use and profit from these methods where it is quite impossible to indulge in posturing.

IV. BREATHING FOR RELAXATION

Although, in a sense, all yogic breathing exercises may be employed for relaxing, as well as revitalization and increased self-control, the suggestions offered in the present section aim directly at the anxiety problems faced by business executives and professional people. Their need for quick, effective relief is paramount. The results available from these suggestions can be noticed immediately. However, they may be temporary, noticeably so. Therefore, special efforts must be put forth to prolong and deepen these results by subtle, attentive, repeated, even habitual, devotion.

No magic is involved in these suggestions, though persons who profit by them cannot help but marvel. An empirical approach is all that is needed. But, like an empirical approach to learning to drive an automobile, one must discover not only how the steering wheel turns the front wheels but also how to keep his mind on the road ahead; for success in the use of suggestions for relaxing requires full-time effort, just as does safe management of an automobile while driving.

First, let us consider two types of techniques which I have not found discussed in Hindu literature. The first comes from China, the other from my own personal experience. They will be called, respectively, "Taoist yoga" and "Archi-yoga."

A. Taoist Yoga

I first became acquainted with the term Taoist yoga and the practice which it names on December 20, 1959. Constant C. C. Chang, Taiwan Normal University, and Visiting Professor at Washington University, St. Louis, attended the annual session of the Southwestern Philosophical Society at Stillwater, Oklahoma, partly to visit with me. He had admired my edition of the Taoist classic, *Tao Teh King,* and was engaged in translating from Chinese into English his own edition of, and commentary on, this same work. On this memorable occasion, Chang confided in me a very ancient, very profound and very simple Taoist relaxation technique. Although the practice involves no secret or esoteric doctrine,

Chang appeared rightly reluctant to discuss it in company where it might be misunderstood and scorned. (Since I have become accustomed to being both misunderstood and scorned and have developed considerable insensitivity to such attitudes, I am willing to expose this idea here with much less caution.)

The Taoist relaxation method consists, naturally, in something very simple: "Listen to your breathing." Nothing more is needed, except persistence and patience in such listening. One must persist; otherwise his attention redevotes itself to anxieties. One must be patient, for impatience here merely adds to anxieties; patience is itself an attitude which undercuts the roots of anxiety. The healing and revitalizing as well as relaxing effect of attending to one's breathing may be observed by giving it a trial. Such attention makes one realize that he exists as a breathing being, that breathing involves inhalation *(yang)* followed by exhalation *(yin),* that these succeed each other in a natural, rhythmic, continuing and reliable order, and that when he devotes himself to Nature's Way *(Tao)* all goes well. Not only does one who attends to his breathing tend to take a deeper breath but he also gradually prolongs it, and in the process quiets his fluttering mental activities as his mind harmonizes itself with the slower, and slowing, rhythm of his breathing. By listening, he must focus his attention on the sound; thereby he withdraws it from whatever has been disturbing, exciting and fatiguing his mind. Of all the ways for seeking relaxation, none can be more harmless than this. No outside help, no drugs, no devices, no special skills, no muscular effort, no training period, no involved instruction are needed for successful use. It can be used anytime, anywhere, by anyone who has a few moments to spare.

Unfortunately, most of those who begin to try out this Taoist technique will give up too soon and drift into the conclusion that their experiment was a failure. How long does one have to listen to his breathing? Why not as long as he feels fatigue? If the method is to be effective, he must persist until he feels the effects. At any rate, he should keep listening until, to finish Chang's brief statement, "you finally do not hear it." Listen to your breathing with undivided attention until you do not hear it any more. When you have persisted with patience until this happens, your anxieties should be considerably lessened. There is nothing, of course, to prevent you from arousing them again, when you turn your attention back to their initiating objects, persons or activities. But one who has pacified himself with such a relaxing pause should have a bit more reserve energy to cope with his task. And one who resorts to this technique often can proceed with his day's maneuvering, enjoying a degree of confidence that he can escape from business frenzy when and as he wishes. The traditional Taoist seeks self-containment; this technique requires nothing more than opportunity and will to escape from the demands made upon self by externals, and ability and will to listen to one's own self-made sounds until they can be heard no more. Whether one then sleeps or finds his attention occupied by other things, the surrendering of his attentiveness to the sounds of his breathing has occurred without further mental disturbance.

Perhaps I should apologize to Chang, since all of the foregoing explication is my own interpretation. He said merely, "Listen to your breathing. Then finally you do not hear." This intuitively clear, common-sense advice can only be distorted by complex elaboration. Chang demonstrated with a slow breathing cycle and with a manner in which an enveloping quiescence was intuitively sensed. One who cannot grasp what is simple can hardly expect to comprehend the same when it has been made complex. Hence my apologies to Chang and to the reader. If the reader fails in his own Taoist experiment, he need apologize only to himself.

B. Archiyoga

Archiyoga is like traditional hatha yoga in being concerned with breathing, with deliberate attainment of relaxation and revitalization, with self-knowledge and self-control relative to breathing cycles, and with voluntary effort to modify some acquired breathing habits. It differs from them, however, in several ways. Three kinds of differences will be noted first. Other differences will become clear as we discuss details.

(1) Whereas traditional methods place emphasis upon attainment of rest in and through the full pause *(abhyantara kumbhaka)*, its efforts are directed toward the use of the empty pause *(bahya kumbhaka)*. However, as we shall see, this involves a seemingly slight but very significant difference.

(2) Although traditional techniques serve, and are intended to serve, as means, they emphasize enjoyment of the peace experienced during a pause as an end-in-itself. Such experienced quiescence functions not only as the goal, even if only a sip of it, but also as power to produce further quiescence. Implicit in Hindu ideals is the view that good ultimately triumphs over evil, peace over war, and quiescence over disturbance. Such overcoming occurs naturally whenever the power of a more ultimate reality, inherently more stable and restful, has opportunity. But effort may be needed to withhold or retard our ambitious, aggressive, anxiety-producing tendencies. If one can actually participate in the nirvanic goal, he will so appreciate its intrinsic worth that he will be moved to reduce the power which his will to act, including his will to breathe, has in preventing him from full and continuing enjoyment of Nirvana.

Archiyoga, on the other hand, emphasizes use of the down-stroke and empty pause as a means to restoring natural breathing. The end-in-itself quality of momentary pauses and the subtle power which ends-experiences have in molding our motives is in no way denied. But the primary purpose, more Taoistic than Hindu, is to eradicate nervous breathing and restore natural breathing—a distinction which has yet to be clarified.

(3) It recognizes a need for doing battle with our desires —a subtle psychical battle. So does traditional yoga. But the traditional battle centers about holding one's breath as long as possible during pauses so that immediately apprehended peace may be enjoyed. Archiyoga can win its battle only by surrendering all will, volition, intention or ambition of a conscious and deliberate sort so that there is spontaneous, automatic, unconscious, will-less breathing, which nature provides so noticeably in little children, cud-chewing cows, purring cats and in any living being immersed in deep slumber. Traditional yoga also can win its battle only by surrendering conscious will, but it aims to surrender to pacifity (passivity) rather than to animality. Hindus do not deny animality, but they tend to regard the locus of the control sought as spiritual rather than as animal. In Archiyoga, man's animal nature is believed to embody self-restorative powers whenever his autonomic nervous system can regain full control from his voluntary nervous system. Thus, these two different emphases regarding ways of conceiving the battle to be fought result in a subtle, but fundamental, difference in method.

C. Nervous Versus Natural Breathing

Although the terms "natural" and "nervous" must already have some relevant meaning for the reader, specific effort to sharpen the distinction denoted seems needed. Observe or recall how an infant awakens gradually but wide-eyed from a sound slumber, or how you yourself begin to stir during an undisturbed, lethargic awakening from a deep sleep. One's first responses tend to express some inner tendency which does not require significant modification of the harmonious and wholesome gestalts of regular breathing patterns. One may move a finger or toe, or arm or leg, without interfering with the wave-like movements, to and fro, of the ponderous and unimpeded rhythmic cycles. At the first dawn of consciousness, no problem occurs and no interest is aroused. As long as no specific issue attracts attention, one may be aware of the movement of his chest or toe without being aware that it might be different and without any concern about its becoming different. At first, one merely observes whatever emerges into his consciousness without any attachment of interest in it as such.

Eventually, however, attention becomes arrested and focused upon some problematic object or activity. Whether it be related to a native hunger, a sudden pain, a startling fear or mere curiosity, when one attributes importance to, and attaches interest in, anything, he naturally directs further attention to it. Then, if one is able, he musters his whole body and mind under the control of his attention and adjusts them to it and also to readiness for further adaptation to it. Then follow grosser muscular movements of arms, legs, torso, back and neck which do require shifts in muscular responses that interrupt the free-flowing of natural breathing rhythms. Some tensing of muscles becomes necessary and, when such tensing continues or grows more intense, some nervous tension develops because, as soon as one moves his muscles in the way he wants to, his voluntary nervous system comes into operation.

We do not notice our nervous condition as such, because our attention is directed at some object or activity. The more strained our muscular and attentive responses, the more strenuously we focus attention upon the objects and the less able we become to observe such strain in ourselves—until fatigue forces us to locate our disability in order to deal with it. Then we realize that something is wrong, even though we do not know what. If we try to will our way out of fatigue, by attending more insistently to it or to something which we believe will cure it, we may simply aggravate our condition. For although some measures offer temporary relief, such as a drink, smoke, reading, movies or going for a ride, they may merely postpone or magnify the problem of recuperation of strength, nervous and muscular. If a person can discover how to refrain from willing and how to return to a condition of natural breathing, he may recuperate much more quickly and completely.

A person does not have to act in order to become nervous and subject himself to nervous breathing. He need merely prepare to act. In fact, he need merely think about acting, imagine himself acting, dream of acting. However, only a little interestedness in things and prospects does not tax our energies normally. Our bodies produce enough energy for amazing amounts of problematic struggling and zealous anticipation. The supply is so great that we can work for hours upon hours restricting our natural breathing with nervous interference of regular breathing rhythms. We manage to get enough air anyway, most of the time. It is only when we develop feelings of fatigue that nervous breathing becomes a problem. One who can relax his attention every few minutes may continue all day without noticeable drain of strength. But when one must keep his mind, and his whole bodily orientation, constantly adapted or readapted to persistingly demanding problems, he may be forced to interfere with his natural breathing for prolonged periods. The source of such interference can be external to self (in the predicaments which one faces) or internal to self (unrelenting ambition that keeps one plotting, worrying and preparing every minute). Fear of failure or inordinate pride, especially when deep-seated in one's makeup, contribute to persisting anxieties that require nervous breathing which shortens breath habitually.

Knowing about the distinction between natural and nervous breathing is not sufficient for our purposes. Some who become acquainted with the distinction still look outside themselves for a cure of ills. If the sources of anxiety are indeed outer, then a vacation from them may help. A day at a quiet beach does wonders. Some succeed in using Sunday as a day of rest. But when taking a vacation means travel, with its own sets of problems, excitements, tensions, one may need to get back on the job "so he can rest up from his vacation." Some look externally for instruments, such as drugs or liquors, to induce sleep, or push themselves to an exhaustion which demands sleep immediately. The technique proposed here involves not merely knowing about the distinction but also ability to apprehend intuitively the difference within oneself.

How do you detect the difference between nervous and natural breathing? Not by looking elsewhere, though there can be no harm in observing your bodily movements in a mirror to study breathing rhythms and their interruptions. Attention must be directed inward. Even if you do not listen to your breathing, you must, nevertheless, attend to it and to the movements which we call "breathstrokes." Attention should be directed, not to particular muscles or postures, though use of standard yogic breathing exercises and postures may indeed help, but to the experience of relative rest and anxiety upon approaching the bottom of your breathstroke. Although one will be conscious of the whole breath cycle, concern should be focused primarily upon that aspect of experience to be found at the bottom of the breathstroke. Thus, in your imagination, direct attention toward the "bottom of your lungs." You do not need a clear picture of your lungs or any breathing mechanisms for this purpose. Rather, try to devote undivided attention to an approaching empty pause and to the noticeable power which induces initiation and pursuit of the upstroke. For it is in this area or period or pause that the clue to the Archiyoga technique must be located.

The downstroke need not be complete. One may pause anywhere in the downstroke, and indifference to completion of the downstroke is itself a favorable ingredient in success. However, if one has previously forced himself to take several complete breaths so that the supply of oxygen in his blood has become temporarily in surplus, he should be better prepared for success. Removal of distractions and performance of preliminary muscular stretching exercises may be needed. Although one needs, at first, to give deliberate attention to the problem of relaxing, he must seek to become indifferent, not just to his other problems, but to the problem of whether or not he shall breathe at all. Those who have become thoroughly saturated with anxiety complexes may be incapable, at least at first, of becoming willing to be indifferent to breathing. Not only does breathing persist instinctively, but willing is also instinctive; and under conditions of stress and strain nervous or willful breathing becomes instinctive or "second nature." How then can one deliberately become indifferent to his own interested nature, and, still more paradoxically, how can he become interested in becoming indifferent to his vital interest in breathing?

It is this quest for indifference to breathing which constitutes the battle for relaxation that Archiyoga is designed to help you win. One does not achieve this kind of indifference to breathing by directing his attention elsewhere but by focusing it wholly upon such breathing itself. Natural breathing is indifferent breathing. It is breathing in which your voluntary nervous system plays no significant role. It is breathing in which volition, at least volition as a conscious, attentive, directive force, has no influence, directly or indirectly. It is natural because forces within your own inner nature, or, more specifically, in the demands made by your circulatory and respiratory system for more oxygen, take place naturally, without any act of intention. Nervous breathing is its enemy. Archi-yoga consists in the theory and practice of this battle whereby one deliberately seeks to develop an attitude of indifference to breathing so that natural breathing can take over the whole job. The result, when natural breathing can be prolonged until physiological revitalization recurs, is a profound rest.

D. The Battle for Rest

The purpose of the following pages is to present an outline of some typical stages to be expected in a recommended experiment.

1. First, some preliminaries. You should place yourself in a relaxed position. The Supine Posture, yet to be discussed (see Chapter IV, Section IV), is perhaps the best. This means you should lie down in a most comfortable condition. Many will find a carpeted floor best, though some will prefer a couch or bed. In winter, or cold weather, a bed with covers is better. At night, when you use this method to induce sleep, you will naturally want to be in bed. You may be in a seated position (in the office, while being transported, or in a lounge) or even standing (when waiting in line, in an elevator, or for a delayed companion). Results in these latter positions must be expected to be merely temporary.

Also, an intentionally induced series of deep breaths is advisable. The longer the series the better, perhaps. Preparatory muscular stretching posture exercises may be necessary for maximum benefit. These exercises should be sufficient in amount to assure considerable elimination of tensions controlling your muscles. Specific attention to relaxing particular muscles, a procedure to be described in Chapter IV, Section IV A, may be necessary at times.

2. Deliberately attend to your breathing cycle. Notice its regularity. If irregular, try to make it regular. Observe the upstroke, the full pause or transition from upstroke to downstroke, the downstroke, the empty pause, its duration and the process of transition from downstroke to upstroke. Continue to observe each of these for some time. Then increasingly focus attention upon the downstroke, its fading into the empty pause, and the gradual, subtle takeover by whatever power causes the upstroke. Do not speculate upon the nature of the power, what causes it, how it operates, for such speculation will distract attention from the immediate problem and make dealing with it more difficult. Merely observe the presence of such power in action: its initiation, growth, expansion and full control in forcing the continuation and completion of the upstroke.

3. Gradually lengthen your breath cycle, especially by prolonging the empty pause. Do not force such prolongation by an effort of will, but accomplish the result by assuming an attitude of indifference. That is, as the downstroke approaches its termination, take an attitude of not caring how long a time will be needed for termination, how long it remains terminated, how long the empty pause continues, or whether the upstroke ever begins again. The upstroke will begin again anyway. Physiological needs for oxygen in the blood and alveoli affecting a group of nerve cells in the medulla, a pace-maker tissue, naturally force initiation of an upstroke whenever the need becomes great enough.

You will notice that initiation of the upstroke occurs without your willing it. Your indifference to it does not hamper it in any way. In fact, it will occur even against your will, as you can note from trying, if you do not already know from previous experiences. Continued observation of fading downstrokes, duration of pauses and unwilled initiation of upstrokes, each successive cycle taking just a bit longer, and each observation being made with a trifle more indifference regarding the results, may bring the desired result—complete restoration of natural breathing.

4. However, when one's system is saturated with anxieties, results may be very slow in coming. Repeated reintrusions into consciousness of impulsive tendencies of one sort or another, urging interested control of breathing, take over again and again. You will have to observe how your tendencies toward nervous breathing continue to reassert themselves. Nervous breathing allows the downstroke to complete itself only by a "holding on," so to speak, to the whole process of transition to the upstroke. Nervous breathing may be experienced as a kind of mothering of your breath, involving a kind of anxious fear which refuses to let the breath cycle get completely out of control through an attitude of indifference. The anxiety pervading your whole being manifests itself in part as a care not to let your downstroke get out of hand. It may be experienced as a subconscious but evident concern that your breathing does not diminish into nothingness, fade away, or drop into a bottomless abyss. Yet this very caring, this subconscious mothering of your breath, is the most important part of the very anxiety which must be conquered.

5. The battle to be observed is whether you can permit the powers initiating and forcing the upstroke to arise spontaneously, free from voluntary control, or whether you submit to the pressures of habituated anxiety-controlled nervous breathing to function as if insisting on controlling the whole transition process. This is a subtle battle and you may have to observe for long periods before you develop ability to discriminate between being interested in restoration of upstroke and being indifferent to it. However, you may be able to discriminate intuitively on your first try. You may or may not observe the situation as paradoxical. For you must develop an interest in being disinterested. The more interested you become in being disinterested, the more this increasing

interest functions as another anxiety to be overcome, and the farther you are from your goal. The only way you can succeed in becoming completely disinterested is to lose also your interest in disinterestedness. You cannot reason yourself out of such interestedness, for reasoning itself presupposes interest. You must simply submit, by an act of faith, to a trust in your nature. Only then can natural breathing be fully restored. (For a more detailed analysis of the paradoxical nature and problems involved in desiring not to desire, see my *Philosophy of the Buddha,* Chapters IV–VIII.)

Development of ability to discriminate between your feelings of complete indifference and of continued interest in becoming indifferent may be needed as a general kind of ability before you can expect to be able to use it in each particular battle at any particular time. Each deliberate achievement of natural breathing is a specific victory and is not something which can be done once for all. Nevertheless, development of a general ability to discriminate should be a great, even a necessary, asset in winning each particular victory. Acquiring such ability seems needed before establishment of habits of repeated reconquest can be assured.

6. We turn next to suggestions concerning a specific technique. They all center about the phrase: "Let the bottom drop out of your lungs." This command refers not to any actual bottom of your physical lungs, but to whatever you subconsciously think of as underlying the bottom of your downstroke. You may picture a vague or obscure bottom toward which your downstroke tends even though it never quite reaches it. But subconscious faith that some bottom exists serves, like the mothering instinct, as a source of security upon which your anxious self can depend. But since the present method seeks complete surrender of your anxious self to your natural self, even the subconscious presence of a reliable bottom may stand in the way of such complete

surrender. Try letting go of your interest in finishing a down-stroke. Let go completely.

As the breath cycle repeats itself, repeat your act of letting go. Since each turn of the cycle tends to reincorporate something of the pattern of strains to which your anxious life has conditioned it, you must reintend to let the bottom drop out of your lungs again and again. The need for surrendering your willful self, its attachments, its attachment to life, now occurs as a need for surrendering a subconsciously willed attachment to breathing, a will to save it from total extinction. The paradoxical statement of Jesus may be reinterpreted relevant to the present contest: Only he who loses his life, the life of his breath, can save it (have it reborn afresh, free and wholesomely unrestrained). But he who clings to it, refusing to surrender it, finds himself a slave to it, rather than it being a servant to him.

One can conquer nervous breathing only by unnervous surrendering to natural breathing. If nervous control takes over after each surrender, then one must repeat his surrender again and again and more and more completely. Let the bottom drop out farther, more fully, more unreluctantly, more willingly. Development of, and submission to, a constant rhythm of assenting to not caring may be needed and should be expected before natural breathing, a kind of breathing which occurs entirely without caring, can take over entirely.

7. Unfortunately, winning the battle for rest does not assure that the battle will stay won. For as soon as your system rests a bit, becomes even a little refreshed, your ever-active brain is likely to start acting again and your imagination begins working, ideas emerge and interest in these ideas and images becomes aroused, and soon you are dreaming or daydreaming, if not about the same problems then about different ones. Even while you sleep, your dream anxieties may be as energy-consuming as those induced during waking

hours. Even when not overwhelmed by nightmares, one twitches and strains through much of some nights, as evidenced both by how often he wakes up while dreaming and by the tenseness and fatigue of his muscles and nerves when he awakens. Once a dream gestalt takes charge, your attention follows it and you forget your intention to be indifferent. You won a battle, but immediately lost again what you had gained, without even being aware of the loss. You become aware of your loss usually only by again feeling fatigued, annoyingly anxious or obviously nervous. Then you have to do battle all over again. But repeated losing what you have repeatedly won begins to seem like a futile process. What then?

If you dwell upon the futility, you will give up such effort. But if you retain awareness of the fact of winning, repeated winning, you may be convinced that still further effort will be worth while. At this point, one should become aware of the need for developing breathing routines. These are most effective and most likely to result in more enduring rest if combined with posture exercise routines, which will be discussed in Chapter IV, Section XII. Many teachers of yoga prefer to initiate beginners through posture exercises first and then come to the more subtle problems of breathing later. We have chosen to begin by considering breathing methods, but have now reached a point where the need for developing routines for breathing combined with routines for posturing has become obvious. The virtues of the various meditation postures (See Chapter IV, Section XI), as compared with the Supine Posture in which initial victories come easily but may also be lost easily, have yet to be explored. But we believe that business executives and professional people will be more quickly and convincingly introduced to the values of yoga by way of quick initial victories, even if only short-lived, which can be attained in personal experience without so much as stretching a muscle or otherwise disturbing usual habit patterns.

But before taking leave of our discussion of the battle for rest constituting Archiyoga, let us suggest some variations and additions which may prove useful. Although the reader can hardly appreciate the purpose of such traditional techniques for fixing attention, as staring at the navel or tip of nose, he should now be open to suggestions concerning aids for keeping his attention focused in a disinterested fashion which will prevent nervous interests from obtaining control of it again.

1. As a general rule, one should not force a downstroke to completion. But when initial success comes too slowly, one can try forcing a few cycles by expelling all air from the lungs. Such forcing may serve as a limbering exercise which provides freer respiratory muscle movements. If one's breath cycles become shortened rather than lengthened during his process of developing indifference to completing downstrokes, he should take a few deep breaths and try to prolong the breath cycle before each assent to indifference. Although normal breathstrokes should be continuous and smooth, you may experiment with breaking your downstroke into sections —having a series of downstrokes and pauses during what is usually a single downstroke. Each of these short strokes and pauses may be of the same length, or you may lengthen each succeeding one slightly; and you may assent equally to each such short downstroke and pause, or you may assent more fully to each succeeding one, so as to develop a pattern of increasing surrender to indifference with each such series. Then repetition of the series may have the effect of making your surrender to indifference more complete and effective.

2. While developing ability to discriminate between nervous and natural breathing and between complete indifference and continued interest in becoming indifferent, you

may play with each of these by turning your attention again and again from one to the other. If, having won a battle, you lose it too quickly, you should extend the amount of time and attention given to observing the battle while it is being waged. The more time you devote to observing the battle as a game, the more sensitive you become to it, to its existence, to how it occurs, to judging how the battle is going on particular occasions, and how much more effort will be needed before winning an enduring victory. By playing with this battle, you may develop both insight and power as refined as any other kind of perception which you have acquired since infancy. In developing a new kind of sensitivity, you may expect that it will require almost as much effort as was needed for the development, during childhood, of your other first successes in habitual discrimination of, say, how to put your hand to your mouth or how to tell which side of your finger is being touched without looking at the contact. Thus, for those for whom victory has no staying power, prolonged play and development of greater sensitivity may be in order.

3. Anyone who has spent much time observing his condition during an empty pause will have noticed intrusion of pulsations from his heartbeats. Although these may, at first, function as distractions, they may also be put to service in focusing attention in a routine of spontaneously reaffirmed indifference. When deliberately prolonging an empty pause, one may employ such pulsations as counters, delaying each additional pause by an additional pulsation. Furthermore, if one discovers that these pulsations tend to trigger the urges which induce the upstrokes of natural breathing, he may develop a conscious, and then subconscious, confidence that physiological mechanisms exist not only to prompt but also to regularize natural breathing.

Some interaction occurs between the relatively independent pace-making mechanisms controlling the heart and lungs.

In fact, there appears to develop some kind of harmony or harmonic ratio between heartbeat rate and breathing rate. A slowing of breathing rate often tends to slow the heartbeat rate under certain conditions. The intricate, delicate interrelations involved cannot be explored here, but it is well known that yogins can slow their heartbeats somewhat at will through breath control, and business executives and professional people with heart ailments may wish to inquire into possibilities and make their own personal observations. The point being made here is that, when one becomes aware of a need for focusing his attention upon, and keeping it focused upon, enjoyment of an attitude of indifference which assures continuance of natural breathing, he may fasten his attention upon the regularized heart rhythm as a means for regularizing his breathing.

4. Another aid may be found in combining the relaxing at the bottom of a downstroke with the intentional relaxation of an additional muscle, a process yet to be described in Chapter IV, Section IV A. Correlation of two relaxation techniques may have a psychical effect such that each reinforces the other. Just as a mother both sings and rocks her baby to sleep, one may join the rhythms of his heartbeats, his breath cycles, and muscular relaxation series in a psychical lullaby.

E. Comparisons

We will now detail further differences between Archiyoga and traditional hatha yoga breathing methods. As already mentioned, Archiyoga not only centers its efforts in the empty pause rather than the full pause but also concerns itself not with the pause as a cessation of activity, an enjoyed rest, or an end-in-itself so much as a battle for restoration of natural breathing.

The battle is not one aiming at prolonging rest within a

pause, but at eliminating the power which anxious or nervous breathing has in interfering with the restorative powers of natural breathing. Thus, it has no direct interest in either expanding lungs to full capacity or expelling all air completely. It does not urge that a pause be held as long as possible but only that nervous breathing be held in check. Thus, it requires no experimental muscular strains accompanying efforts to prolong pauses, and no chin locks or glottis closures nor any special attention to high, low or middle breathing. It requires no fixed ratios between upstroke, full pause, downstroke and empty pause. Its goal is not immediate enjoyment of cessation of activity but attainment of an attitude affirming indifference to continued breathing. Not prolonged awareness of quiescence but dreamless sleep is its immediate aim. Its ultimate aim is revitalized, vigorous and supple living, and ease in handling daily problems, on and off the job. However, there is nothing to prevent yogins from employing Archiyoga for facilitating inducement of meditative states.

Archiyoga is like traditional techniques in seeking relaxation, in seeking to eliminate desirousness, anxiety and nervousness from controlling our minds and bodies; in seeking healthy, confident and enduring living; in seeking its goal through controlling breathing rhythms and submitting willingly and completely to regularized breathing patterns; in analyzing the breath cycle and focusing attention upon certain parts of it; in joining breathing with posture exercises, and in recognizing a need for deliberate adoption of planned routines to assure continuing success. Archiyoga appears to place greater emphasis upon personal experimentation, though formalized procedures may yet develop, whereas teaching traditions may have beclouded or minimized experimental aspects of earlier yoga.

V. PRANAYAMA

We cannot leave the subject of breathing without making it clear that *pranayama,* as traditionally conceived, involves much more than merely breathing for relaxation. Even though few business executives and professional people can be expected to become interested in exploring these additional features of *pranayama,* at least the reader should know about them. Otherwise he may presume himself to know more than he does about an intricate tradition involving varieties of technical philosophies and mystical identifications, some primarily imaginative and some basically sound.

As explained earlier, the interest of raja yogins in breathing exercises and prolonging pauses is subservient to an interest in attaining Nirvana, a state of totally quiescent being devoid of distinctions and activity which normally can be achieved only beyond this life. In extracting and modifying those aspects of traditional breathing exercises which may be of greatest use to business and professional people, a process already partly accomplished by hatha yogins, we have omitted much that tradition includes under the name *pranayama.* But your author would feel remiss in his duty if he failed to provide some inkling of the more extended meanings of this term.

A. Range of Meanings

Pranayama is a term with a wide range of meanings. Much confusion can result from failing to be aware of this range. On the one hand, it refers to breathing, any breathing, to the process of breathing, or to breathing influenced in any way by one's interest or intention. On the other hand, or at the other extreme of the range, it denotes cosmic power, or the power of the entire universe which manifests itself as conscious living being in us through the phenomenon of breathing.

Kuvalayananda opens his two-volume *Pranayama* with the simple sentence: "*Pranayama* is a yogic exercise in respiration." However, he elaborates (especially in Part II, Chapters VIII–X) upon the history of the evolution of meanings and usages of the term. Although, popularly, breathing is thought of merely in terms of inhaling and exhaling, *pranayama* is often referred to as "the pause in the movement of inhalation and exhalation" (*ibid.*, page 26). After some authors had named each of the four aspects of the breath cycle (the upstroke, the full pause, the downstroke and the empty pause) as four *pranayamas,* an objector is quoted as saying that the upstroke and downstroke "are not independent *pranayamas* but only accessories to *kumbhaka* ('restricted pause') which alone is *pranayama*" (*ibid.*, page 34). Furthermore, some commentators insist that *pranayama* denotes only the full pause, though Kuvalayananda himself disagrees with this view. (See *ibid.*, page 30.) And, although many use the term *pranayama* to name only voluntary restrained breathing, it has been used also to name pauses experienced entirely without voluntary effort. (See *ibid.*, page 44.)

Turning from the history of ambiguities relative merely to analysis of the breath cycle, we next note that each of the Eight Standard Exercises (see above, Section III E) has been called a *pranayama,* as well as their variations. And so, indeed, all deliberate breathing exercises may be called *pranayamas.* Also, breathing rhythms combined with mantra recitations, involving sounds, symbols, meanings and their patterns have been included in what is called *pranayama.*

Remembering the stress which hatha yogins give to yoga as a means to health and longevity, we may next note that the meaning of *pranayama* has been extended to include the health-giving aspects of breathing processes. In this connection, *pranayama* may be thought of as including either, metaphorically, a fire-like burning up of poisons disturbing one's system or, more literally, the process of reoxygenating the blood and restoring physical strength, or both. *Kundalini,* not explored here, imaginatively depicts levels of energy development within the body which grow in power as functions of *pranayama.*

B. Mystical Breathing

More fascinating, perhaps, are the mystical meanings of *pranayama.* By "mystical" we here refer to feelings of identity of self with anything, whether that thing be a part of one's body, an obscure power which surrounds him or expresses itself through him, or the whole universe of being. Many interpreters of yogic mysticism express themselves in fanciful metaphors. The rhythm of one's breathing may seem as but a bit of that rhythm which pervades the universe. The universe of cosmic energy which both surrounds us and pervades us obviously escapes our use when we become fatigued. But, by breathing our way again to strength, we can feel as if the universe itself were buoying us up and providing us with strength. *Pranayama* is then conceived as a process of restoring our vital energy by absorbing it directly from some universal source. Emergence of euphoria with prolonged relaxed breathing seems evidence that *pranayama* is a way of regaining something ultimate in the way of reality and value.

We have yet to analyze the term *pranayama* into its components, *prana* and *yama* or *ayama. Prana,* a common name for breath, becomes, in mystical language, cosmic energy or power which manifests itself in use, and is experienceable not merely as general vitality, with specific expressions through desire, will, a buoyant or appreciative spirit, physical power, ability to endure, influence over others and self-control, but also as intuitively apprehendable when it swells within us while we devote ourselves to healthy breathing practices.

Thus *prana* is power. Proper acts of breathing are ways of appropriating that power. Hence, *pranayama* is a way or process for appropriating power. Even though, in breathing, fresh air from outside the body enters the body and foul air leaves, mystical *pranayama* conceives appropriation of power not so much a drawing in what is outside as a bringing to conscious manifestation an omnipresent cosmic power which exists already latent within oneself as a particular expression of cosmic being. These facts have been cited here not so much for the purpose of inducing the reader to become a mystic as to remind him of the extended meanings of *pranayama*. But it should be mentioned also that those who can and care to pursue some of the mystical aspects of *pranayama* may in fact discover additional ways of achieving relaxation. When a person attains a feeling of oneness with the rest of the universe, his anxiety regarding inimical forces tends to disappear. When one acquires an intuitive apprehension of ultimate power and of his own identity with it, he loses his fear of external powers and develops a trust which is conducive to confident living.

If one conceives the mystical as foreign, he will be disinclined to investigate it. But he should notice that, although differently named and differently conceived, something similar occurs in the conclusions of Western scientists. Cosmic energy occurs in quanta, in atoms and subatomic particles and fields, which are omnipresent and all-pervasive and constitutive of one's body. One can live, act, think, experience and feel good or bad only as available energy permits. One's way of living—including eating, exercising and breathing—determines the quality of one's feelings, the buoyancy of his spirit, and his power to will and do and be. Even though one does not intuitively apprehend the quanta or atoms which constitute his being, he does intuitively apprehend his own feelings of power and pleasure which directly or indirectly depend upon those quanta or atoms. His concern for relaxing and his observations of vitality-restoration functions of natural breathing serve as evidence of his faith that cosmic power manifests itself within him and provides him with his strength. Thus, differences between Western views and those of Hindu yogins are not as great as, on the surface, they seem.

Yama (or *ayama*), the other half of the term *pranayama,* need not detain us long. It is a Sanskrit stem which has developed a cluster of meanings and ambiguously denotes, for example: (1) restraint, control (and some interpret *pranayama* as restrained or controlled breathing with deliberately prolonged pauses); (2) way or process which extends over a period of time (as some emphasize *pranayama* as exercises in which attention to breathing continues for a while); and (3) persisting disposition or enduring nature or tendency to retain strength (and some consider *pranayama* as virtuous habituation to self-realization of self as an inherently self-sustaining superior power). (See my *Yoga: Union with the Ultimate,* Book II, sutra XXX, and Book III, sutra IV.) To interpret *yama* as sustained relaxation, and *pranayama* as a way of sustaining unanxious living through healthy breathing habits, would not be inappropriate.

CHAPTER IV

Posture

Everyone knows, from repeated instruction by parents, teachers, scoutmasters, physical education instructors and physicians—to say nothing about army sergeants and his own personal observations—the difference between healthy and unhealthy posture. Healthy posture involves standing or sitting erect, chest out, shoulders and head held back, spine in a nearly straight line and abdomen muscles tightened. Unhealthy posture is slouchy, with drooping shoulders, head dropped forward, abdomen protruding, back bent and chest contracted. You can notice that, whenever you feel fatigued from executive or professional activities, you have not been standing or sitting erect, breathing regularly or moving your body with deliberate grace.

One may, of course, obtain good posture habits by following courses other than those prescribed by yoga. Some readers are fortunate enough to have established these habits already, or to have a latent basis of habit which recently they have been neglecting. If this volume serves merely as a reminder to help you make use of what you already know, it will have justified itself. However, especially for those who have shirked what seemed an onerous and irrelevant task when younger or who have been otherwise negligent for a long time, a survey of some yogic ideals about posture may yield suggestions with which the reader is now in a mood to experiment. Hindu yogins have been aware of the values of erect posture for health and strength for more than two thousand years. Although elements of formalism may have crept into teaching patterns, practicing yogins exhibit a surprising number of original variations. The vast store of suggestions available should be sufficient to provide at least some minor helps to everyone.

I. WHAT IS POSTURE?

A. The Asanas

The English term "posture" connotes "position" or "pose" and, like a post, is something which remains still or static. The original purpose of yogic postures was to obtain a stable position in which one could keep his body unmoved for hours. In fact, this purpose still remains the ultimate goal of raja yogins who seek samadhi and Nirvana. But during the long development of hatha yoga, multiplicities of exercises have come to be recognized as standard, and the Sanskrit term *āsana* and its English translation, "posture," have been extended to include these exercises as well as both the ultimate and intermediate positions. Traditional hatha yoga has not abandoned the goal of attaining a stable meditative posture, but has added emphasis upon methods for attaining health, vitality and self-control which are necessary prerequisites for success in meditation. In doing so, they have developed many techniques that can be used for purposes of relaxation.

A glance at the meaning of the term *āsana,* now Anglicized as "asana" and "asanas," may prove rewarding. If we look into its etymology, we find that it is so old that its origins are lost in prehistory. In general, it has come to mean "sitting" or "sitting down." It is intimately related to the Sanskrit term *asa,* meaning "seat" or to "the lower part of the body behind," corresponding to our English word "ass," meaning either that portion of the body upon which we sit or a quadruped smaller than a horse upon which we sit and ride. But these meanings appear to be derivative rather than primary. The *ā* in *āsana* is a prefix meaning "to" or "toward," just as the English "a" in such words as "aboard," "aflame," "afore," "afield," also mean "to" or "toward." And *sana,* or *san,* is a stem meaning "quiescent," "peaceful," "sane." Sanity has been depicted in ancient Hindu literature as a condition of perfect stillness, undisturbed by greed, lust, ambition, aggression or violence. The ultimate goal of life is Nirvana, a condition entirely without stirrings of any kind. The quest for sanity has always involved a search for quietude of mind and body.

Thus the primitive and primary meaning of the term *āsana* has to do with attaining peace, returning to quiescence or reaching sanity. The term has retained this meaning in the uses made of it in hatha yoga, for even though one may devote much of his time and attention to movements and exercises, these continue to be regarded as means to a quiet end and not as ends-in-themselves. We make no mistake if we intend to use the now-Anglicized word "asanas" to mean efforts "toward sanity" as well as to refer to the various postures and exercises employed to bring us to such sanity. Our aim, in helping a person quivering with tension and anxiety to regain his original, natural, relaxed self, is, indeed, that of restoring sanity.

Posture, then, for our purposes, is of two general kinds: (1) a stable position, one which can be held, especially for a long time; and (2) an exercise, conducive to relaxation and mental and physical stability, which involves movements as well as holding positions temporarily. Although any sharp division between these two kinds will seem mistaken to traditional yogins, since both function as phases of a single purpose and are performed together with sameness of spirit, some analysis of differences may prove enlightening to readers.

(1) Since a stable position held for a long time was a primary goal of ancient yogins, we find the ancient descriptions of asana emphasizing, if indeed not entirely limited to, still postures. Posture, although one of the "eight limbs of yoga," was barely mentioned by Patanjali in two or three sutras or short phrases: "Posture pertains to steadiness and ease," for the purpose of "effortless alertness and endless attention . . . without disturbance by tensions" or oppositions. (See my *Yoga: Union with the Ultimate,* pages 108–110.) Endless commentaries upon these remarks all agree that the goal of posturing itself is to attain a firm seated position which can be maintained easily and comfortably, without fatigue or irritation or effort, for a long time—from three hours to as much as eight hours. Now it is not a purpose of the present volume to suggest that many readers will wish to hold a seated position for so long a time, unless one discovers, as some have done, that yogic meditation is better than sleep. For those who do seek relaxation through meditation, a firm, stable, seated posture will be found necessary.

(2) Posture exercises, on the other hand, do involve positions taken and held, even if only momentarily. Such exercises may be analyzed into four phases: movement into a position; a stance or retention of the position for a period of rest; movement out of the position; and another rest for a short or long period in some other, perhaps easier or more convenient, position. Posture exercises combine movements and rests and the movements themselves may be more restful when performed slowly and the resting positions may be more restful, for beginners, when not held too long. The same two characteristics of seated postures mentioned by Patanjali, namely steadiness and ease, have been carried over by hatha yogins into posture exercises.

Despite the seemingly strenuous contortions depicted in some representations of yogic postures, they are in fact, or should be, easy to perform. If beginners cannot attain or hold any of the postures without pain or strain, they are not ready for those postures. By slow but steady exercise one grows gradually in capacity. The temptation, and tendency, of zealous beginners to overdo has begotten the warning: Learn to practice yoga only under the guidance of an experienced guru or instructor. We shall suggest several principles to be followed. Pain or strain means "stop" and wobbly or unsteady behavior while moving into or out of a position or while holding a position indicates that you are not ready for this one. Try the easiest postures first. Attainment of steadiness and comfort in the easier ones will prepare the way for others.

B. Purposes of Postures

Although the two kinds of postures just mentioned may appear to have different purposes, the first to keep the body steady for a long period and the second to exercise the body for healthy living, their ultimate goal is the same. For the raja yogin the ultimate purpose is to attain Nirvana and, for the business executive and professional person, the ultimate purpose is relaxed living or at least temporary relief from anxiety. Less ultimate, perhaps, but still general, purposes of postures consist in all of those values of yoga outlined in Chapter II. These are improved physical health (reduction of fatigue, restoration of vitality, maintaining health, longevity, increased suppleness, reduced weight, improved tonicity), improved mental health (reduction of tension, restoration of pliability, freedom from fear, increased serenity and patience, reduction of irritability and greater willingness and generosity), and even more beauty, sex satisfaction, self-knowledge, pride and wealth. These purposes will not be reviewed here.

Rather, we choose to emphasize the more immediate types of purposes which one should have in mind during posture exercises. Although each particular posture and exercise has its own specific virtues or purposes, we may generalize about all, or most, of the standard postures as follows:

Four such general emphases may be kept in mind: (1) The attainment of *erect posture,* both on a particular occasion and recurrently (much as one reaches for another smoke when nervous) and habitually (for constant awareness of a battle among one's habits should be helpful). (2) The *stretching of muscles,* both to give momentary relief from tensions built up through our crouching tendencies and to restore a degree of balance and suppleness to our muscular system. (3) The *stimulation of breathing and blood circulation,* since healthy breathing, healthy posture and healthy blood circulation are all interrelated. (4) The *massaging of internal organs* for improving fitness and tonicity. We may notice, further, that most postures and exercises directly involve control of abdominal and spinal muscles and aim at reattaining a trim, flexible torso.

Perhaps we need a reminder that the purpose of yogic postures is not athletic in the sense of muscle building. Neither the yogin nor the executive needs great muscular strength. Of course, if desired, one may use yogic exercises for the purpose of developing muscular strength. But one who concentrates on this purpose often minimizes the other purposes, and when he fails to become athletic or showy, gives up yogic exercising for the wrong reasons. Typically, one with athletic interests seems to indulge in vigorous exercises first—chinning, tumbling, running and then breathing more rapidly as he gets out of breath. Yogic exercises, however, when properly performed, are slow, steady, graceful and continuingly comfortable. Athletic exercise normally uses energy which the body is expected to restore when it rests from exercising;

one purpose of yogic postures is to increase one's store of energy while exercising and by means of exercising.

Recently I noticed an article in a popular weekly magazine on how to "possibly stretch your height by a half-inch or more." It was not the "long-legged look for which American women are famous" nor the curvaceous lines of the professional dancer who posed for pictures of how to "lengthen the muscles of hips, knees and lower legs" which attracted my attention. Rather it was the typical American advice concerning one posture exercise which seemed, on the surface, similar to the yogic shoulderstand. The advice: "Bicycle [move your legs round and round in the air as if bicycling] until tired." The yogic ideal reverses this advice. It would say: *Hold the posture steady until rested.* The article continued its advice: "A hot bath will ease the soreness." Yogic relaxed stretching does not require easing of soreness because one does not properly exercise so violently or so long that soreness develops. There is no objection to a hot bath, certainly, which may provide its own kind of relaxation. But to advise exercising *until tired* is antithetical to yogic ideals.

II. PRINCIPLES FOR POSTURING

A. Keep Goals in Mind

The main principle, from which the others may be seen to follow, is to keep the goals in mind. When the goal is relaxation and not show, or improvement of health and not athletic prowess, then use of posture exercises will be thought of as possibilities and not as requirements, or as directions which serve as guides for efforts and not as standards of perfection from which one ought not to fall short. As Jesus viewed Sabbath observance and other rules, so we should think of yogic exercises as "made for men, not men for" exercises. Some of the more difficult postures cited in the following exceed the capacity of many hatha yogins. Achievement of the asanas, except perhaps the easiest, is not essential to the practice of yoga or to the attainment of some of the goals of yoga, even of hatha yoga.

A person who feels unsuccessful merely because he has not stretched as far as others mistakes the purpose of yogic exercises. He misinterprets the goal as something to be found in the forms of the postures themselves, whereas the goal for executives and professional people is relaxed, healthy living. One who attains relaxation through moderate exercise thereby attains the goal he seeks. The standard postures serve as means to an end. They should not be mistaken as ends-in-themselves. When one keeps these more modest goals in mind, he is less likely to be disappointed in his yogic efforts.

B. Avoid Overdoing

The foregoing general principle leads, as a matter of course, to certain perhaps less general principles which themselves yield rules that may, for convenience, be stated negatively, even though positive results are intended.

1. First and foremost is the necessary admonition: Do not force or strain yourself. The goal is relaxation, not strain, so straining to reach the goal tends to be self-defeating. Any forcing may be harmful, temporarily or permanently, both to muscles or bones or internal organs and to one's willingness to try for further benefits. Thus the first rule is: *Take it easy.*

2. The next rule for beginners is similar to the first. Do not become fatigued performing exercises. That is, do not spend too much time doing new exercises at first. Only after one has acquired some experience regarding his muscular conditions and capacities by several shorter periods does he become able to judge how much time he can profitably devote to posturing during any one exercise period. Although

a period of from fifteen to thirty minutes once or twice a day may eventually become one's standard, as a beginner he should either exercise for shorter periods or spend more of the time in resting. So a second rule is: *Take your time.*

3. A third rule for beginners is: Do not try to perform all of the postures during any practice period. Although one seeking relaxation may, and should, give some attention to stretching all of his muscles, efforts to develop additional suppleness through trying any of the more difficult standard postures should remain modest. For anyone who has set his mind upon becoming skilled in posture performance, we suggest that it may be better to become adept in a few postures than to try them all at once and fail in most of them. Hence, another rule: *Leave some for the future.*

4. A fourth suggestion is: Do not begin with the hardest but with the easiest postures. Some postures strike us as amazing. Some difficult postures seem easy. Although one can hardly refrain from trying out some of the difficult poses, he should anticipate that he cannot do them. He should work away at improving himself in those which appear easiest for him. As he achieves just a bit of improvement in the easier ones, he will begin to sense for himself how fast or how slowly he can proceed and how far he may expect to go eventually toward mastering the standard postures. Hence: *Begin with the easiest.*

5. A most disappointing experience for the beginner is to find that, after making some progress in stretching a particular muscle, he has to begin all over again the next day. Most people who have tried bending over and touching their toes have, after some effort, improved their reach. But, after resuming and re-establishing their daily crouching positions accompanied by typical tensions and anxieties, their muscles tend toward permanent contraction again. So the same effort required before has to be repeated. Forewarned by recalling

this kind of experience, a person may be less disappointed. In the long run, one may gain some relatively permanent increased suppleness from repeated stretchings of the same sort. But in the beginning: *Be patient.*

6. People differ. Bodily abilities and needs vary with age, sex, size, weight, physical proportions, muscular development, heart ailments, hereditary conditions, adaptability. Persons with long arms and short legs can touch their toes more easily. Some persons arch their backs more easily. Some can bend their legs more easily. Some have slimmer waist lines which permit most torso-bending postures to be carried farther. It is a mistake for anyone to believe that he ought to be able to attain the standard postures whenever his personal conditions in fact prevent or greatly inhibit such attainment. One's posture goals should be personal and not measured by the traditional peaks. Hence, a sixth rule: *Be noncompetitive* in your posture goals and efforts.

7. Many postures can be obtained only *after* relaxing. Anxiety, and the nervous and muscular tension accompanying it, tends to prevent you from attaining them. Any degree of ambition regarding achieving a standard posture may retard such achievement because ambition tends to transform itself into anxiety; the more frustrated you become, the more nervous and anxious and tense you become. Thus the more zealously one exerts himself, the more he may be defeating himself. Postures which can be attained only after relaxing tend to permit more-than-normal stretching and may yield a more lasting result. But an anxious approach itself serves as an effective barrier to success. Hence, a seventh rule: *Be unanxious, be calm* in your approach to every practice.

8. Not merely the approach but also the continuing conduct of practice needs to be calm. Before, during, between and after exercise one should rest. (a) Before an exercise one should rest, by means of breathing exercises, a bath, a nap

or by using the Most Relaxed Posture *(Savasana)* which we shall discuss first. (b) During an exercise, one should proceed slowly enough to coordinate his breathing with his muscular movements. And he should relax, even if only momentarily, in the position which he comes to hold. Many yogins place special emphasis upon the pervading power of rest which comes, even if only briefly, during the pause while one is holding any one of the standard positions. As exercises, many positions are not intended to be held for long periods. But one should try to extend the period of relaxation in a balanced position whenever a posture can be held longer. (c) Between each of two or more exercises, one may do well to rest again in *Savasana.* (d) After one has completed his exercise period, he should pause a bit and feel a restful spirit pervading his attitude. Especially, one should not start walking or running immediately after he has twisted his legs or back into an unusual position. In sum, one should relax before exercising, during exercising, between exercises and after exercise: *Relax during practice.*

C. Consider Conducive Conditions

Some conditions promote yogic efforts, some hinder and some may be definitely dangerous.

1. Yogic instructions almost universally urge us not to practice yogic exercises immediately after eating. One may, of course, use modest breathing exercises and the Most Relaxed Posture, but these are not exercises requiring muscular or nervous effort. You are familiar with the warning to swimmers: Don't go in the water until two hours after eating. The same applies to yogic exercises, even though one is in less danger. The heavier the meal, the longer you should wait.

2. Emptying of bladder and bowels before exercising is desirable, when possible. The contents of stomach and intestines may inhibit many of the stretching movements which

involve contractions of the abdomen. However, some posture exercises are especially conducive to promoting bowel movements. One of these, called *pavanmuktasana,* has many varieties and consists in drawing one or both knees up to the chest and binding them to it with your arms. This may be done either in a sitting position or while lying on your back. As you practice various exercises, you will doubtless discover which seem most reliably conducive to your purposes.

3. One should avoid exercises, especially the more vigorous ones, when sick or soon after illness or after fatiguing work. Women, of course, need to use caution before, during and after menstruation periods and during pregnancy. A person with heart difficulties, poor muscular coordination, or any other disease should use care in selecting exercises. One person may aggravate his illness; another may improve it. Some breathing exercises, the Most Relaxed Posture and a few of the milder stretching exercises may be beneficial to anyone at almost any time.

4. The floor, ground or bed on which exercises are performed should be suitable. Conditions will vary somewhat with a person's size and weight, age and vigor, and assurance of muscular control. Most exercises are best performed on the floor. But a floor without a rug or pad is likely to be too hard. Yogic tradition calls for cleared ground, a spread of kusha grass, a tiger skin and a cloth. But these suggestions reflect primitive forest conditions. Modern living provides a plethora of alternatives. A well-carpeted floor may be both the best and the handiest for many. Except for a few of the most relaxed postures, a bed is likely to be found too soft. A person needs a firm foundation for his postures and movements, but one which does not injure his skin or bones.

5. The exerciser should have room enough. Especially for headstands, shoulderstands and rocking or rolling exercises, one should have sufficient room so as not to bump into furni-

ture or walls or toys. A beginner should allow himself plenty of extra room while trying out new positions. If he falls, bumping into furniture may be dangerous.

6. Clothing, if any, should be suitable. First of all, one should discard all tight-fitting clothes which bind his body or hinder his movements. When posturing is pursued privately, a minimum of clothing seems advisable, though personal tastes, climate and other factors are always to be considered. Some, especially women, will prefer personally fitted elastic costumes. The existing varieties of design for such costumes have already become very numerous. One should, if possible, discard his glasses. Clothes with pockets should be emptied of all hard materials such as pens or keys. Fear of soiling clothes or of ruining a press serves as a deterrent to satisfactory results.

7. For those who practice indoors, a well-ventilated room is advised, though one should avoid drafts, and refrain from exercising in excessive heat or cold. Repugnant odors, pollens and dust which prevent easy breathing should be avoided if possible.

8. Finally, one should seek not only a place freed from noisy distractions and interruptions but also a time when he is free long enough to pursue his exercises in peace and without anxiety. When one fears being interrupted at any moment, the air of anxiety created thereby inhibits his practice. Few persons will find ideal conditions for yogic efforts, but knowing these rules may aid a beginner in quest of a suitable time and place.

D. Do Not Give Up Too Easily

The twin faults of most beginners are overdoing and underdoing. Just as we have outlined above some ways for avoiding overdoing, so now we offer suggestions for preventing underdoing.

1. One may be misled by the suggested rules, Take it easy, Take your time, Relax during practice, etc., into thinking that yogic postures require no effort. Most of them do demand sustained conscious attention and effort. The first rule: *Don't be lazy.*

2. Secondly: *Don't give up too quickly.* Those who rush into yogic experiments and overdo soon reach their limits. Many are astounded at their incapacity and become disappointed immediately. Those who push themselves too zealously tend to strain and pain their muscles right away, or exercise too long and vigorously so they suffer from aches the next day. If one resolves to heed the forewarning that he should proceed very slowly but persistently, he is less likely to give up too easily.

3. Thirdly: *Don't give up before you have established a routine.* Until you have selected a continuing pattern of exercises most suited to your needs, reserve a regular time each day for experimenting. Try out several different exercises over a period of several months, before either settling upon a most efficient selection or quitting. Regularity of practice periods is a must for anyone seriously desiring success.

4. Finally: *Don't give up before your exercises show significant effects upon your daily carriage,* whether walking or sitting or working, and upon a more relaxed and more graceful manner of handling your business or professional problems. Do not give up until you feel that you are as healthy as you can be. By then you will know how much your health depends upon your exercises. And then you will not consent to abandoning them.

E. Retain an Experimental Attitude

One may, at first, try to conform to traditional patterns and take the traditional postures as his tentative goals. But as one proceeds, he will find new alternatives that have not been suggested to him which may please him better. Some of the traditional postures will seem trivial and may be passed by. Others will be impossible to achieve and should be forgotten. Each new capacity which one attains will open new avenues for exploration. Anyone aware of the history of the development of the postures now considered standard must know that much experimenting has been done and some of the postures now most highly recommended were not mentioned in earlier instructions. Although one should regard those postures which have stood the test of time with some appreciation, he may expect to add variations of his own, some of which may, if he becomes a teacher, attain a respected place in future tradition. A rule, here, if one is needed: *Do not perform traditional posture exercises merely according to rule,* but retain an experimental attitude. If you keep the ultimate purposes of yogic practice in mind, you will be able to judge whether and to what extent old and new postures best serve those purposes.

III. KINDS OF POSTURES

A. How Many Kinds?

Any attempt to discover an "official" list of standard postures must end in failure. But some remarks about the complexity of the problem should reveal something of its nature.

1. If the word "posture" is taken in its most general sense, then there are as many postures as there are positions the body can take. The number will be determined more by one's patience than anything else, because the number of varieties is almost infinite unless one limits himself to merely the grosser forms.

2. If one turns to early Hindu literature, scattered references provide examples, but shed little light upon how many were eventually to become recognized by hatha yogins.

3. The early *Hatha Yoga Pradipika* lists and describes fifteen postures used by famous yogins: *Svastikasana, Gomukhasana, Virasana, Kurmasana, Kukkutasana, Uttanakurmakasana, Dhanurasana, Matsyasana, Paschimottanasana, Mayurasana, Savasana, Siddhasana, Padmasana, Simhasana* and *Bhadrasana.* However, it points out that one need not practice all of them.

4. A tradition has developed around the number "eighty-four" which has continued to be accepted and quoted by orthodox hatha yogins. The *Gheranda Samhita* speaks of Siva describing eighty-four hundreds of thousands of postures of which eighty-four are the best. Danielou (*Yoga: The Method of Reintegration,* pages 146–149) gives "a complete list" of "the eighty-four postures," but it provides little insight for beginners; many of the postures seem no longer significant and many currently popular ones are not included.

5. The *Gheranda Samhita* continues: "Among these eighty-four, thirty-two have been found very useful." These are: *Siddhasana, Padmasana, Bhadrasana, Muktasana, Vajrasana, Svastikasana, Simhasana, Gomukhasana, Virasana, Dhanurasana, Savasana, Guptasana, Matsyasana, Matsyendrasana, Gorakshasana, Paschimottanasana, Utkatasana, Samkatasana, Mayurasana, Kukkutasana, Kurmasana, Uttana Kurmasana, Uttana Mandukasana, Vrksasana, Mandukasana, Garudasana, Vrsasana, Salabhasana, Makarasana, Ustrasana, Bhuganagasana, Yogasana.* Although regarded by many as authoritative, this work limits its list largely to those postures related to sitting. The currently popular headstand and shoulderstand postures may have been introduced later. The history of hatha yoga postures is one which begins with emphasis on seated postures and proceeds in the direction of more dynamic, more extreme types of stretching.

6. Current books on yoga asanas differ greatly in both the numbers and kinds of postures to which their authors give

notice. Yogic instructors also have their favorites; whether they teach quantities of beginners or lead devotees toward the meditative goals of raja yoga makes a difference in their preferences. And, we must add, contemporary yogins do not agree always upon how a particular posture should be named or how to interpret the traditionally named asanas.

7. The number of kinds will doubtless tend to become personalized, for as each person finds those which seem most useful to himself, he is likely to discard and forget many of the others. As new kinds of postures become favorites of individual teachers and come to be passed on to others, the number changes again.

B. How to Classify?

When confronted with such a maze of kinds of postures, a teacher naturally seeks some simpler way of grouping them to get a manageable mental picture of the task ahead.

One of the most obvious ways, and one likely to appeal to beginners, divides them into groups according to whether the performer is sitting, standing, upside down or lying on the floor. However, this classification soon proves inadequate, since both variations of static positions and dynamic exercises tend to lead from one of these groups to another. Some postures which at first appear as sitting postures, e.g., the Lotus Posture, may be performed lying face down (as *Matsyasana,* the Fish Posture), or upside down (as *Sirsha Padmasana,* the Headstand Lotus Posture), or standing up on your knees (as *Parvatasana,* the Mountain Posture), and each of these also has distinguishable variations.

Other attempts—such as dividing them into static or dynamic, or into those intended to be held for a long time and those to be held only momentarily—are too simple. Organizing postures according to the animal names suggested by them (cock, cobra, bull, camel, peacock, tortoise) is too artificial; not all postures have animal names; and, except perhaps for convenience of remembering, this is useless. One may alphabetize them for convenient reference, but the order in Sanskrit differs from that of English equivalents and some postures have two different names in Sanskrit and some two or more in English. (See List of Asanas and List of Postures at the end of this volume.) One might classify them according to primary purposes, such as meditation, relaxation, massaging of internal organs, stretching, increasing blood circulation in the brain or promotion of bowel movements; but much overlapping exists here and different postures may perform the same function better for one person than for another. The beginner might wish to find postures classified according to ease and difficulty, but those easiest for some often prove most difficult for others.

We have adopted, somewhat arbitrarily and partly for intellectual convenience, a classification based mainly upon the various ways in which the body bends. Perhaps most obviously, the body bends forward, as when we bend over to touch our toes; and we may do this whether standing or sitting or even sitting with our feet up in the air. Second, one may bend his body backward, not as far as forward, but more so perhaps than he realizes; one may bend backward while standing, while lying on his stomach, while standing on his head or even while lying on his back. Third, one can bend his body sideways, either to the right or to the left; this too may be done while sitting or lying down or standing on one's head, but most yogic treatises limit this kind of bending to the standing position. Fourth, one may twist his trunk to the right or left. Fifth, one may bend any or all of his appendages (arms, legs, head, fingers) in various ways, though yogic tradition seems to direct most attention to the legs. Sixth, deliberate massaging of the abdominal organs by drawing the abdomen inward and upward may take several forms and may occur in either standing or sitting positions. Seventh, several different postures may be used for meditation. Finally, we come to series of postures and how they may be arranged into patterns and routines. This classification, too, will prove unsatisfactory for anyone who seeks to be exhaustive, since many of the exercises not only involve bending in two or more directions at the same time but also move serially from one kind of bend into another.

C. Outline for the Following

In accordance with the foregoing classification, we shall treat some of the main postures in series, as follows: 1. Relaxation Postures (Section IV) ; 2. Back-stretching Postures (Section V) ; 3. Front-stretching Postures (Section VI) ; 4. Side-stretching Postures (Section VII) ; 5. Spine-twisting Postures (Section VIII) ; 6. Appendage-limbering Postures (Section IX) ; 7. Abdomen-massaging Postures (Section X) ; 8. Meditation Postures (Section XI) ; 9. Posture Routines (Section XII) .

The present chapter is devoted almost entirely to explaining and illustrating standard hatha yoga postures. We will postpone personal suggestions regarding some easy stretching postures and quick relaxing techniques that may be used at the office or when only short periods are available (which we have called "little yogas") until the final chapter on Aids to Relaxation.

IV. RELAXATION POSTURES

We shall distinguish three relaxation postures through which one may obtain a maximum of muscular and nervous relaxation. These consist, basically, of lying flat on one's back (*Savasana,* or the Most Relaxed Posture) , lying flat on one's front *(Advasana),* and lying on one's side *(Dradhasana).* Each has its variations.

A. The Most Relaxed Posture

We begin consideration of standard postures with the one which is surely the easiest possible and probably the easiest imaginable. It consists, first of all, in lying flat on one's back, face up, with arms at the sides. All one has to do, or so it seems from outward appearances, is to lie perfectly still. Eyes may be closed or open, but if open held still; or, rather, they should be held still whether open or closed. But closing the eyelids tends to promote freedom from external disturbance. One may, during the initiating of this pose, roll his eyes, first together in one direction, then together in the other direction, and then in opposite directions, if he chooses, before relaxing his eye muscles and focusing his eyes upon some stationary object or fixed spot on the ceiling.

The apparently complete stillness, achieved after one has finished his initial deliberately motivated relaxing efforts, suggested to early practitioners the name "corpse" for this posture. The Sanskrit term for corpse, Anglicized as either *sava* or *shava,* is used to name this asana: *Savasana* or *Shavasana.* It is also called *Mrtasana,* a term etymologically related to "mort" (death) and "mortal." Formally, the most appropriate English name for it should be "the Supine Posture," though I have found no translators using this term. But since, functionally, it is the posture through which one may obtain the greatest relaxation, we shall designate it as "the Most Relaxed Posture." (See Plate 1.)

Much more is entailed in this posture than simply lying flat on your back with legs stretched out and arms at your sides and without a pillow. You should seek a most comfortable position; normally your legs will be moderately close together and your arms near your sides; other variations will be noted later. Although you may practice this posture on a bed or couch, a floor with carpet, rug or blanket is usually found more satisfactory. The foundation should be firm, but the surface should not irritate your skin or bones. Clothing, if any, should be loose. You should take a few deep breaths to stretch your lungs a bit and to assure an adequate supply of oxygen. You may precede this posture with breathing exercises. Then resume a slow, regular breathing rhythm. Needless to say, a quiet place is most conducive to success, as is freedom from breezes which may wiggle your hairs or tickle your skin.

The relaxing technique associated with this posture consists primarily in deliberate attention to each of the noticeable muscles of your body. After lying comfortably on the floor, and adjusting, even stretching, each of your limbs, direct your attention first to the muscles of a single portion of your body. It is customary and convenient to start with a toe, such as the big toe of your right foot. Without wiggling the toe, think of the tenseness in it and deliberately release that tension. Then think of the next toe, and the next, in the same way. Then think of the muscles in your feet, both top, bottom, and each side; then in your heel, and ankle, and calf, and knee, and thigh and hip. Then direct your attention to the other big toe, and the toes next to it, in the same order. Then proceed to think of your abdominal muscles, chest muscles and back muscles. Then relax the muscles in your right thumb, right index finger, etc., and then your palm, wrist, forearm, upper arm and shoulder. Do the same for your left hand and arm. Then attend to the muscles in your neck, the back of your head, chin, cheeks, lips, tongue, ears, forehead, and eyes, until all of the muscles that come to your attention have been relaxed. Although the order in which you do this may not be significant, it will prove important to have an habitual order so you will not be disturbed by doubts of which muscles to attend to next.

You should notice, as you proceed, that with the relaxing

of some muscles a tendency toward relaxing of others already begins and that although you attend to specific muscles in one finger, for example, your whole hand begins to feel relaxed. As you progress up or down the body, a relaxed feeling may seem to envelop it entirely. If you desire to go to sleep, you need not be concerned about attending to all muscles or all portions of the body before going to sleep. Drop off any time. If you intend to remain awake, taking only a short semiconscious nap, you may then prefer to continue all the way intentionally.

If, for any reason, you do not attain the desired feelings of relaxation with a first series of attentive acts, you may wish to try again, either running over exactly the same series or going into more detail. For example, instead of relaxing with one act of attention all of the muscles of your right index finger, you may attend in detail to each of its three segments and three knuckles, and to the muscles on the bottom, top and sides of each segment and knuckle. Knowledge of muscular anatomy is not necessary for the purposes of this technique, though if one has such knowledge, he will work out his own attentive-series pattern accordingly. If one is extremely tense, he may vary the normal procedure and move each muscle slightly, trying to stretch it, even if only very minutely.

Two additional suggestions may be found useful. First, one may correlate his attentive acts with his breath cycle, so that he relaxes one muscle with each exhalation. If he gradually slows his breathing cycles and thus his attentive acts, he may note an additional tendency toward drowsiness. Secondly, this is an excellent time to practice Archiyoga, either during the attentive series or at its end.

Some warning may be needed. It may seem like a lot of trouble to attend to relaxing each and every particular muscle, especially if you can think of so many of them.

Obviously the result is accomplished by an act of will. Why not, then, by the same act of will, relieve tension in larger portions of your body all at once, or, even, all of your tension, or omnitension, all at once? Try it. You will notice that such relief is impossible, whereas the slow, steady, step-wise procedure works. Rapidity in shifting your attention from one muscle to another tends to deter relaxation. The very impatience expressed in a will to attain relaxation quickly is, in fact, a subtle kind of avarice which itself needs to be suppressed. Only by becoming willing to submit your will to taking as long a time as it is going to take to achieve relaxation can you begin to relax at all. The very slowness with which you proceed to shift your attention, after actually experiencing a feeling of relief in one muscle, contributes to the cumulative effect which eventually overwhelms you in a mood of total peace.

No mention has been made, thus far, of the position of the hands and direction of the fingers relative to the sides of the body. Your hands may fall naturally into a most comfortable condition as you lie on the floor. Thus your hands may lie in such a way that your fingers point upward, or toward your body, or downward, or in any intermediate direction. However, I would like to suggest an additional little yoga often overlooked by some yogic instructors. Since your hands function constantly for handling, holding, grasping or clutching, they tend toward closure most of the time. You use your grabbing muscles to handle doorknobs, drawer pulls, pens, paper, books, instruments, cutlery and drinking glasses—to say nothing of shaking hands, typewriting or smoking. Whenever you become anxious, your fingers tend to clench into a fist. The habitual tendencies embodied in your finger muscles tend to close your hand as you lie down to relax. Deliberate effort to stretch your fingers—by putting your palms together and bending your elbows out, or by bending each one back individually, or by spreading them apart from each other on the floor—before you begin your attentive series should prove useful. But, additionally, I suggest that you point your fingers downward while in *Savasana* so that the weight of your hand will help keep your fingers extended and thus further relaxed during the posture period.

Although, in *Savasana,* your arms normally remain near your sides, some variations in arm positions may be noted. Your hands may be stretched out on the floor above your head, which position is then called *Yastikasana,* the Stick Posture (see Plate 2), or stretched out from your shoulders. Other angles or directions are possible, but normally the angles for both arms and legs remain symmetrical. (See Plate 3.) One may even feel a need for having his legs separated and for having the direction of his arms parallel to those of his legs. Comfort, however, and not formal rules, should serve as guide.

When should one practice *Savasana*? Obviously, as an aid to going to sleep, it may be practiced in bed after one retires at night. It is excellent for a nap after lunch, for an afternoon yoga break, or before leaving the office to battle with rush-hour traffic, if you happen to have a spot of floor or couch available for private quietude. It may help cure insomnia, although severe cases require several repetitions. Of course, we can generalize that this posture may be used whenever one needs relaxing. When no privacy or floor is available, one may be able to adapt his attentive series to other postures and conditions, such as sitting in an office chair or in a train or taxi; but one can hardly expect to obtain the full effects of *Savasana* from such circumstances. One ought not try to use *Savasana* upon arising in the morning, for his attentive series may put him back to sleep again.

We should note an ambiguity in the use of the term *Savasana.* On the one hand, it refers not merely to the supine position but also to the attentive series with its relaxing effect. On the other hand, it refers to the supine position and to rest with or without the attentive series, especially when used as a resting pause between other postures in a posture series. Which meaning is intended should be clear from the context. We shall refer to *Savasana* as the Most Relaxed Posture in both of these senses.

B. The Prone Pose

The Prone Pose *(Advasana)* is like the Most Relaxed Posture (*Savasana* or the Supine Posture) in being a resting position. But it differs primarily in the fact that one lies flat on his front instead of on his back. Again your arms are at your sides and again, so far as the positions of your hands and fingers are concerned, you may wish to give attention to stretching them and directing them toward the floor. (See Plate 5.) Your head may lie on either cheek and you may change from one cheek to the other as you wish. The attentive series may be adapted to *Advasana* and its variations.

Variations include (1) extending arms out from shoulders, (2) extending arms above head on floor (or at any other comfortable angle, with feet also spread apart, perhaps at angles parallel to arms (see Plate 6), and (3) folding arms and resting your head on them, on either cheek. (See Plate 4.) This latter variation is called *Makarasana,* the Crocodile Pose or the Dolphin Pose.

C. The Side Pose

One may prefer to relax while lying on his side. Shri Yogendra, in his *Hatha Yoga Simplified* (pages 125 and 93), describes and illustrates *Dradhasana* as "lying on the right side of the body in a state of relaxation with the right arm under the head, as if for a pillow." The right arm is bent so that the head rests on it near the wrist. The spine is kept as straight as possible. The left leg is directly above the right one and the left arm lies straight on top of the body with its hand resting on the left thigh. *Dradha* means "firm," and this may be called the Firm Pose though, since firmness is desired and expected in all postures, this characteristic hardly differentiates it significantly from other postures. This position for relaxation may be preferred by those with large stomachs or nasal difficulties. Lying on the left side with the left arm under the head is a natural variation.

V. BACK-STRETCHING POSTURES

Although the anxiety-ridden executive may have more to gain from front-stretching postures, since he already stretches his back somewhat as he bends forward during his daily activities, we will begin our several series of limbering exercises with back-stretching series. We do this, partly because these series can be approached most conveniently from the Most Relaxed Posture so that a beginner can make frequent use of this posture during the series, and partly because the beginner may be able to grasp the series conceptually more easily and to begin making noticeable progress with less difficulty and danger than with the front-stretching series. The back-stretching postures emphasize lengthening the muscles of the back half of the body, including those of the neck, shoulders, trunk, buttocks, thighs, calves and heels. They also massage the organs in the abdomen and thorax by pressing them within a contracted area.

Back-stretching series will be grouped, somewhat arbitrarily, according to different starting positions. The postures of our first group start from the Most Relaxed Posture and this group will be called the Supine-starting Series. Exercises of the second group begin from a prone position and this group will be called the Prone-starting Series. Postures of the third group both begin and continue in a standing position and this group will be called the Standing Series.

A. The Supine-starting Series

Five series, all beginning from a supine position (flat on back with face up), together with an advanced series extending the fifth, will constitute the six distinguishable sets of postures included under the present heading.

The first three all terminate, ideally, in a closed jackknife condition where the line of the trunk and the line of the straightened legs come as close to being parallel as possible. This terminating condition is called, in Sanskrit, the *Paschimottanasana. Paschima* means "behind," "back" or "posterior," and *uttana* means "stretched out." Hence *Paschimottanasana (paschima-uttana-asana)* means a "back-stretched posture," and could serve as a generic name for all of our Back-stretching Postures. However, the name has become a proper name for a specific posture, namely that in which one's head touches the knees while legs are flat on the floor. The name may be extended to this same head-to-knee position when one lies on his back (the termination of our second series) and when one sits on his buttocks (the termination of our third series). This same head-to-knee position terminating a standing-posture series, however, has a different specific name, *Padahastasana.*

The first three series will be named after their starting movements, namely, the Head-first Series, the Feet-first Series and the Head-and-Feet Series. The fourth series ends in a shoulderstand and will be called the Shoulderstand Series. The fifth ends in a condition which resembles an ancient wooden plough and has come to be called the Plough Series. The sixth is a highly advanced series which presupposes and begins with the fifth series and includes several postures, each of which may be regarded as terminal, but we shall use the name of a most extreme posture and call it the Noose Series. Each of the postures in these series may have its own variations.

1. The Head-first Series

The reader has already practiced sitting on the floor and trying to touch his toes. Thus he is already acquainted with most of this series. If he begins, as recommended, from the supine position, he will raise his head first, keeping both legs straight on the floor and holding his trunk in such a way that his spine is as nearly straight as possible. The position of the arms is optional; they may be stretched above the head, extended out from the shoulders, folded on the chest, placed on the floor beside the thighs, or extended horizontally out in front. The latter position is more likely, especially if the upper part of the body is heavier than the legs. One may put a weight upon his feet when imbalance prevents raising the trunk first without raising the feet; however, in orthodox posturing, no props are used. Although exercises normally proceed better without shoes, one may find heavy shoes an expedient aid in performing this exercise. One may begin from a sitting position if imbalance makes this starting position impossible for him.

Between the horizontal and vertical positions, the trunk may be stopped and held at any number of degrees. The forty-five-degree angle is, perhaps, an arbitrary stopping and holding position, though one who concerns himself with formal poses may wish to consider this as a distinct posture. (See Plate 7.) So also with the degrees of the angles from a vertical position (see Plate 8) to a forward-bending position. But, except for another precisely forty-five-degree angle position (see Plate 9), one is likely to be concerned with pressing forward as far as he can and with repeating the forward movements so as to stretch his muscles a little farther each time.

PICTOGRAPH CHART NO. 1

BACK-STRETCHING POSTURES

A. Supine-starting Series

1. The Head-first Series

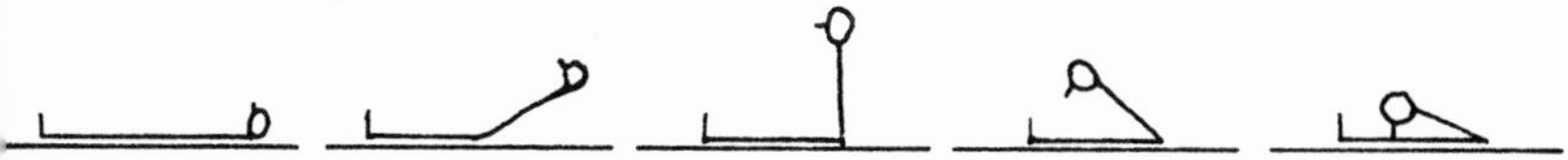

2. The Feet-first Series

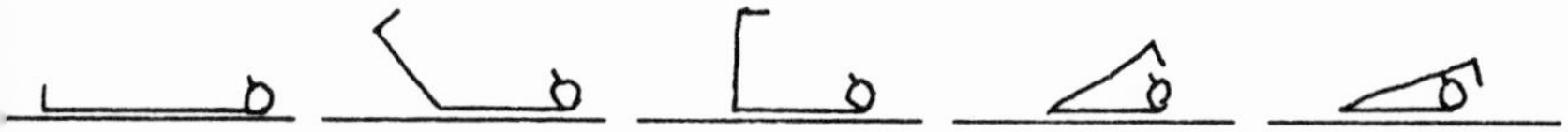

3. The Head-and-Feet Series

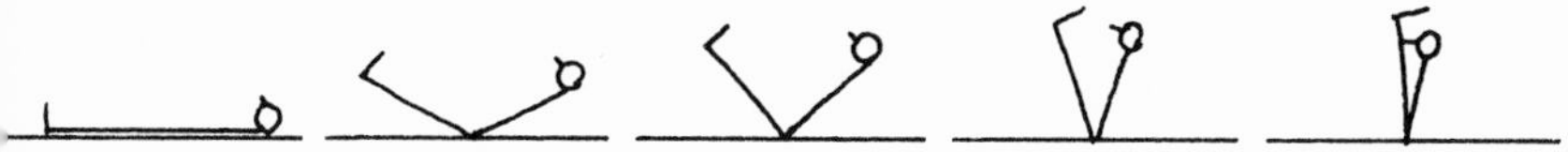

4. The Shoulderstand Series

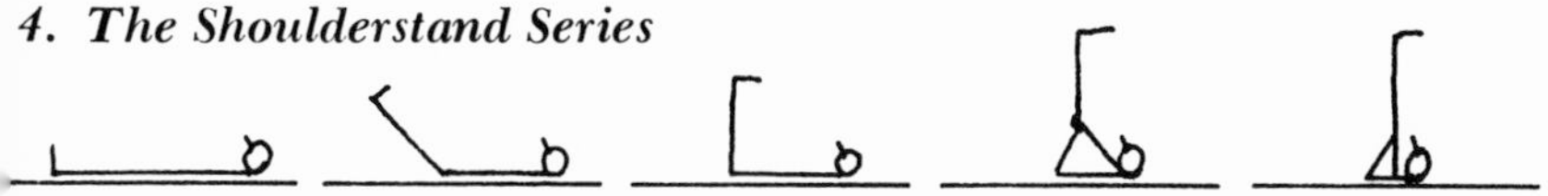

5. The Plough Series

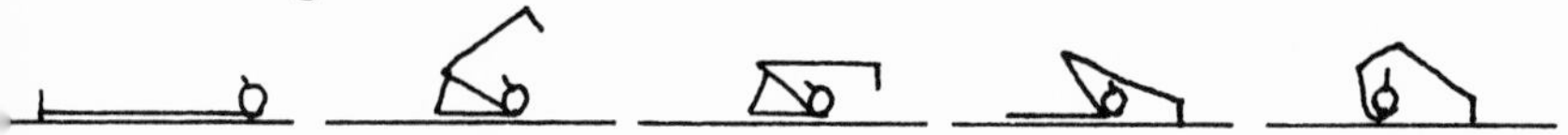

6. The Advanced Noose Series

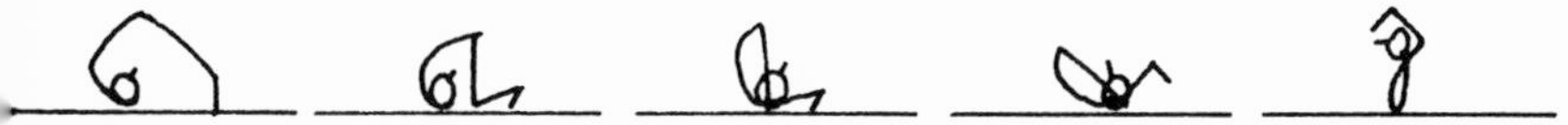

Few people should expect to achieve the limit in which the head rests upon his knees. (See Plate 10.) The limit is a goal in the sense that one can go no farther in this direction (unless he puts his head on the floor between his knees). But the true goal is the relaxation obtained from stretching the muscles, and not the limit theoretically possible. Certainly beginners should not expect to approximate the limit. But one should know what these possibilities are and have them in mind as a direction in which to go but not as a standard which, if not reached, causes a feeling of frustration. Only after months or years of practice may one begin to approach the limit, and his chances of doing this are less when he begins his efforts late in life after muscles, tendons and joints have already stiffened into a relatively permanent mold.

One who approaches the limit will find some options open to him and some aids and traditional forms of interest. Although one begins and carries through this series mainly by the use of the abdominal muscles, they are normally insufficient to bring this series to its ideal limit. One may, in pressing forward to touch his toes, extend his hands above and beyond his toes for several inches. This is obviously a good procedure for increasing the stretching. But tradition advises catching hold of the big toes with the index fingers and pulling the trunk forward and downward a bit. Although one may hold his arms straight, tradition carries this posture series further. One may then drop his elbows to the floor and keep them touching the floor. In this position one may also have more leverage to draw his head closer to his knees. The next stage calls for placing one's forearms also flat on the floor beside the legs and grasping the ankles or heels, whichever is most convenient, with the hands. This position also provides leverage as needed. Although the limit is regarded as reached when one touches his head to his knees, some extremely supple persons can put the head between the knees.

Variations of these limiting positions include some leg-stretching postures, which we have yet to examine. (See Section IX.) Swami Vishnudevananda (see his *Complete Illustrated Book of Yoga,* Plates 61–63) varies this series by keeping one leg stretched forward and bending the other leg so that (a) his heel is set in his crotch (Bernard calls this *"Maha Mudra";* see his Plate VII) or (b) his foot is placed on his thigh, both fingers holding the extended big toe. He can also stretch an arm behind his back and hold the big toe of the foot lying on his thigh. But these are unusual achievements which must remain beyond the hopes of most beginners.

2. The Feet-first Series

The reader has also already practiced lying on his back and raising his feet in the air. This excellent abdominal-muscle exercise may be extended into a back-stretching exercise simply by drawing the legs farther and farther toward the head. Again, one may distinguish formally and hold as postures those positions in which the legs are halfway between being on the floor and in a vertical direction and halfway between a vertical direction and touching one's head. (See Plates 11, 12, 13.) Again, the limiting position (see Plate 14) is not something which a beginner should expect to attain. Furthermore, it is not even a traditionally recognized posture, for efforts in this direction turn naturally into the Plough Series, to be discussed below. However, any posture involving the feet may be called *Padasana,* "Foot Posture"; and since *Uttana,* a term of many meanings, such as "stretched out," "stretched up," "endeavoring to rise" and even "upright," may be used to describe leg positions, the postures of this Feet-first Series in which the legs are raised from the floor may be called *Uttana Padasana.*

Variations advisable for beginners include raising only one leg at a time. Considerable practice of such variations for days, weeks or months may prove useful before one seriously tries to stretch both legs very far in the direction of the head. One may also pull his legs toward his trunk by taking hold of his big toes, as in the previous series, or by wrapping his arms around his legs to draw them closer. Ambitious persons may place a light weight (e.g., a pillow) upon the legs as they approach the head, but this kind of effort is fraught with dangers, especially if the weight is hard or heavy. Again, heavy shoes may be used to promote the downward movements of the legs. But caution is needed. Do not overstretch or strain.

3. The Head-and-Feet Series

Our third series begins by raising both head, or trunk, and feet, or legs, at the same time. This series combines the movements of the first two series and is, in some respects, much more difficult. The beginner may wish to postpone this series until later, especially if his abdominal muscles are not well developed or if the weights of his trunk and legs seem greatly out of balance. This series cannot be performed merely by raising the head and legs while the back of the trunk continues to lie on the floor. One should try to keep his spine straight and balance himself on his buttocks. One may need to shift his arms so their weight will aid in achieving a balance. When in traditional form, called *Vajroli Mudra,* one's hands remain flat on the floor below and beside the thighs.

Formally, we can distinguish four stages. In the first stage the angle of the legs to the trunk is the same as in the first stages of the first two series (135 degrees) but whereas in the first the trunk was raised forty-five degrees from the floor and in the second the legs were raised forty-five degrees from the floor, here the amounts by which both legs and trunk are raised from the floor together add up to forty-five degrees. (See Plate 15.) In the second stage, the angle between the legs and trunk is about ninety degrees, as in the second stages of the first two series. (See Plate 16.) If one modifies this position so that he rests on his sacrum instead of his buttocks and catches hold of his legs with his hands and sways like a boat on water, it may then be called the Boat Pose or *Navasana.* In the third stage, the legs-trunk angle is also the same as in the third stage of the first two series, though few people will reach this far. (See Plate 17.) If one can spare his hands from balancing services, he may then put his arms around his legs to draw them closer to his trunk. In the fifth stage, theoretically, one's legs and trunk are both vertical and parallel to each other, though in practice this ideal can hardly be attained. (See Plate 18.) Swami Vishnudevananda illustrates this stage with a head-on-knees and index-finger-grasping-big-toe posture similar to that terminating our first series except that both hands and feet are high in the air. (*Op. cit.,* Plate 56.)

4. The Shoulderstand Series

This series, which evidently was not among the earliest hatha yoga postures but which has become well known and widely practiced, is one of the easier series, despite its formidable appearance to beginners. Starting naturally from a supine position, one may raise his legs (see Plates 19 and 20) in exactly the same manner as in the first two stages of our second, or Feet-first, series. (See Plates 11 and 12.) As he goes into the third stage, however, he should raise his hips and prop them up with his hands, resting his elbows on the floor. His weight may be mainly on his elbows, though some of it will be on his shoulders and head. (See Plate 21.) One should practice this position repeatedly before trying the next stage and should develop both firmness of the position of elbows, shoulders and head upon the floor and of hands upon the hips and steadiness in holding the legs in the air. It is unwise to continue in this position long if one feels very wobbly. In the final stage, one should bend his trunk into a vertical position, so that his spine and legs form a straight line. He will have to lower his hands from his hips to his ribs. (See Plate 22.) Most of his weight will then rest upon his shoulders, although pressure against the neck and head may be great. The elbows remain on the floor and under pressure, but their function becomes more that of keeping the body in a vertical position than of bearing the weight of the body, as in the second stage.

A beginner should hold a shoulderstand position for only a short time—a few seconds, for example—and should rest in a supine position before trying it again. As one obtains more experience with this position, he may wish to hold it longer, for several seconds at a time. Sivananda (in *Yoga Asanas,* page 159), who has been a lifelong professional yogin, says of the fourth stage: "On the first day do it for a minute. Gradually increase the period to three hours. After six months wrinkles on the face and grey hairs will disappear." This advice and these claims seem extravagant. And, even though his illustration depicts a position somewhere between our second and third stages, few people can find three hours a day for this position and if they did could hardly expect to "conquer death." Besides, there may be dangers as well as benefits from this position.

Persons who have any doubts about their physiological condition should consult their physicians regarding prospects. Those with high blood pressure or heart diseases, brain, ear, eye or sinus troubles, or hemorrhagic diseases, for example, should use extreme caution. Benefits include a stimulating readjustment of all the cells of the body with a reversal of gravitational pull upon all their parts. Increased flow of blood and increased blood pressure in the brain may improve its functioning, and aid recall, reasoning and problem-solving ability. Such increase may also stimulate the thyroid and other ductless glands in neck and head. Drainage of sacs in the intestines and other organs, where sedimentary deposits have accumulated, may be improved. Temporary relief from hemorrhoid pains may be obtained. Details of physiological benefits and dangers remain beyond the scope of the present volume and should constitute a special branch of medical investigation. But that benefits and dangers are involved should be obvious.

Further general cautions about the position may be needed. One should be careful not to tip over in any direction and fall to the floor. An unusually soft floor surface may be indicated for beginners with any doubts about their abilities in this matter. One should especially avoid falling in the direction of his head, for he may break or bruise his neck. Any unsteadiness or wobbliness in one's approach to the position is a sign for extra caution. When coming out of the position, one should do so gradually, for speed may result in harmful jarring of the body.

Many variations of postures in this series are possible. The position of the toes is optional; one may point them skyward if he is feeling muscular and vigorous and seeks a full stretch, or he may relax them flat-footedly if he seeks a moment of rest while holding this position. One may, of course, separate his legs, either sideways or in scissors fashion, and may exercise by bicycling them or swinging them around in circles. Additional cautions are needed for these feats. Many of the leg-stretching exercises to be discussed in Section IX can be performed in this position. One may bend both of his legs forward toward his head, approaching the Plough Posture, to be discussed next, or bend his legs and spine backward for an additional stretch. If one can achieve and maintain a sufficiently balanced poise, he may lower his forearms to the floor and place his hands flat on the floor. He may even put his arms upward, placing them on his thighs. (See Vishnudevananda, Plate 43.) But these extensions remain beyond the capacity of most beginners and are presented here only as suggestions and as evidence that possibilities seem practically inexhaustible. One need never become bored with asanas.

Thus far we have neglected terminology. Two names traditionally attach to this series. The first, *Viparita Karani,* consists of two words, *viparita,* which means simply "inverted" or "reversed," and *karani,* which may mean either "doing" or "making" or, less commonly, "form." On the one hand, *Viparita Karani* refers to the process of inverting oneself from a feet-on-the-ground to a feet-in-the-air position. (As such, it could refer to the headstand series also.) On the other hand, it has come to name the position, especially the position held during our fourth stage, where much of the weight is placed upon forearms and elbows. Although I have never seen the term used, one might speak of *Viparitasana* in naming this fourth stage. The second term, *Sarvangasana,* is a compound of *sarva,* meaning "whole" or "all," and *anga,* meaning "body." This often translates into English as "The All-Members Pose," indicating that all portions of the body are involved. One may wonder at this name, since all members of the body seem involved in many postures. However, since many postures neglect the arms whereas in this posture they play a fundamental role in obtaining and maintaining the position, I suspect that the "all" may signify inclusion of the arms, neck and shoulders as well as the buttocks and legs. Although the name *Sarvangasana* refers specifically and primarily to the position held during our fifth stage, it is sometimes used to name the variations and even the process and fourth stage when involved in arriving at it.

5. The Plough Series

Our fifth series begins in exactly the same way as the

previous three, by lying in a supine position and raising the legs first. As in the second and fourth series (see Plates 11–14 and 19–22), the head remains on the floor throughout, and the legs are raised to the vertical position. Then this series partakes of aspects of the second and fourth series, by both moving the legs beyond the vertical position and using the arms and elbows as supports for the hips, at least for beginners. One may stop with his legs about forty-five degrees above his head (see Plate 23) and again with his legs in an approximately horizontal position, parallel to the floor. (See Plate 24.)

One does not reach the plough position until his feet touch the floor above his head. (See Plate 25.) Few beginners should be expected to be able to do this until after months of practice. In the third stage, one will continue to use his arms, hands and elbows for support, though in the fourth and fifth stages, the weight is shifted increasingly to the shoulders (this series is, in some respects, a variation of and an extension of the Shoulderstand Series); after the arms bear no weight, they may be placed flat on the floor either in a direction away from the head (the traditional form of the completed Plough Posture), or out from the shoulders, or in the direction of the feet. (See Plate 26.) Some fold their hands on the crown of the head, keeping their elbows on the floor, to provide steadiness in the fifth stage.

Beginners again should heed the cautions and note the benefits just outlined for the Headstand Series. Since the pressures upon the abdomen and lungs from increased compacting of the space containing them, and pressure upon the blood in the brain, increase, diseases and discomforts endangered or aggravated by these pressures should warn one not to engage in this series. Persons who have had trouble with slipped spinal disks should consult their physicians before trying this one; but many persons will find this exercise, conducted with modesty and due caution, conducive to spinal improvement. Normal persons desiring brain stimulation, abdominal massage and further stretching of spinal and leg muscles, however, should find this one of the healthiest of exercises. Possible excessive pressure upon the abdomen during this exercise warrants repeating the advice about waiting for a long period after eating and emptying bowels and bladder before performing it. Since the lungs also come under pressure, suitable breathing exercises seem advisable during the preceding rest period. The position should be held, at first, for only a couple of seconds; later one may extend the period as he becomes accustomed to the pressures, shortness of breath, and extent of his abilities.

Ambitious beginners may appreciate some typical aids. If one finds himself continuing to be unable to touch his toes to the floor after much practice, he may try to touch the floor with one foot at a time, leaning a bit to one side or the other, if he has sufficient control over his balance. One may even regard the position in which his legs are separated as far as possible, after both touch the floor, as a variation from the normal Plough Posture in which the legs are kept close together. Another bit of advice, which may be unnecessary, is that one move continuously into the plough position without stopping at any of the formally demarkable stages, and that the weight of the legs, as they move in the direction of the floor above the head, may spring the legs farther than if they are moved merely by voluntary effort. The faster the legs move into this position, the more power inertial pressure will exert in stretching the back and leg muscles. Extreme caution should be exercised at this point, however, for too much strain may cause damage.

A further suggestion is that one may roll from approximating the Plough position toward the limit of our first series, and then back again. By doing this several times, an exerciser develops a rocking motion which gives his back and leg muscles a double stretching, one as his fingers approach or extend beyond his toes, as in the first series, and the other as his feet extend beyond his head and approach the floor above it, as in the Plough Series. This exercise not only is good for abdominal muscle development, and promotes muscular limbering further as one approaches the limits of the two series, but also gives him a feeling of mastery over his muscular balance and may promote a euphoria which outweighs any feeling of frustration at not carrying these traditional postures to their ideal limits.

One should be satisfied with attaining *Ardha-halasana* or a Half-Plough Posture. *Hala* means "plough," or "plow," and *ardha* means "half." Those who complete the Plough Series may speak of the final position as a *Purna-halasana* or Full Plough Posture. In the fourth stage of our series, after the toes touch the floor above the head, the angle of the back may not yet have reached a seemingly vertical position. But the fifth and final stage has not been reached until this angle is either vertical or bent somewhat in the direction of the feet on the floor. That is, in the final position, the feet move as far from the head as possible. (See Plate 26.)

6. The Advanced Noose Series

Beginners are advised to ignore this series which may be thought of as originating not from a supine position, but from the Full Plough Posture. It consists of several advanced positions, each of which may be regarded as an end-in-itself. Each has its own distinct name. The naming and organization of this series as a series is our own, but its rationale can be grasped both from the following descriptions and, especially, from carrying the series through in practice.

The first stage is simply the Full Plough Posture terminating our fifth series, which we have just finished describing.

The second stage consists in dropping the knees to the floor, slowly, and bending the spine still further, if this is possible. The legs, from knees to toes, will be flat on the floor, and the arms, normally, will be extended, flat on the floor, in a direction opposite from the legs. (See Plate 27.) The position of the knees in relation to the head is wherever they happen to fall. This position may differ somewhat with people of different body builds. One should not expect to remain in this position very long—at least in the beginning.

The third stage is like the second except that the knees are drawn toward, even up to, the shoulders. (See Plate 28.) Then the knees or upper calves will cover the ears. Hence this has come to be called *Karnapitasana* or the Ear-covering Pose. *Karna* means "ear" and *pita* (apparently a contraction of *pihita,* "closed," or a variation of *pida,* "obscured") means "closed" or "covered." The Sanskrit title is sometimes used loosely enough to include our second stage and variations such as the one in which the arms are placed around the legs, one arm around each leg, an action which may aid in pulling the legs toward the shoulders. (See Vishnudevananda, Plate 53.) Some persons extend the term *Halasana* (the Plough Posture) to include these two stages.

The fourth stage involves rolling over on the back, while keeping one's head between his knees or calves, and then placing his arms, or rather shoulders, in the crooks of his legs. (See Plate 29.) The hands may be either flat on the floor beneath the hips (see Bernard, Plate XXVII) or clasped around the buttocks (see Vishnudevananda, Plate 71). The lower legs are crossed at the ankles and thus locked, while the back of the head rests upon one of the crossed legs. This posture is called *Pasini Mudra* or the Noose Posture, a title evidently suggested by the seeming strangling of the head by the legs. The term *mudra,* meaning "form," is an alternative for the term "pose," "position" or "posture," although it tends to be used to name variations rather than primary types of posture. If one cannot get himself into this posture from the *Karnapitasana,* he may do so through a series of leg-stretching exercises in which he gets one leg at a time behind his head. Vishnudevananda illustrates a series of exercises for this purpose. (See his Plates 61–71.)

The fifth stage is like the fourth except that one rolls himself up so he sits on his buttocks with his hands on the floor to keep balanced in this position or on his buttocks, if he can balance himself otherwise. (See Plate 30.) The arms, or shoulders, remain in the crooks of the legs and the head remains locked by the legs crossing at the ankles. This may be regarded as a noose posture although, since it also appears similar to a turtle tipped on end, it may be called the Raised-Tortoise Posture, *Utthita Kurmasana.*

B. The Prone-starting Series

Two kinds of series will constitute what we here call the Prone-starting Series." The Prone Posture (see Plates 4–6) is, like the Supine Posture, another relaxing position, but one in which the front of the body is directed downward rather than upward. This posture consists in lying flat on the floor, with legs, abdomen, chest and arms all touching the floor. The head may rest on the floor, if the arms are stretched out beside the body, out from the shoulders, or above the head; or the head may rest on the arms folded under it. One normally rests his head on one or the other of his cheeks. These two kinds which start, or may start, from the prone position will be called the Hips-first Series (you may prefer the Buttocks-first Series or some other appropriate descriptive term) and the Headstand Series.

1. The Hips-first Series

This series, simple to conceive but difficult to perform,

consists in moving from a position in which both the spinal column and the legs are parallel to the floor to a position in which the legs and spinal column are both vertical to the floor and parallel to each other. One must make an effort to keep both of his legs perfectly straight and parallel to each other and to keep his spinal column straight at all times. Five stages will be distinguished.

The first consists of lying in the prone position, but one will need to adjust his arms in preparation for the rather strenuous effort needed. The beginner may have to put his hands on the floor close to his chest and experiment with raising his torso as in regular push-up exercises. But ideally he will have his hands stretched out in front of him on the floor, his elbows bent only a little and his toes pulled up under his feet as far as possible.

The second stage, here formally described, is a position that is more likely to be passed through than held for any length of time. By putting pressure on his toes and the palms of his hands, one bends in the middle, lifting his hips from the ground until his body forms an angle similar to that in the second stages of the first four series described above. (See Plates 7, 11, 15, 19.) Ideally, the arms should be kept straight and should form a straight line with the trunk of the body throughout the series.

The third stage consists in bringing the body into a right angle (see Plate 31), again as in the third stages of the first four series outlined above. One will have to move either the positions of his feet or of his hands or both in order to bring them closer together on the floor. His feet should be flat on the floor by now. Although one should try to move smoothly and continuously between positions, he may have to move his hands or feet one at a time.

In the fourth and fifth stages, the hands and feet are brought closer together, first (see Plate 32) to an angle similar to that in our first three series above (see Plates 9, 13, 17), and finally (see Plate 33) as close to each other as possible. In the final position, the head will be touching the knees (see Plate 34), just as in the final positions in the first three series above. (See Plates 10, 14, 18.) Some persons will end with their hands in front of their feet, some will place them beside their feet and some may even put them behind their feet. But one may grasp his ankles with his hands, either keeping his arms straight (see Plate 34) or bending his elbows behind his knees.

One may then reverse this series and return in a similar way to his original prone position. This series does not, as such, constitute a part of hatha yoga tradition, so far as I know; not only is it an analogous variety of back-stretching exercise, but something like it occurs in the traditional, and very ancient, *Surya Namaskar* series which begins and ends in standing positions. This series will be discussed when we come to Posture Routines in Section XII.

2. The Headstand Series

Two basically different kinds of headstands need to be distinguished, one in which the body is supported on the elbows and the other in which it is supported on the hands. In both, of course, most or all of the weight rests directly upon the skull of the head, while the arms are needed for steadying the body. Either of these two kinds of headstands may be used for purposes of the following two series; but the former seems to be both more traditional and more popular with hatha yogins, and our descriptions and illustrations will be limited to it.

The Sanskrit name for head or skull is *sirsha* and the term *Sirshasana* (or *Shirshashana*), meaning Head Posture, is used for all of the stages of both series and their variations regardless of which kind of headstand is used. Many English trans-

BACK-STRETCHING POSTURES

B. Prone-starting Series

1. *The Hips-first Series*

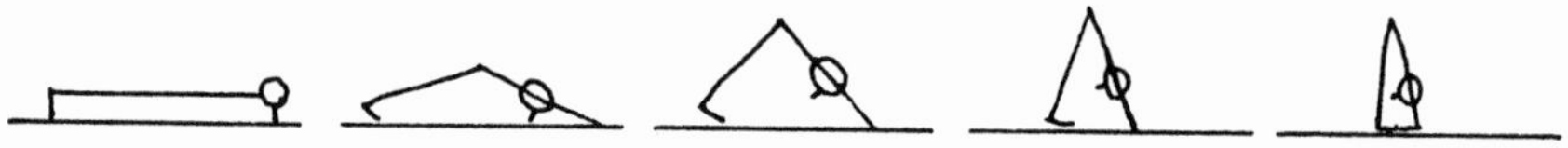

2. *The Headstand Series*

a. The Straight-leg Series

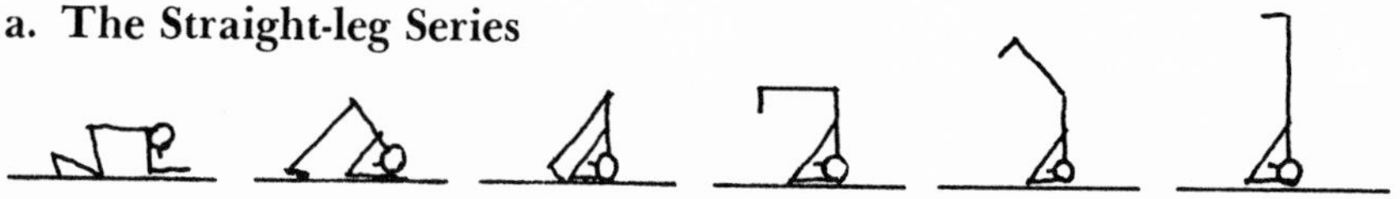

b. The Bent-leg Series

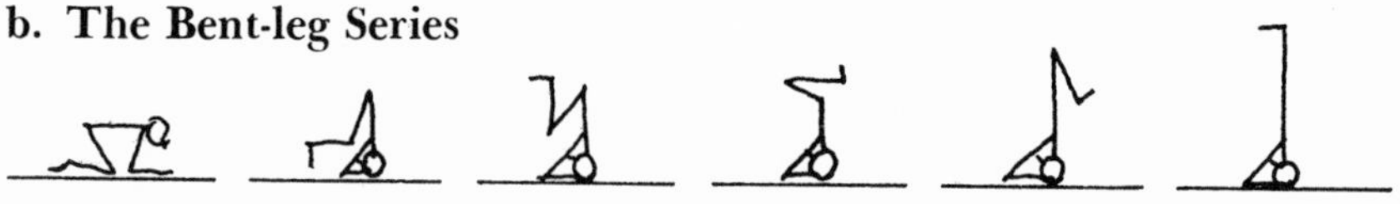

lators have adopted the term Topsy-turvy Pose, and a recent joke about the late Jawaharlal Nehru's practice of standing on his head for a while each morning suggests: "Perhaps he has to. This may be the only way one can see things straight in a topsy-turvy world."

Two different kinds of Headstand Series should be kept in mind also. Although neither of these is primarily a back-stretching exercise, both belong to the class of forward-bending exercises. The first of these is more clearly a back-stretching series since the legs are held straight throughout, and its stages are, in many respects, quite analogous to stages in all of our back-stretching series. We call this the Straight-leg Series. In the second series, one devotes most of his attention to problems connected with balancing, rather than to keeping his legs stretched and straight. We name this the Bent-leg Series. This second series apparently is the older and more traditional of the two, and many beginners may find it easier. These two series can easily be confused and, as we shall indicate below, they may be deliberately combined.

Although one may begin these series from a prone position—for one should rest both before and after such exercises—he may also begin from a standing position. Many will prefer to think of themselves in a starting posture only after they have reached a position in which they rest on elbows and knees. At any rate, for pictorial convenience, we shall omit further reference to the prone stage here.

a. *The Straight-leg Series.* In our first stage, one gets up, or down, on his knees and elbows, with both feet and hands also touching the floor. (See Plate 35.) In this series, his knees are farther away from his elbows than in the second series. Thighs and upper arms both tend to be vertical; the back is horizontal, or it would be if one's upper arms and upper legs were the same length. The head, neck and spine should form a straight line.

In the second stage, one lowers his head to the floor, cups his hands around his head, raises his buttocks, straightens his legs, keeping his head, neck and spine still in as straight a line as possible. Formally, this stage constitutes a posture in which the spine and legs form a right angle (see Plate 36), as they do in the third stages of each of our first four series and in the immediately foregoing Hips-first Series. Actually, persons with different body proportions—such as long or short legs, long or short trunk, long or short neck—must take them into consideration in judging what is proper for them at this stage.

The two elbows and the head form a triangle which plays a most important role in the Headstand Series. The elbows should not be too close together, or the body will tip too easily toward one side or the other. The elbows should not be too far apart or they will provide insufficient leverage to support the body and be unable to steady the body sufficiently as it moves backward and forward. One may begin by aiming at something like an equilateral triangle, and then adjust the distance between his elbows as his own personal experience indicates. Earlier in his attempts he may need more backward-forward support and later he may prefer more sideways support.

The fingers of the hands cupped around the head may be interwoven to provide firmness, but at the same time sufficient play should be allowed so they will not be pinched when the head moves toward them under the shifting weight and position of the body as it proceeds into the third stage. (See Plate 37.) The feet remain on the floor in this stage, though only the toes need touch it directly. One may have to slide, or otherwise move, his feet somewhat toward his head in order to obtain the desired form. This position is not held long and may be sought as a particular posture only by those interested in perfecting all of the formal steps.

The third stage is attained by shifting the weight of the

body entirely off the feet and entirely onto the head and elbows. The feet are thus raised from the floor. Formally, the spine takes a perpendicular position and the angle of the legs, which are kept straight, to the spine is the same as that in the fourth stages of the first three Supine-starting Series and the first Prone-starting Series. Actually, one must concern himself primarily with attaining a stable balance in all directions at this stage, and approximate the formal ideals as best he can. Both the relative and absolute sizes and weights of the legs and trunk will determine necessary variations in different persons. Those who are fat and those who are thin may find themselves faced with quite different problems here. One may not require being cautioned about needed adjustments of fingers and hands as he moves into this position; pinching will serve as its own warning to start over again. But one should be cautioned about his neck. If his body is heavy and if he has not recently had experience with putting the weight of his body on his neck, he should use discretion. The head, neck and spine should be kept in a straight line; otherwise the neck may buckle and break.

The fourth stage is reached when one has raised his legs to a horizontal position. (See Plate 38.) This movement will involve some shift in the vertical position of the trunk. The angle, which ideally approximates the right-angled postures of the third stages of our first four Supine-starting Series and our first Prone-starting Series, can hardly be kept. Although one must continue to experience pressure on his elbows so long as he is in the process of shifting his weight between stages, he should progressively seek a balance in which very little weight falls upon them. So long as there is any danger of falling over backward, however, one should keep some of his weight on them. A person should have had some experience with rolling out of a headstand onto his back before he can do this series with perfect safety. A person with a heavy trunk and short light legs should approximate a vertical position more closely than one with a lighter trunk and longer, heavier legs.

In a fifth stage, the legs are lifted further toward a vertical position but formally stop halfway between horizontal and vertical lines, forming an angle like that in the second stages of the first four Supine-starting Series and in the second stage of the first Prone-starting Series. Actually, there is little virtue in stopping in this posture, except for those desiring to demonstrate to themselves perfection of control and postural form. Legs are kept straight, as in all stages of this series.

The final stage is reached when one's legs attain a vertical position and line up perfectly with the spine and head. Almost all of the weight is directly on the center of the crown of the head. One does not sway after attaining perfect balance. Toes may be pointed upward, continuing the feeling of perpendicularity, or the feet may be held in a flat or horizontal position. The latter may be more conducive to relaxation. Beginners should hold this position only a very short time, but those who have become experts and seek to attain more of the benefits to be outlined below may wish to retain this position much longer. In coming out of this posture, one may inversely attain each of the formal stages or lower his legs continuously. He should not drop them suddenly, however, but try to maintain a smooth, continuous, gradual descent and touch the floor gently. His neck should be kept in line with his spine in the descent also, or danger of breakage will recur. In this series, the legs are kept straight during their descending stages also.

b. *The Bent-leg Series.* In the first stage of this series, one's knees are placed closer to the elbows, and the trunk is more likely to assume an horizontal position when the thighs rest on the calves. (See Plate 39.)

One attains the second stage by way of raising his thighs—

both buttocks and knees. One may, but we are neglecting to, distinguish a stage in which he has raised his trunk as far as he can without lifting his feet from the floor. Legs continue to be bent. Our second stage is attained when one gains his balance after his feet have been lifted from the floor. In this posture, the thighs may rest against the chest and the lower legs remain in a position approximately parallel to the floor. (See Plate 40.) A beginner may need to experiment with his ability to maintain his balance in this position during several exercise periods before proceeding further.

The third stage consists in shifting the lower legs from a horizontal to a vertical position. (See Plate 41.) The thighs remain somewhat close to the abdomen, and the exact position here may vary with personal taste and body proportions. But, formally, the relations between the calves, thighs and trunk is such that they appear to form the letter N when the body is viewed from its left side. The weight of the body need be shifted only slightly between the stages in this series, and balance is more easily maintained than in the Straight-leg Series. The legs remain bent throughout this series until its final stage.

In attaining the fourth and fifth stages of this series, one keeps the angle of his lower legs to his thighs about the same as in the third stage. He merely extends his knees away from his trunk until the line of his lower legs is horizontal in order to attain the fourth posture, and then raises his knees until they are directly in line with his spine to attain the fifth stage. In this fifth posture, the legs may be either held at a formal angle, reversing the angle of the upper legs in the third stage, or dropped limply as one seeks repose in this position.

The series terminates as a formal series when the lower legs are raised into a vertical position so that the whole body forms a straight perpendicular line. Both the Bent-leg Series and the Straight-leg Series terminate in the same posture. (See Plate 42.) One may reverse this series also through its formal stages or simply drop his feet slowly and continuously to the floor, retaining a bent-leg position throughout.

Turning to variations, we may note, first of all, that these two series may be combined, and in various ways. One may proceed to the final headstand posture through the Straight-leg Series and return through the Bent-leg Series. Or he may proceed first through the Bent-leg Series and return through the Straight-leg Series, thus using the combination as a genuine, even if only moderate, back-stretching series.

Other variations which should be reserved for advanced practitioners will be noted later, such as those involving the Lotus Posture and leg exercises yet to be explored. Simpler and easier, however, are postures in which, from the final stage of the Headstand Series, one spreads his legs, either out sideways, as far as he can, or into a walking stride, also as far as he can. He may experiment with bending his legs in various ways from these straight-legged positions. Finally, we may note here that one may arch his back during some headstand postures, but this notation anticipates positions to be reviewed under the Front-stretching Postures.

Benefits and dangers from headstands are similar to those from shoulderstands already discussed above. In addition to the modest back-stretching exercise, one will note especially an increase in the flow of blood to his brain as well as augmented breathing efforts and temporary improvement of blood circulation. Although one must judge the results from his own personal experience, common claims include improvement of memory and intellectual ability and even, in some cases, improved eyesight. Also, increased blood pressure in the sinuses and nasal passages may aid those with hay fever or colds, in the ears may restore partial loss of hearing, and in the throat may improve vocal tone. Although for formal perfection and personal convenience this asana is performed with a minimum of clothing, it is one that is more easily adaptable to office conditions than many of the others. One may have to modify the formalities when wearing his office clothes, but he may nevertheless obtain the benefits. Any executive who can maintain short periods of privacy between appointments may develop the habit of doing a headstand several times a day, as a substitute for stimulants. Although caution and practice are needed, this asana is one of the easier to master and one of the most effective for relaxing purposes, despite appearances to the contrary to those who have not tried it.

C. The Standing Series

The two following series are called Standing Series not merely because the exerciser begins and ends each series in an erect posture but also because he remains standing on his feet throughout the series. The legs never bend at the knees and the body bends only at the hips. Both spine and legs remain straight during the bending processes as well as when the body is fully erect.

The reader already well knows both the values of, and needs for, standing erect, unless he has progressively forgotten. The values have been pointed out in his physiology, health and physical education classes, and the results of proper stance as against slouchy posture have been evident from his own experience, unless he has failed to take the trouble to notice them. Straightening the spine and neck conduce to chest expansion and drawing in the abdomen and a tightening of all muscles controlling standing balance. Circulation improves along with deeper breathing and one's general tonus seems more lively. Unless one holds his erect position with tension and rigidity, he is likely to find erect posture more relaxing and restful than stooped posture.

These facts were known to yogins centures ago and standing erect became one of the standard postures.

Any standing, stable or firm posture may be called *sthasana*, and any upright standing, as opposed to sitting or lying, posture may be called *sthitasana*. Any position involving the feet *(pada)* may be called *padasana*. Sivananda (*Yoga Asanas*, page 108) refers to an erect standing posture with hands kept at the sides as a "whole" or "perfect" standing posture *(Purna Padasana)*. (See Plates 80 and 43.) A common way of practicing erect standing is with the hands folded on the chest in a prayer position *(Prarthanasana)* (see Plate 180), to say nothing of other variations of hand positions.

We arbitrarily adopt the descriptive terms "bend down," "one leg up" and "combined" to name our series of standing postures.

1. The Bend-down Series

In the first stage, one stands erect, not only firmly and stably balanced, with chin up and back straight, but with special attention to the various muscles running from top to bottom of his back—from head to heels. (See Plate 43.) He should hold this position until he feels relaxed in it, for any tension present in the beginning stage may prevent successful attainment of the remaining stages. The arms may be kept at the sides or raised together either to a vertical position above the head or to a horizontal position in front of the shoulders. They will be lowered gradually in the direction of the toes. In any case, the arms should be kept straight also.

In a second formally notable posture (see Plate 44), one may pause with his trunk at an angle to his legs which is the same as that already noted in the second stages of the first four Supine-starting Series and of the first Prone-starting Series and in the fifth stage of the first Headstand Series, or halfway toward a horizontal posture.

PICTOGRAPH CHART NO. 3

BACK-STRETCHING POSTURES

C. Standing Series

1. The Bend-down Series

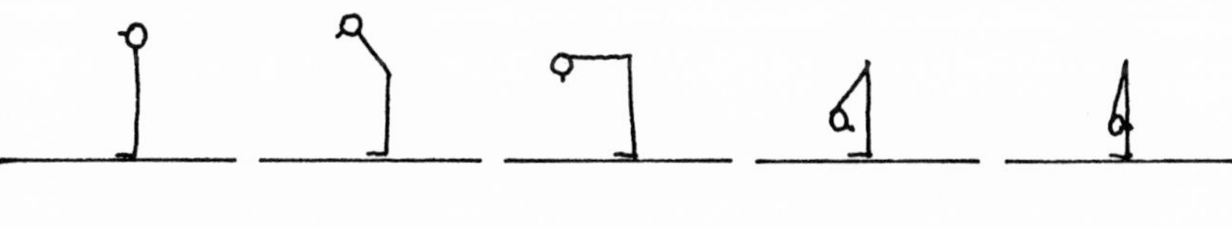

2. The One-leg-up Series

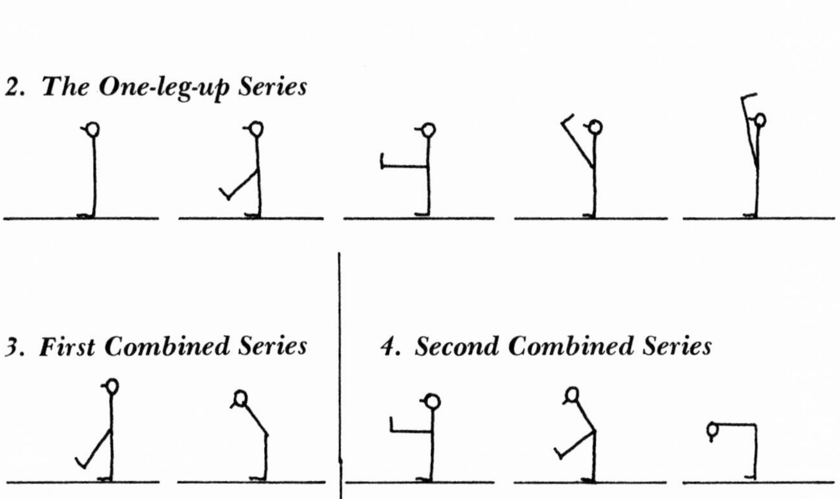

3. First Combined Series

4. Second Combined Series

5. Third Combined Series (Advanced)

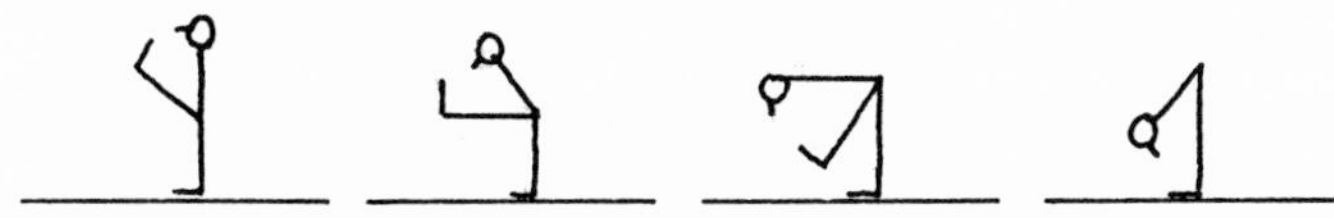

6. Fourth Combined Series (Most Advanced)

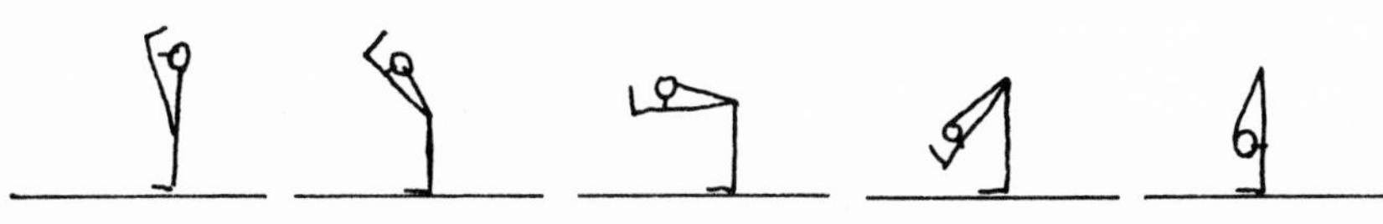

In the third stage (see Plate 45), the trunk stops at a horizontal position, in which the trunk and legs form a right angle, as in the third stages of our first four Supine-starting Series and of our first Prone-starting Series and in the fourth stage of our Headstand Series. If the hands are also extended in the same horizontal direction, one may experience more stretching of his posterior muscles.

The fourth stage consists in dropping the trunk further until it forms an angle halfway between horizontal and vertical lines. (See Plate 46.) For most persons, especially beginners and those with "mature" abdomens, this is likely to be the final attainment. Younger and thinner persons should be able to go on more easily toward touching their toes.

The fifth and final stage is reached when one's fingers touch his toes, although many variations need to be noted here. A very limber person may go on to place his fingers and then the palms of his hands on the floor in front of his feet, and then he may move the palms to the sides of his feet and, even, place them on the floor behind his feet. Another formal feature of this standard posture, called *Padahastasana* or the Hands-and-Feet Posture, is the touching of the knees with the head. Thus, in effect, this kind of standing posture is much the same in form and function as the fifth and final postures of the first three Supine-starting Series and of the first Prone-starting Series. Consequently it is sometimes referred to as a Standing Back-stretching Posture or *Sthita Paschimottanasana.* When formally perfect, one's index fingers are hooked around his big toes, his legs are straight, his spine is as straight as possible under the circumstances, and his head touches his knees, either in front of them or between them. A variation of this pose consists in grasping the ankles with one's hands (see Plate 47); in this case either the arms may be straight or the elbows may be bent in such a way that they will extend toward or beyond the backs of the calves.

One may return to his full or starting position, gradually

and continuously, or he may again stop at each of the formally demarked postures. He should remain in the final pose only very briefly, at least when first attaining it, and he should have attended to breathing and empty-abdominal conditions as noted already in discussing our first back-stretching exercises. One should deliberately relax again in his standing position if he has developed any tensions or strains during the exercise. Ideally, one performs this whole series in a relaxed state of mind and with a minimum of muscular strain. The goal is a loosening and making more supple the neck, spinal and leg muscles, not muscle building.

2. The One-leg-up Series

The opposite of a bend-down series is a bend-up series, but since one cannot bend up without taking his feet from the floor, and thus falling, he will have to do his standing bend-up exercises one leg at a time. Although a person might bend up if he had a bar to hang from, and repeat all of the just-outlined poses in reverse, yogic tradition has refused to employ any instruments whatsoever, except mat and loincloth, since the aim has been to achieve that kind of complete self-control in which one is absolutely freed from all dependence upon externals.

Any posture in which special attention is given to one foot or one leg may be termed *eka pada,* meaning "one foot" or, by extension, "one leg," in contrast to postures placing equal emphasis upon both legs which are termed *dva pada* or *dwi pada,* meaning "two feet" or, by extension, "two legs." Those unfamiliar with Sanskrit often mistakenly take *Eka-Pada-Asana* or *Ekapadasana* to be the proper name of a single posture, whereas it functions as a proper name only in specific contexts. All of our five following standing series are *eka pada,* as are one-leg postures in lying, sitting or upside-down series.

In the first stage, one stands erect, relaxed and balanced, as in the first stage of the Bend-down Series. (See Plate 43.) Calmness may be even more important in this series, since moving and shifting one's weight while standing on one foot creates many problems not experienced when standing more firmly on two feet. One should never engage in strenuous stretching exercises while nervous or tense because he is more likely to strain himself and do damage to his bones, joints and ligaments. A person is not ready for stretching exercises until he is able to approach them with a considerable degree of patience. Hence, it is usually better to begin exercises from a supine position than from a standing position, unless one has ability to relax himself while standing before beginning. This first stage, then, which tends to be skipped by those filled with anxieties, may be the most important one so far as fullest utilization of standing series is concerned.

The second stage consists in raising one leg from the floor, thus placing all weight on the other leg. This is easy and everyone who can walk can do it. But the need for giving attention to balancing the body on one foot until wobbling or swaying ceases is important. Those persons who already have developed perfect balance will confront no problem here and may attain firmness and calmness immediately. But all who find themselves unsteady when standing on one foot face considerable work in this stage; they may have to practice for months or years to obtain the needed steadiness of stance for continuing this and the following series. When one who attains calmness and relaxed self-control during the first stage loses them during the second stage, he should direct his efforts toward reattaining them in this stage before proceeding farther. Formally, one's leg will be held at an angle midway between the vertical and horizontal lines of the body. (See Plate 48.)

The third stage is reached when the raised leg rises to a horizontal position. (See Plate 49.) Needless to say, one should try to retain or increase the inward pressure upon his abdomen as his leg rises, which he sought during the first stage when standing erect. Most people can, with practice, attain this stage, though problems of balance increase as one's leg is extended. The position of the arms will trouble some. Unsteadiness may lead to waving the arms about in quest of balance. But one has not attained self-control until he can hold his arms steady also. One may choose stable hand positions from among many options. He may keep his hands at his sides, place them on his hips, extend them up in the air or out from the shoulders sideways or forward. Except when hands are on hips, his arms should be kept straight. A well-known variation consists in taking hold of the big toe of the raised foot with both hands, and grasping it lightly with the thumbs and index fingers. This variation has been called *Hastapadangustasana* or the Hand-foot-stretching Posture. Difficulties in keeping the spine and legs straight tend to develop here, but an effort to keep them straight should be made.

The fourth and fifth stages, which few can expect to attain, consist in raising the leg higher, first to halfway between horizontal and vertical, and then all the way to a vertical position. One may raise the leg alone, with arms in the previously selected position, or keep his fingers on the big toe, if possible. Some may wish to put their arms around the raised leg in approaching the final stage to draw it closer to the head. The head will touch the knee or lower leg if the series is brought to final completion.

Lowering the leg should be orderly, smooth and under perfect control—not sudden. Maintenance of perfect balance during the descent is desired. Although some persons may be able to perform this series better with one leg than another, just as they tend to be right-handed or left-handed, one should take turns and try to exercise both legs equally during any exercise period.

3. Combined Series

In proposing and depicting the following Combined Series, we go beyond anything which we know about in yogic tradition. But the relationships of the postures in this series to those already considered and their usefulness as standing back-stretching exercises are so obvious that no violation of the purposes of the tradition is involved in suggesting these extensions. Each of the four following Combined Series consists simply in joining the two second, third, fourth and fifth stages, respectively, of the preceding two series in such a way as to obtain the relaxed standing posture of the first stages and, as the series advance, presuppose any intermediate stages.

The First Combined Series consists simply in beginning with the second stage of the One-leg-up Series, in which one leg is raised halfway from vertical to horizontal positions (see Plate 48) , and then bending the trunk forward as one lowers the raised leg to the floor. Thus one ends this two-stage series in the same posture as the second stage of the Bend-down Series. (See Plate 44.) Anyone can do this, though, as in learning new dance steps, one may profit from practicing it a bit before proceeding to the next series.

The Second Combined Series begins with the posture taken during the third stage of the One-leg-up series (see Plate 49) and proceeds to the posture held in the third stage of the Bend-down Series. (See Plate 45.) When the raised leg is horizontal, it forms a right angle with the trunk. As the leg is lowered, this right-angle position is maintained. One may stop at a formally designated midway stage. (See Plate 53.) He cannot fail to notice the stretching pull on his back and leg muscles. Again he should be cautioned not to overdo but to proceed gradually. One may reverse this series or simply proceed to stand erect as in reversing the Bend-down Series. If he chooses, he may start with his fingers clasping his raised big toe and carry this position through the stages of the series, but this is likely to be beyond the ability of most attempters.

The Third Combined Series, which is so far beyond the capacity of most people that it is merely something to think about as an indication of direction for possible further extension, begins with the fourth stage of the One-leg-up Series and proceeds to the fourth stage of the Bend-down Series through two distinguishable formal postures. The raised leg forms a forty-five-degree angle with the trunk, and this angle is kept as one progressively bends down through the three stages.

The Fourth Combined Series, attainable only by long-time devotees of suppleness, starts with the fifth stage of the One-leg-up Series (see Plate 50 or 51) and ends with the fifth stage of the Bend-down Series (see Plate 47), by going through three intermediate stages. (See Plates 52, 53, 54.) One can hardly fail to notice analogies between angles of the trunk to the leg on which one stands in all of these standing series and the angles depicted in earlier series.

Although we have defined the Combined Series as beginning with stages in the One-leg-up Series and proceeding to stages in the Bend-down Series, one might differentiate a second set of combined series by reversing these respective directions. At any rate, if one has followed the exposition thus far, he has begun to see why tradition has it that there are eighty-four hundred thousand postures and also why some sensible limitation must be adopted by each person. One need never become bored, however, with yogic posturing, since the possibilities of new varieties of series seem practically endless.

Perhaps we should call attention to what is obvious, namely, that the simpler stages of the standing series are among the postures most conveniently available for office use. Unless one wears clothes that are too binding to permit stretching, one may bend down while standing even in conditions of minimal privacy. Few business executives or professional people fail to find some moments of privacy in which they can employ the principles involved in these postures. Even those without private offices may find themselves alone in an elevator or restroom. One may pause on a stairway to raise a leg or bend his trunk. Additional hazards of falling down stairs must be taken into consideration, but the usual handrail may provide a safety factor. No one, surely, can say that he can find no opportunity for practicing yoga during office hours. Developing habits of bending down and raising a leg several times daily may in themselves be sufficient to maintain or improve health and relaxation, especially when accompanied by additional breathing exercises.

VI. FRONT-STRETCHING SERIES

When body muscles extend in so many different directions, an attempt to classify muscle-stretching exercises into those emphasizing muscles of the back and the front and the sides is quite arbitrary. Yet, for conceptual convenience, the gathering together of those exercises which direct attention primarily to ways in which the body bends should prove very useful. When the body bends forward, the muscles along the back of the body become stretched. When the body bends backward, the muscles up and down the front of the body stretch. When the body bends toward either side, the muscles of the other side stretch. At any rate, our classification, no matter how artificial, divides the posture exercises in this fashion. By Front-stretching Postures we mean those in which effort is made to bend the body backward, regardless of whether the body is face down, face up, standing or upside down. Although some overlapping is hardly avoidable, we have tried to defer treatment of those bending exercises which give special emphasis to the legs and other appendages until Section IX, even where back stretching or front stretching may also be obviously involved.

Just as in describing what we meant by "back," so we must say, in defining what we mean by "front," that we refer to all of those muscles which have their location mainly in the front of the body. Interior muscles obviously become involved. If an author could depend upon his readers having a detailed knowledge of muscular anatomy, the whole system for classifying exercises could be different. Front here includes front of the neck, chest, abdomen, pelvis, upper and lower legs, knees, ankles and even feet. Not all of these parts of the body participate equally in each of the exercises, but all of the exercises included in the present section tend to involve all of these parts somewhat.

A. Prone-starting Series

Whereas our Back-stretching Postures section began with the Most Relaxed Posture and a Supine-starting Series, we find convenient reversing the organization here and beginning our Front-stretching Postures section with a Prone-starting Series. Although we might have used the obvious procedural titles, Head-first Series and Feet-first Series, here also yogic tradition already has a well-established, simple and easily identifiable set of names for most of the postures and series to be examined. English translations have become quite standardized and these standardized names are becoming part of common parlance.

1. The Cobra Series

Bhujangasana, the Cobra (Snake or Serpent) Posture, is so named because, in its perfected form, the body's outline simulates the appearance of the front part of a cobra with its head raised from the ground. We distinguish three stages.

First, one should rest in a prone position (see Plate 4) and breathe regularly and relaxingly. Preparatory to the second stage, one should move his arms from his usual resting position in such a way that his hands rest flat on the floor near or beneath his shoulders. Persons with different arm-length ratios relative to their trunks and suppleness of spine may vary the precise location of their hands in relation to the shoulders after a bit of experience. As one's spine becomes more supple through bending exercises, this location may shift somewhat. The elbows will be bent and held close to the sides of the chest. Another preparatory portion of the first stage consists in raising the head from its resting position, expanding the chest, throwing back the shoulders and raising the elbows in readiness for placing weight on the hands.

The second stage, which is as far as beginners should expect to get, consists in raising the chest off the floor and holding the head erect by means of putting pressure on the hands. (See Plate 55.) The abdomen, from the navel downward, continues to rest on the floor, as do the hips, thighs, knees and tops of the toes. The elbows remain bent, though not as much as during the preparatory first stage. Even though the head faces straight forward in the formal Cobra Posture, one should also bend his head as far back as possible to provide maximum stretching effects. The precise distance which the chest is raised from the floor is partly a matter of personal capacity. Beginners should seek to raise as far as possible, or rather as far as convenient, without discomfort or apparent danger to the spine. When compared with our third stage, which requires much more stretching, this stage may be called *Ardha-Bhujangasana* or Half-Cobra Posture. However, the name *Bhujangasana* (Cobra Posture) commonly applies to all of the postures in this series.

PICTOGRAPH CHART NO. 4

FRONT-STRETCHING POSTURES

A. Prone-starting Series

1. The Cobra Series

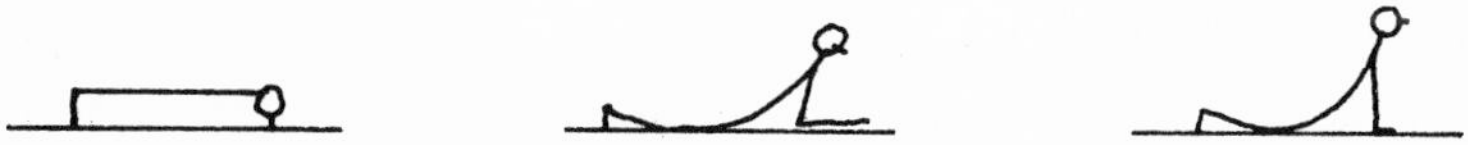

2. The Locust Series

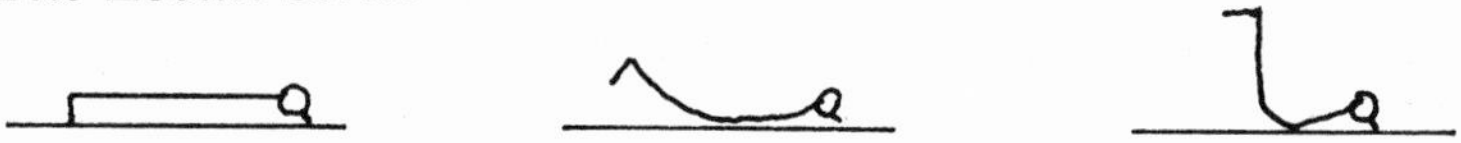

3. The Bow Series

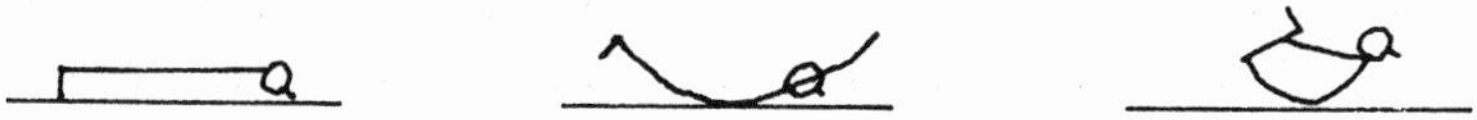

4. The Rocking Bow Series

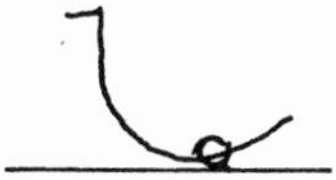

5. The Peacock Series (Advanced)

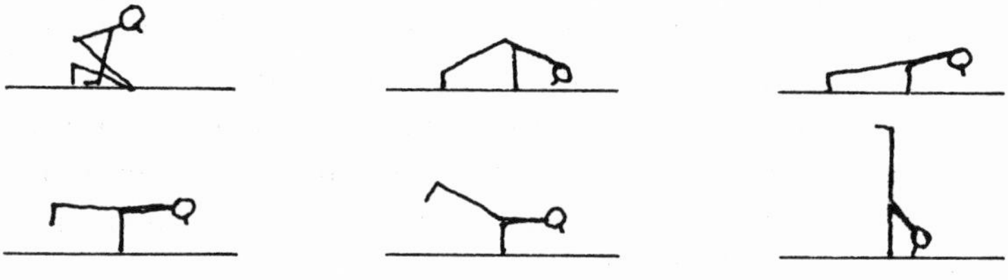

6. The Cow Posture

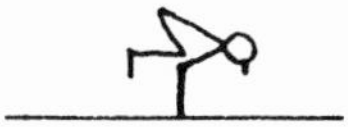

7. The Scorpion Series (Advanced)

The third stage, which like the second should be approached slowly, is reached ideally as the lines of the spine and legs approximate a right angle. (See Plate 56.) The legs remain flat on the floor up to the groin. The arms become straightened, though teachers differ as to whether they should be perfectly straight or retain some slight bend. Shoulders are kept back and the head is bent back as far as possible. One may even face the ceiling, though in the formal pose one faces straight forward. One should attend more to the process and progress in bending the spine. Some believe they can notice when each additional vertebra comes under pressure during the process of bending upward and backward. Moderation and persistent caution is needed in all back-bending exercises, especially as they become more extreme. As a variation, one may straighten his arms and raise his whole body on hands and toes while retaining all other aspects of the Cobra Posture. Another quite different variation calls for keeping the Cobra Posture but raising the hands off the floor. Still another consists in bending the knees, kept on the floor, and touching the back of the head with raised toes of both feet.

This posture is another available for office use. One does not need to remove his clothes in order to obtain some of the benefits of this exercise, even though he may have to adjust them after he is finished. A few such postures, in which one proceeds slowly both into and out of each, interspersed with short periods of rest and controlled breathing, should prove quite refreshing. We have neglected throughout to discuss synchronization of breathing and posture exercises, but here especially is one exercise in which coordination of lung expansion and back bending may be found particularly convenient and beneficial.

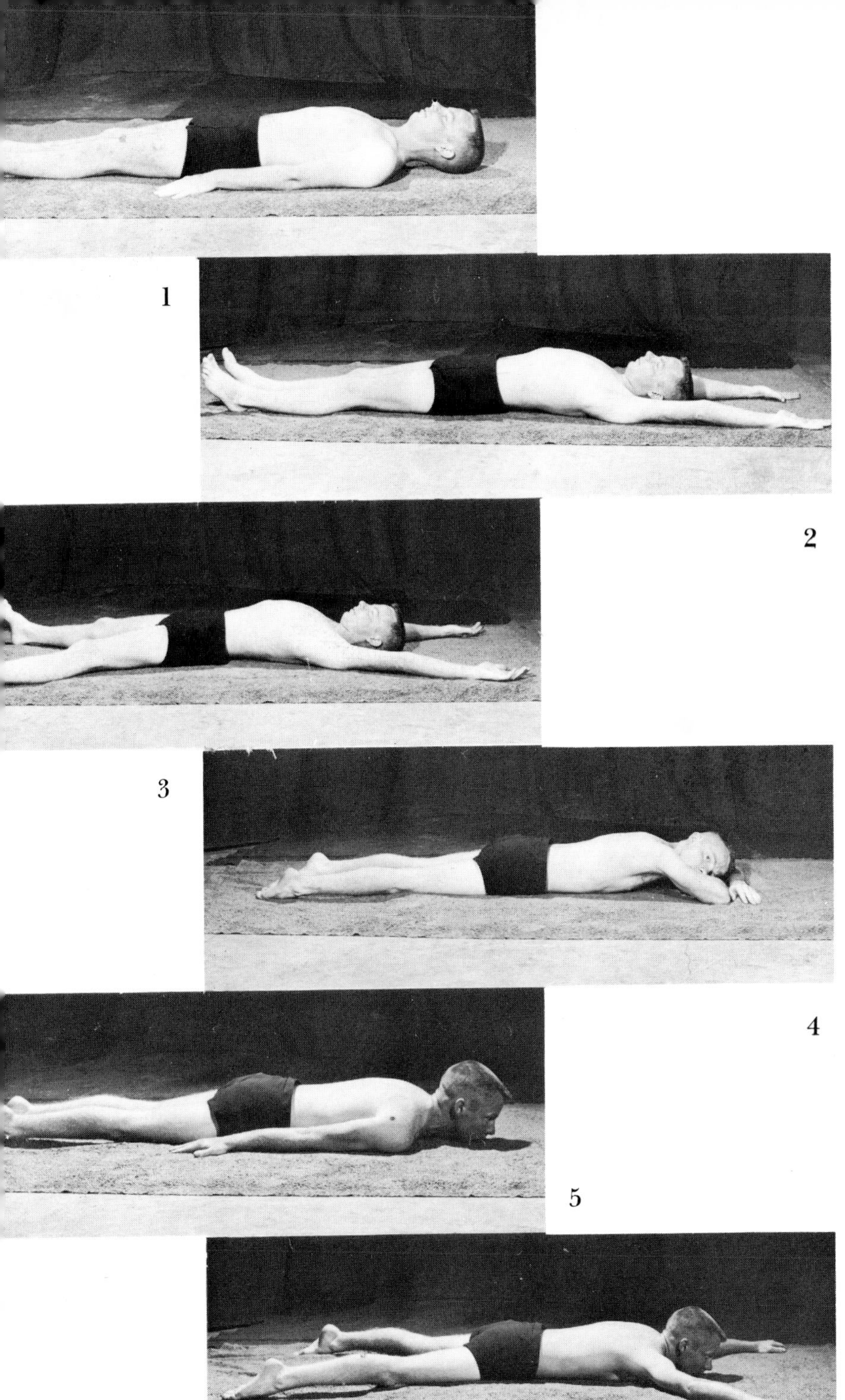

1

2

3

4

5

6

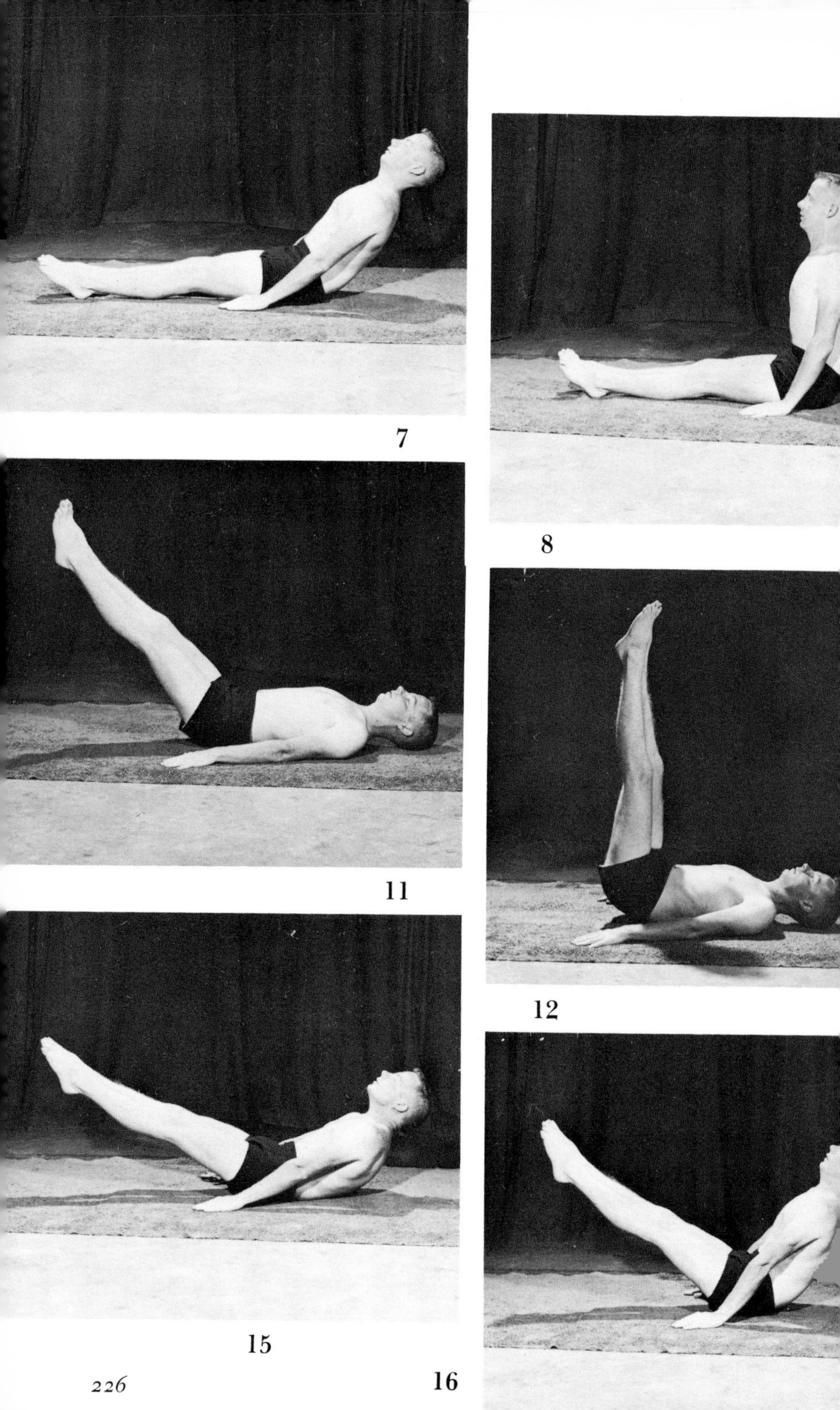

7

8

11

12

15

16

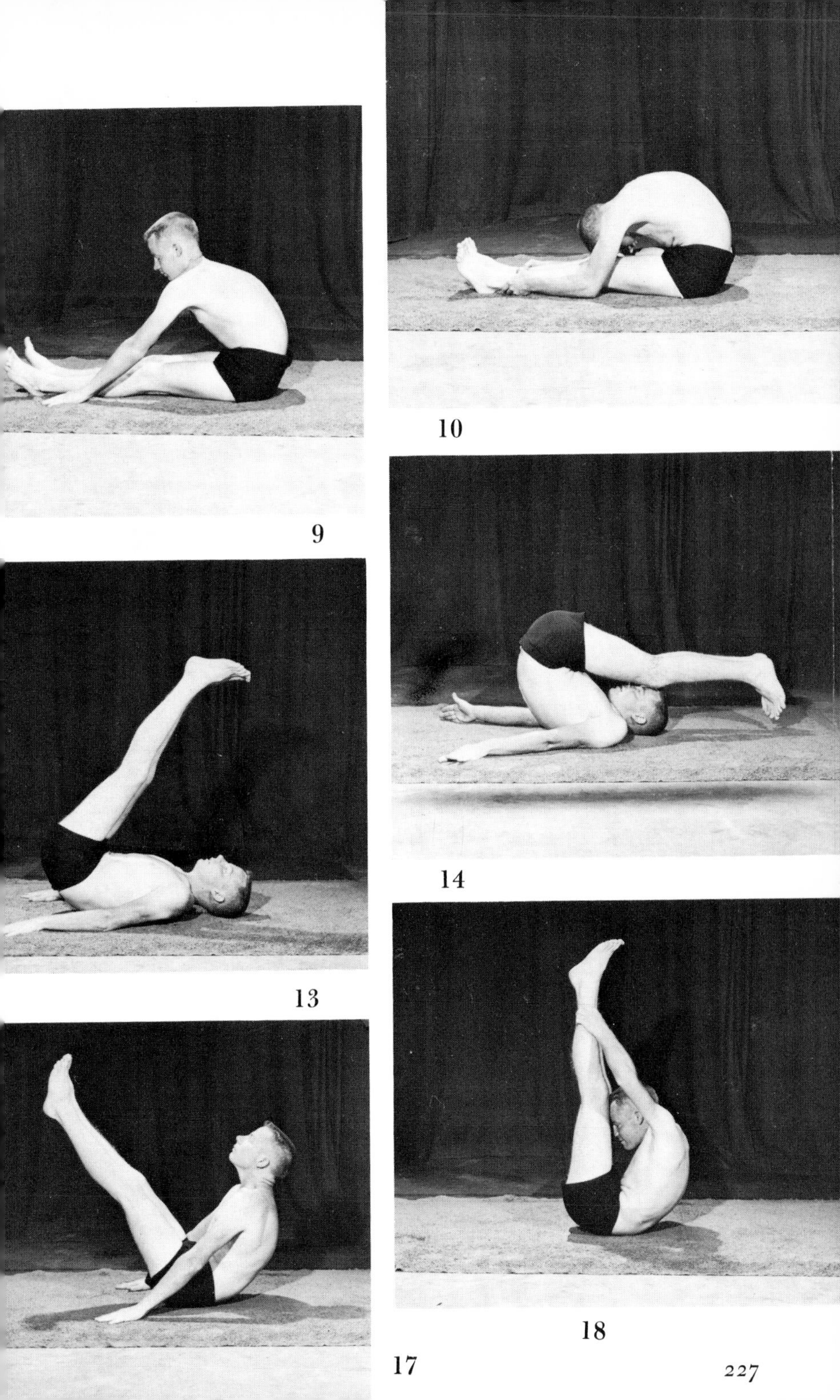

9

10

13

14

17

18

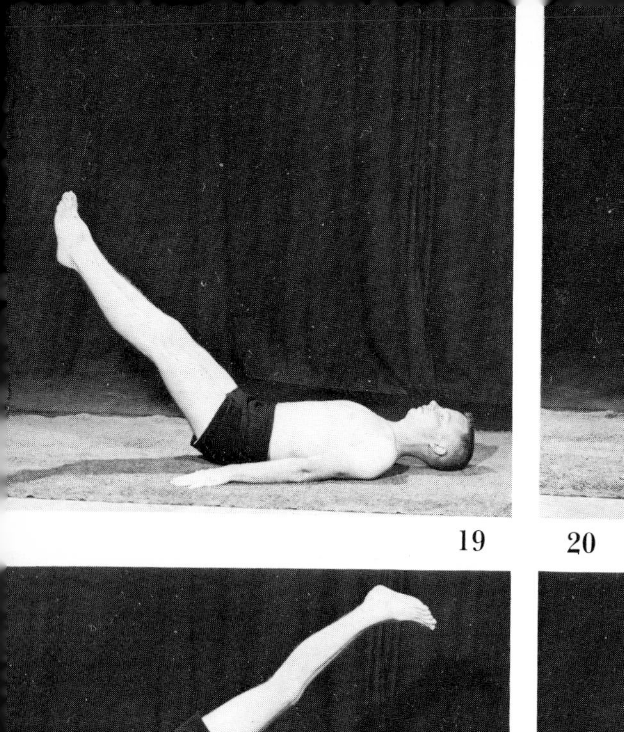

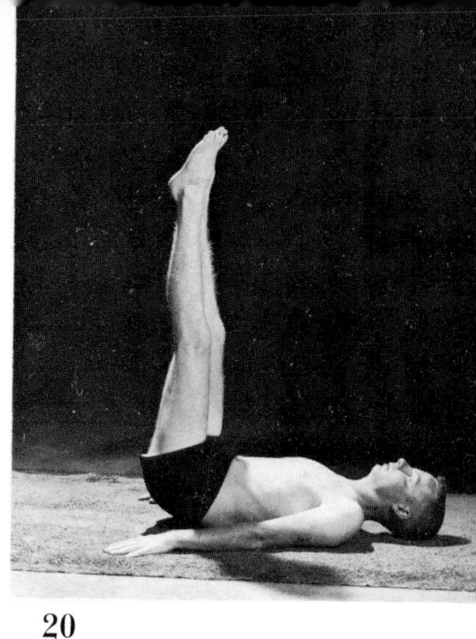

19 20

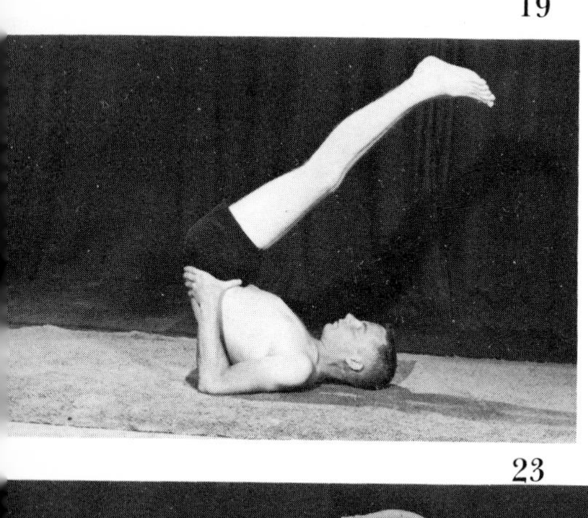

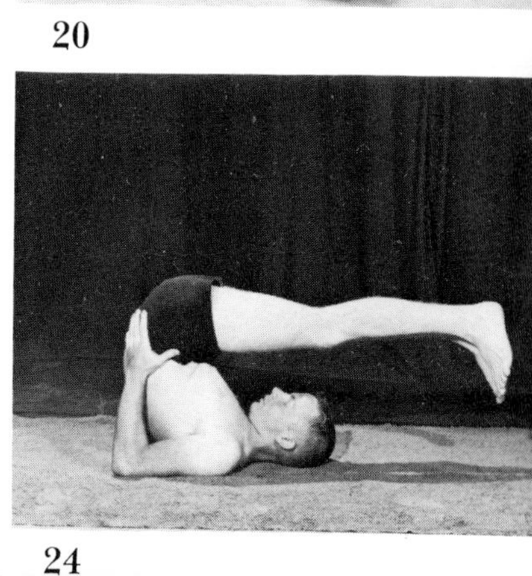

23 24

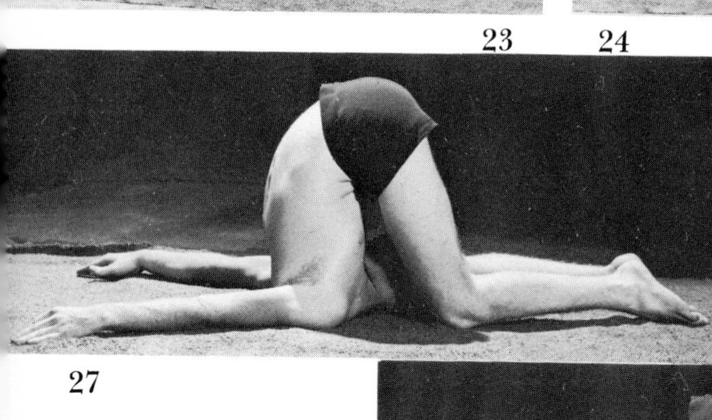

27

28

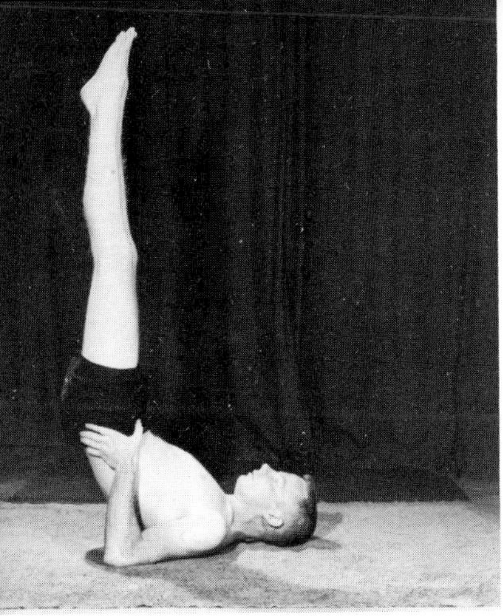

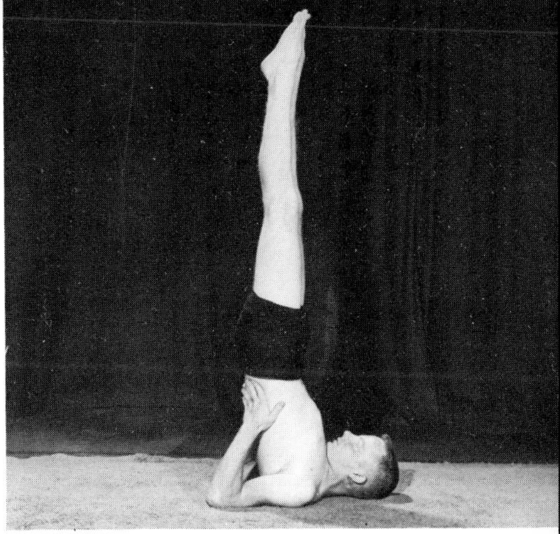

21 22

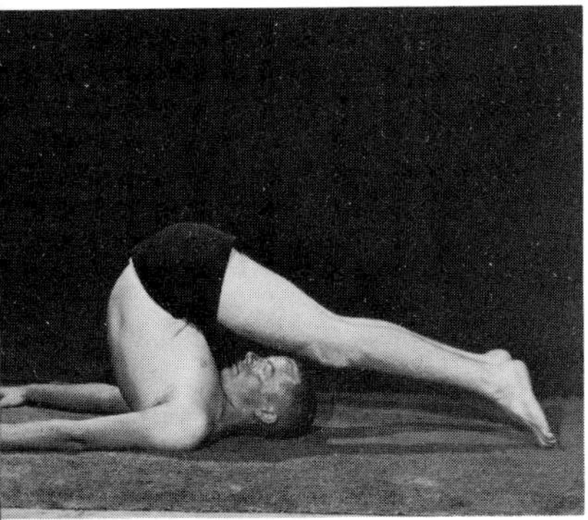

25

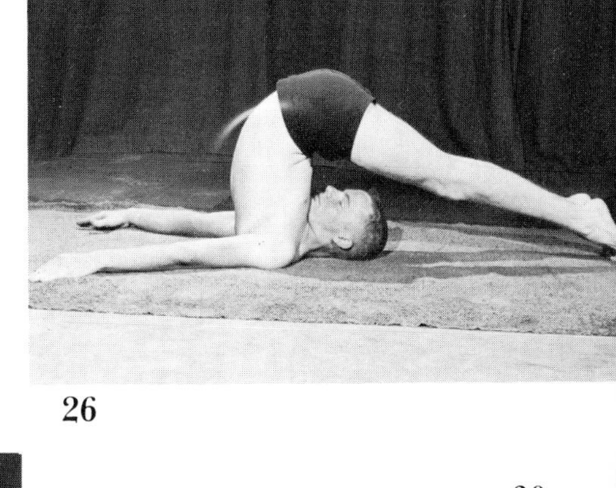

26

30

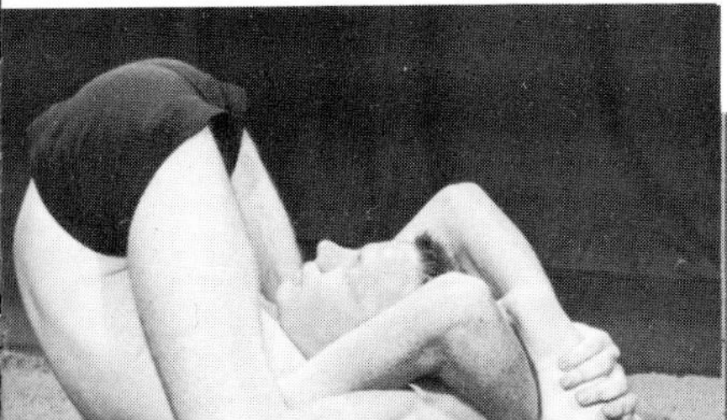

29

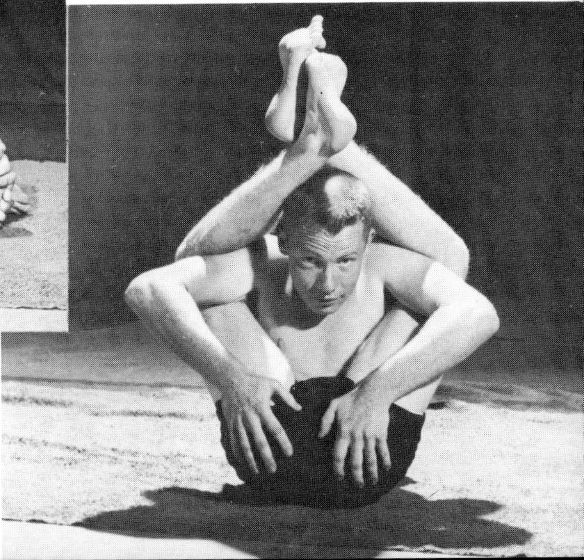

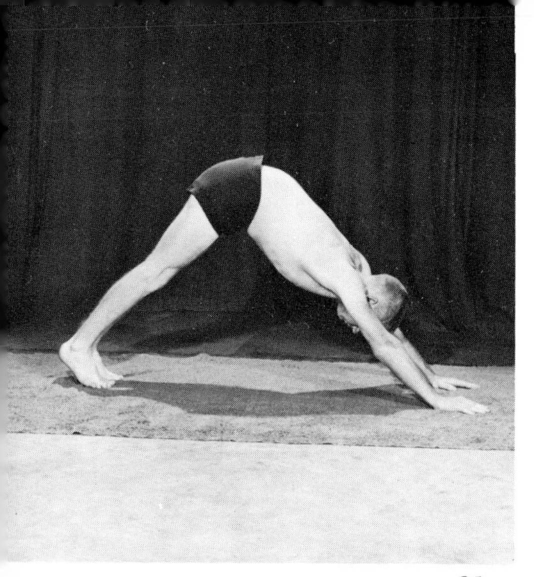

31

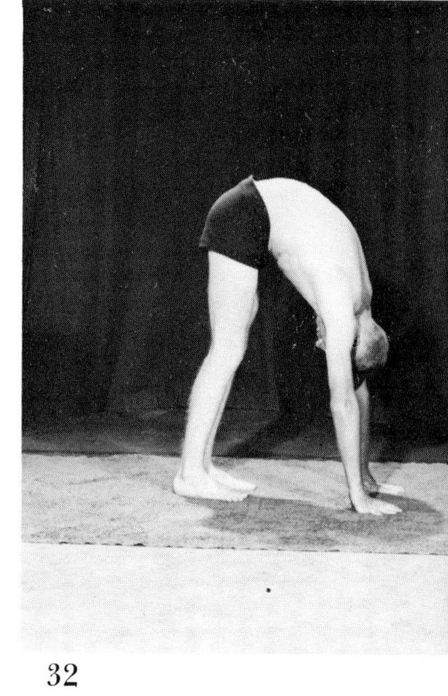

32

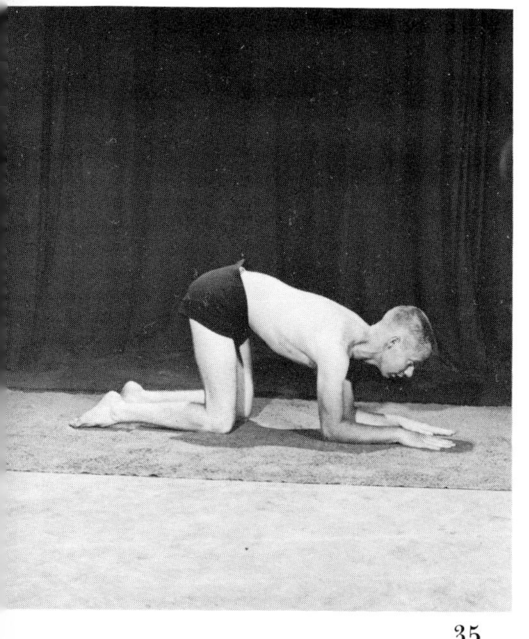

35

36

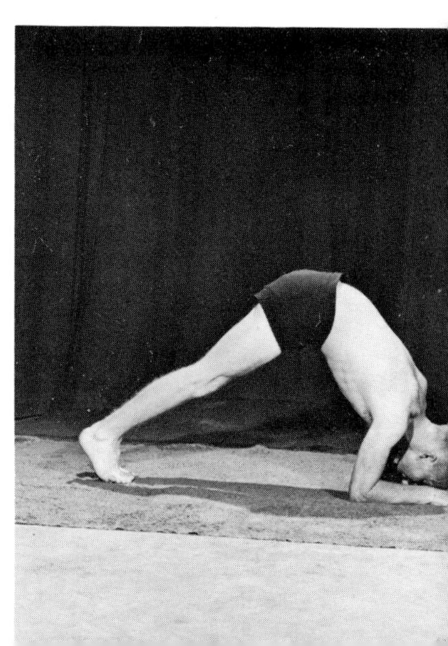

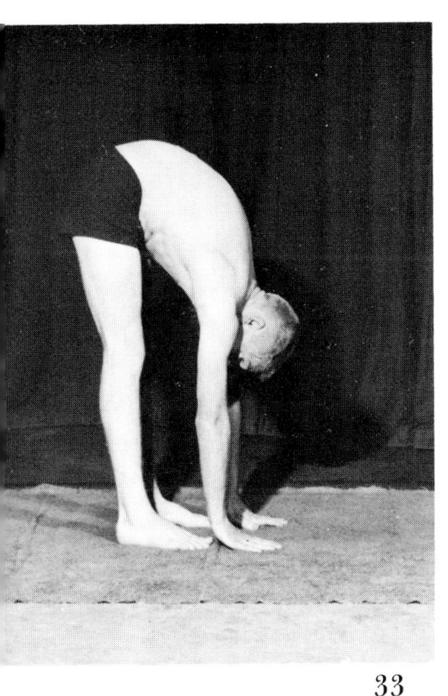

33

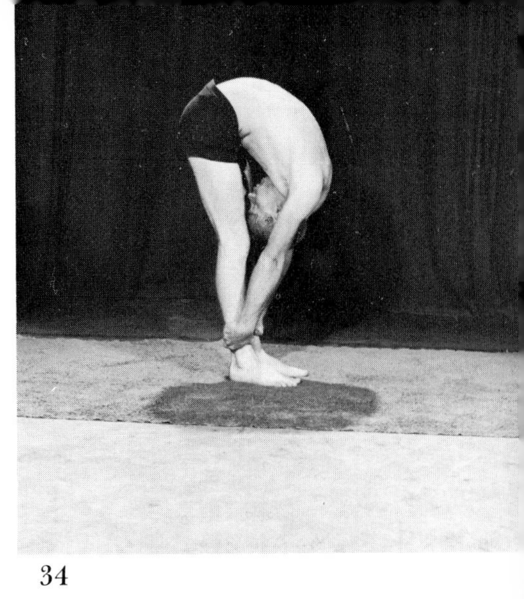

34

37

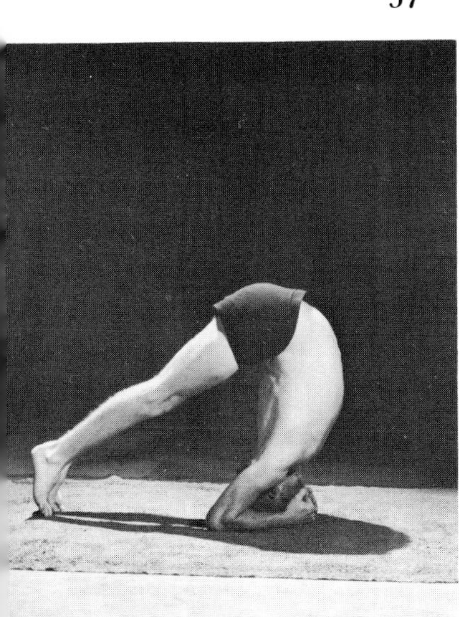

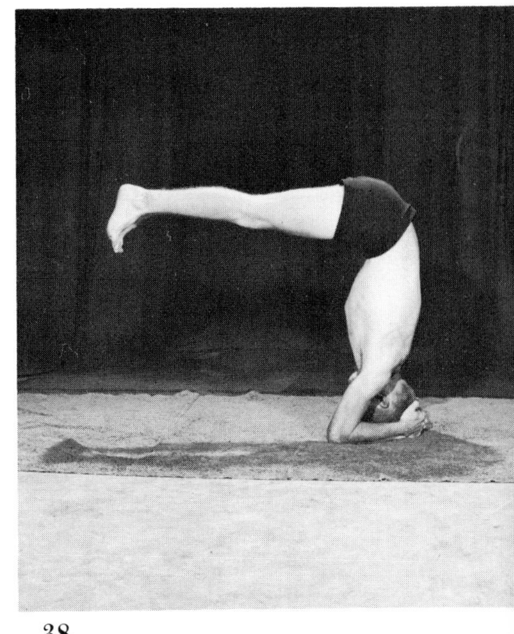

38

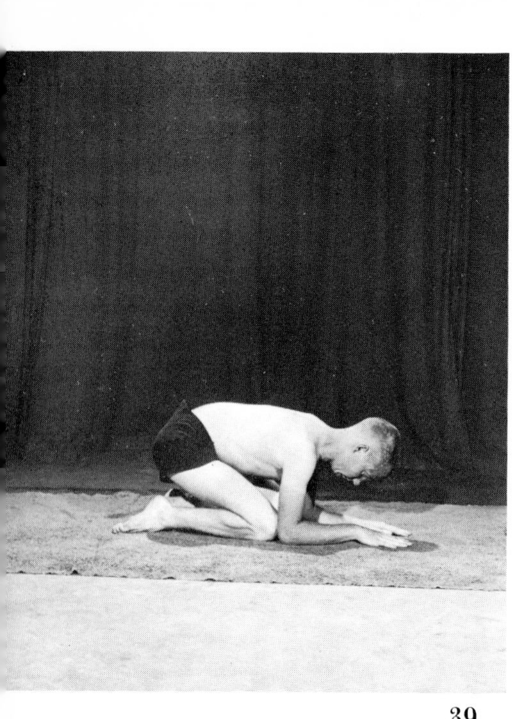

39

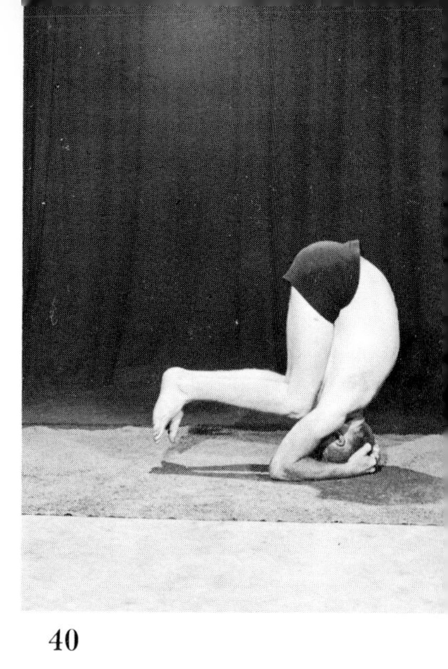

40

43

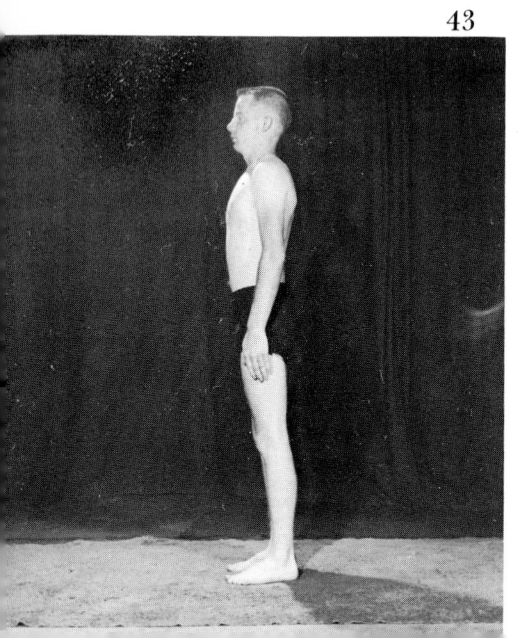

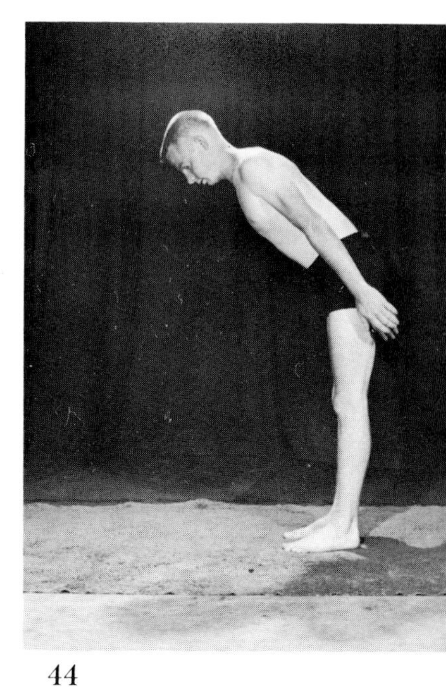

44

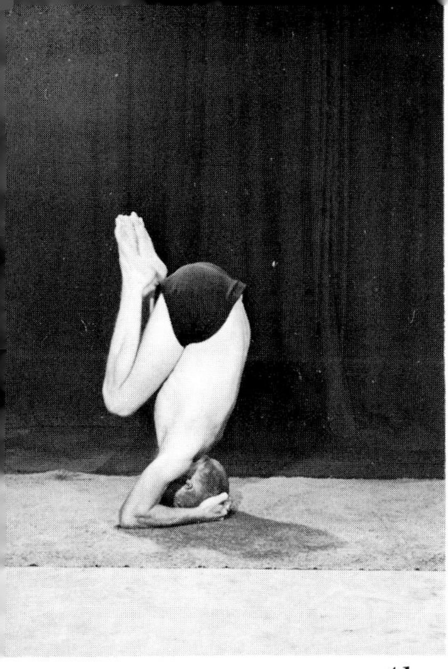
41

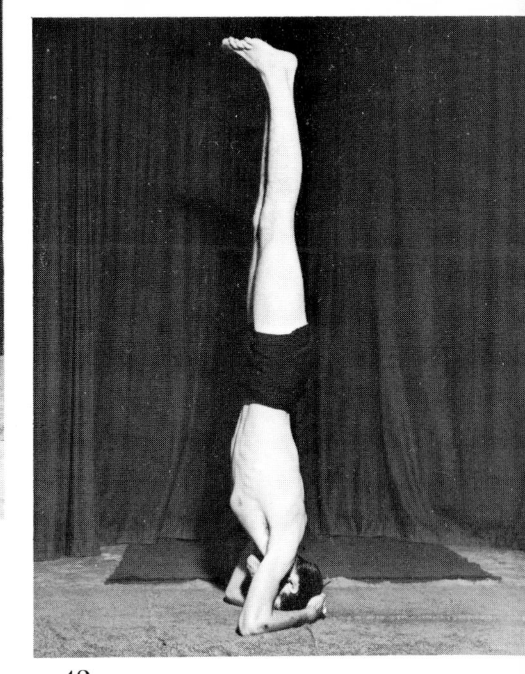
42

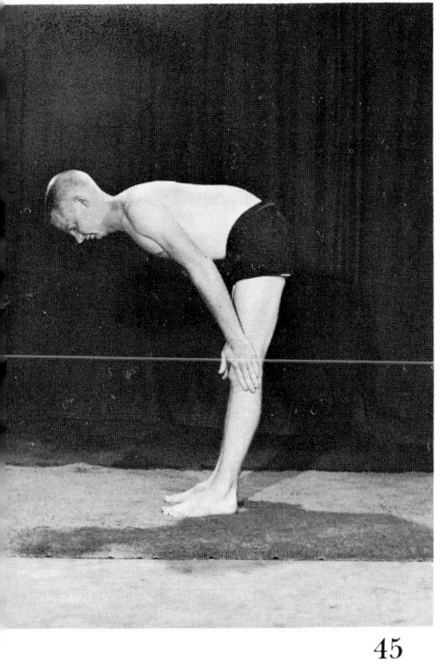
45

46
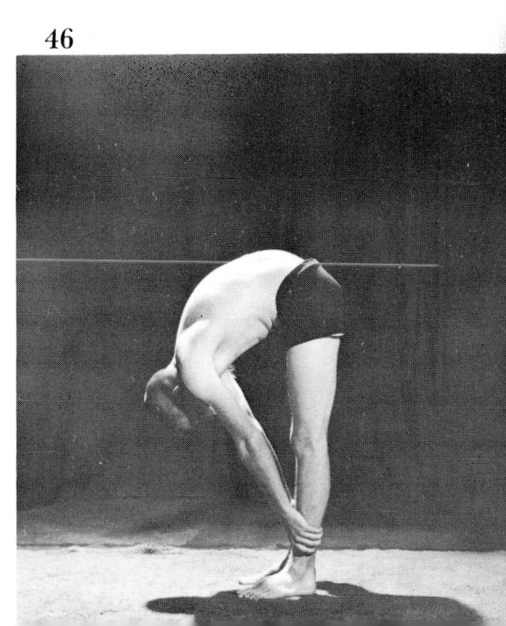

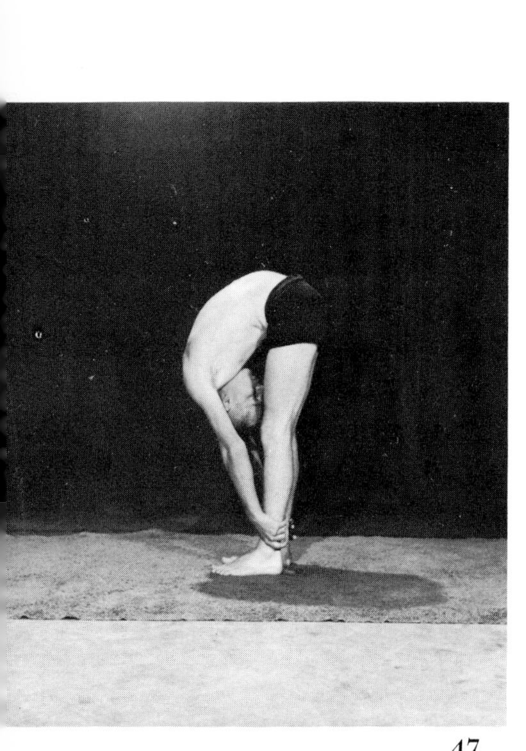

47

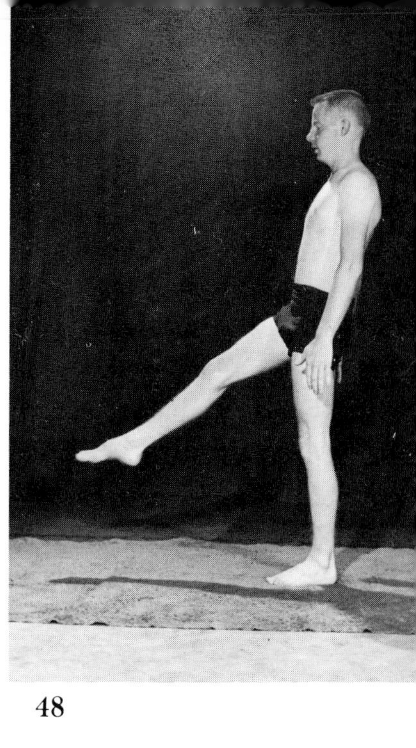

48

51

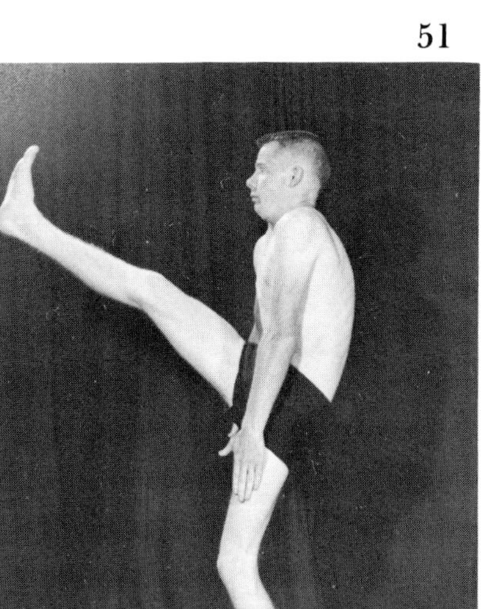

52

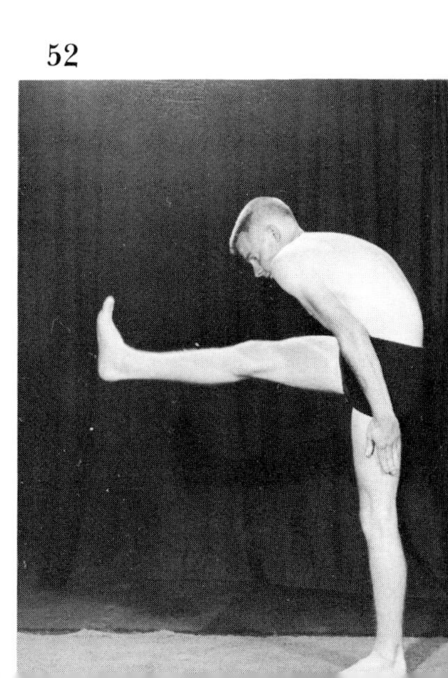

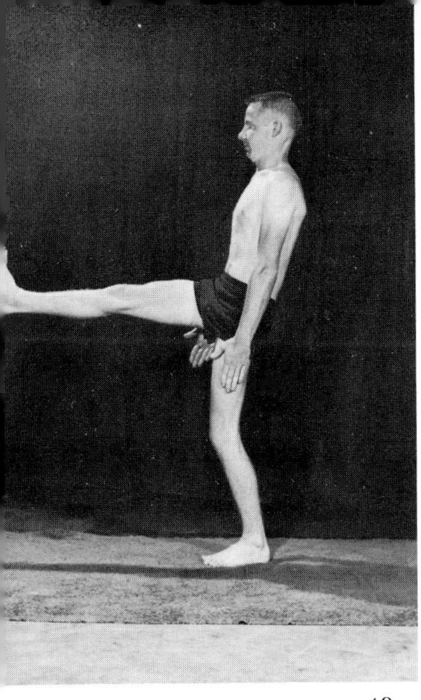

49

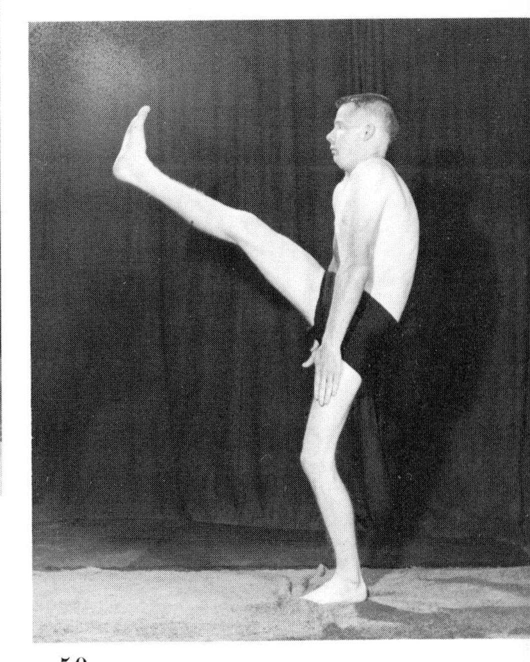

50

53

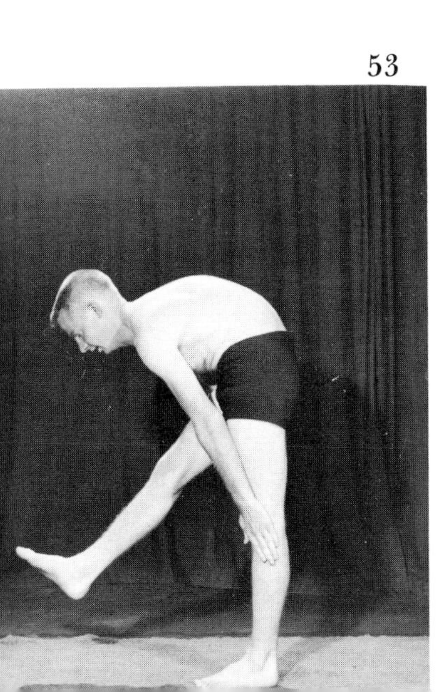

54

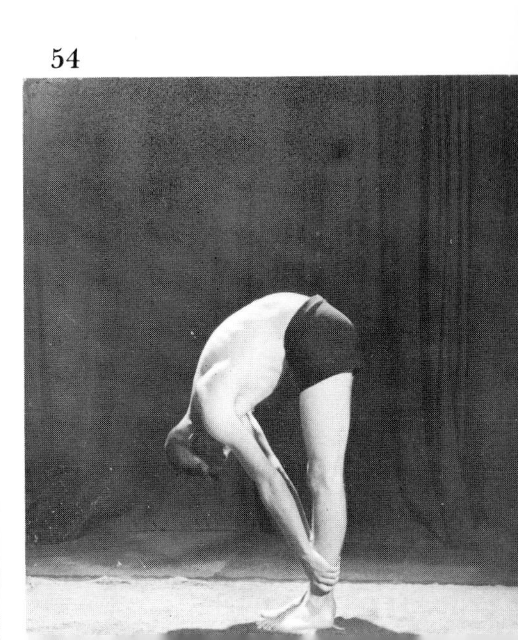

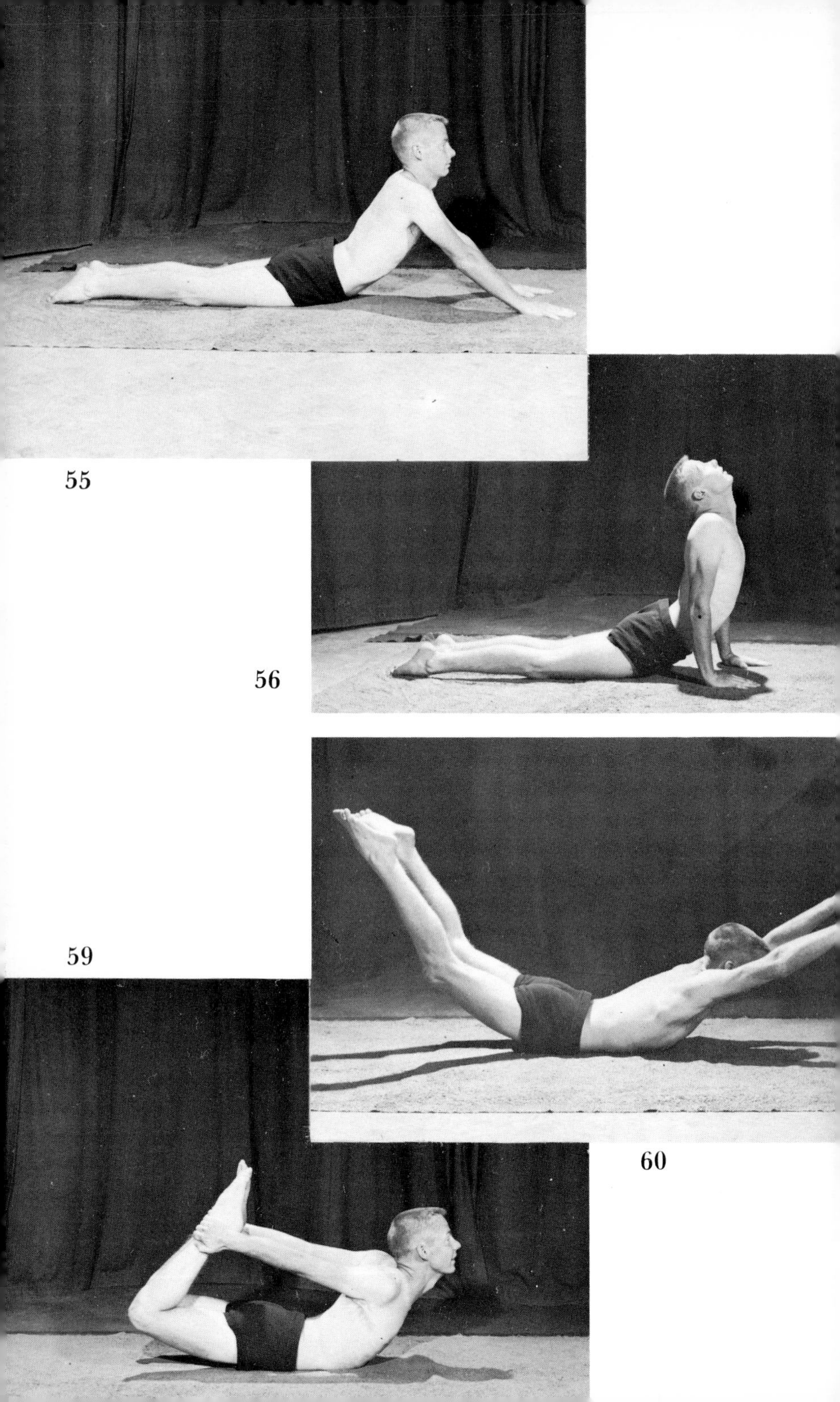

55

56

59

60

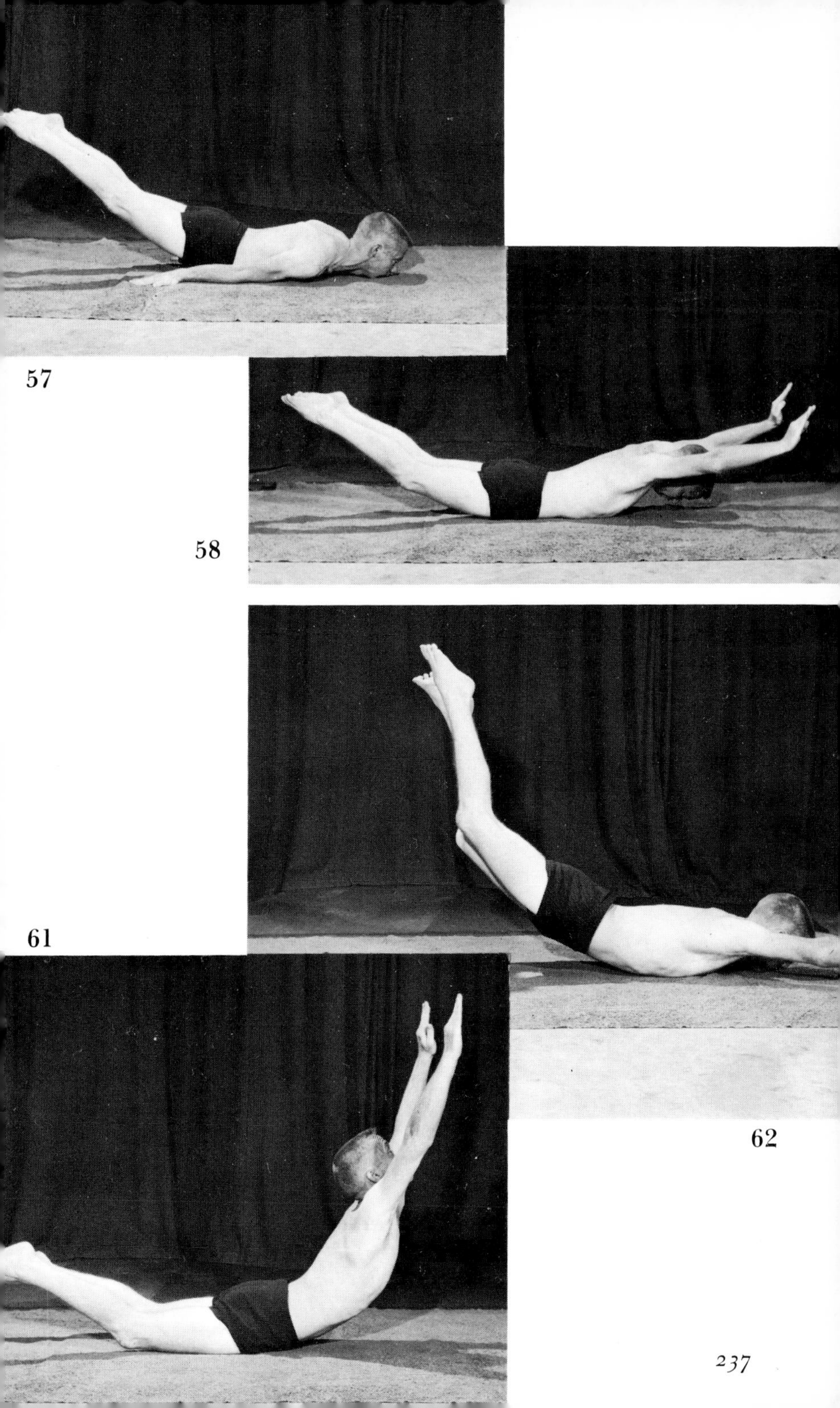
57
58
61
62

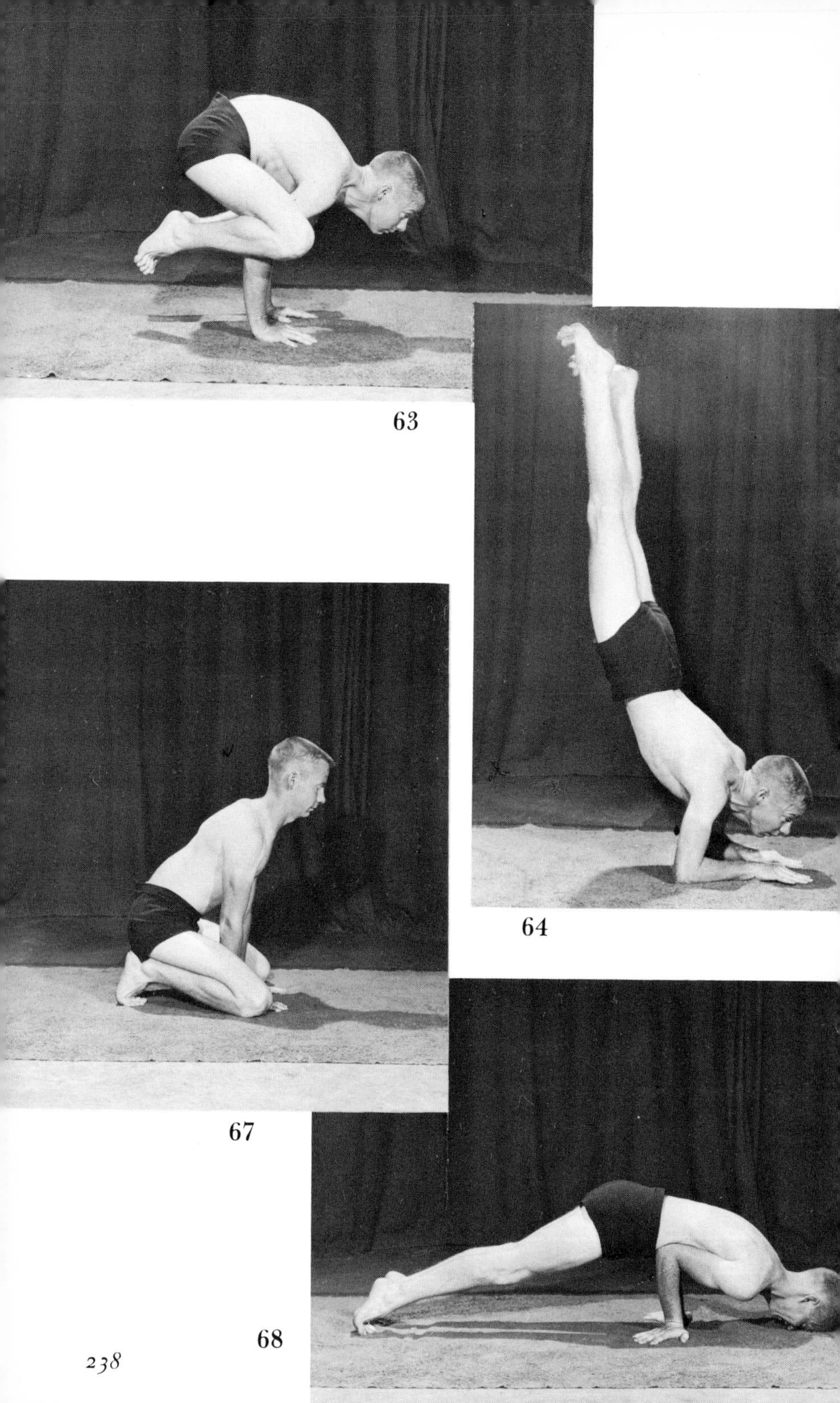

63

64

67

68

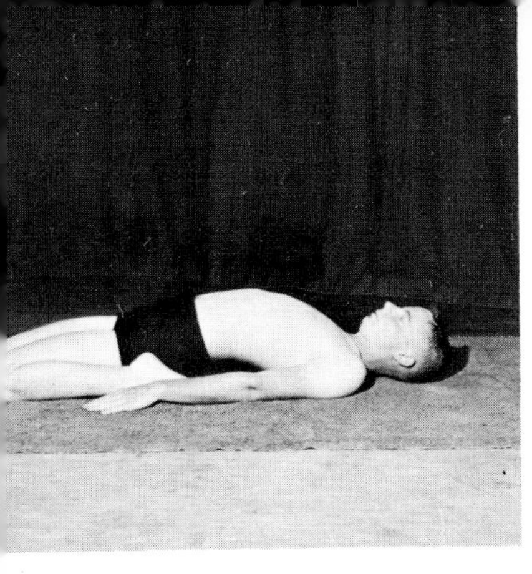

65

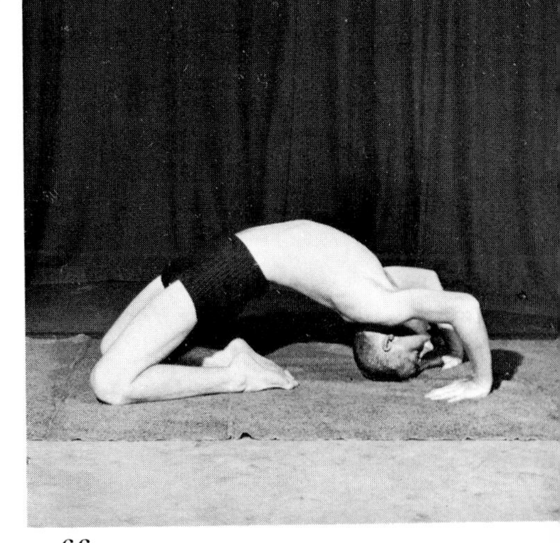

66

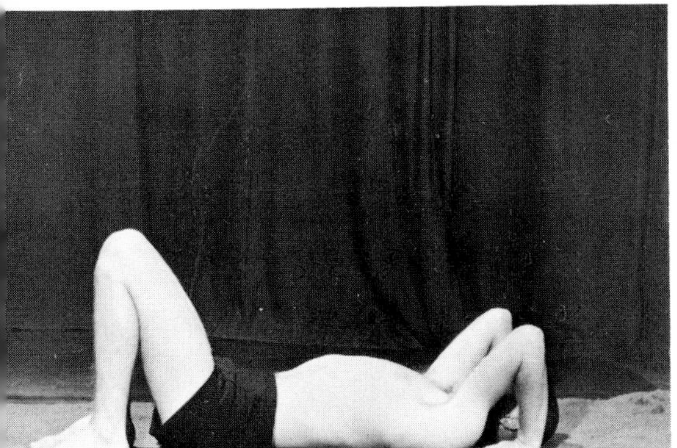

69

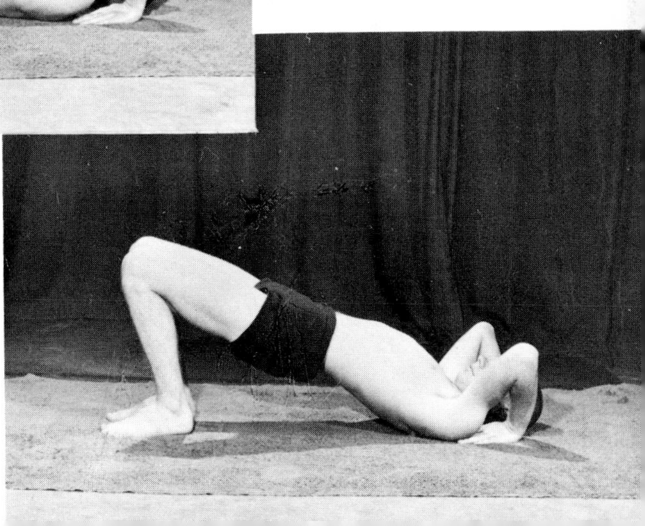

70

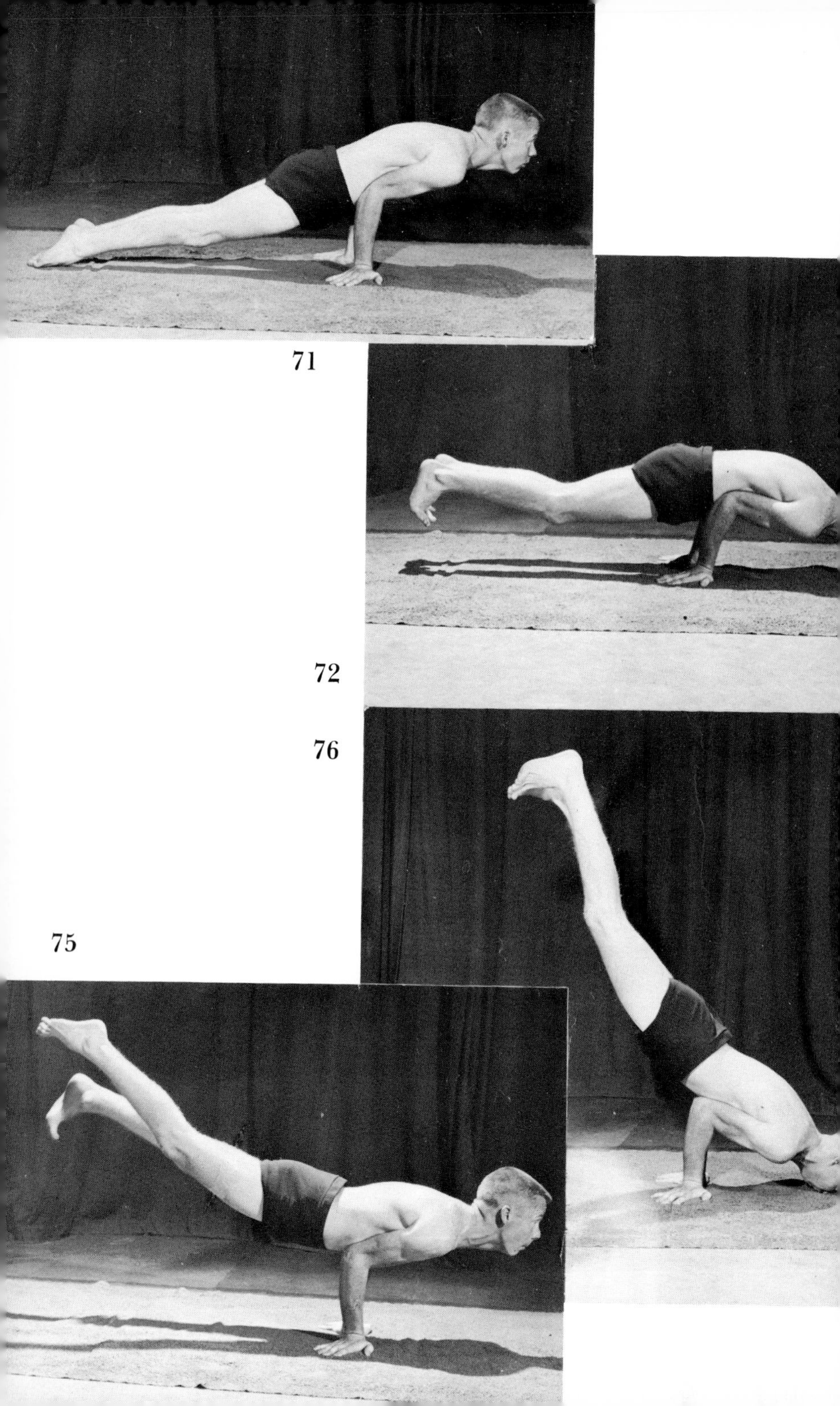

71

72

76

75

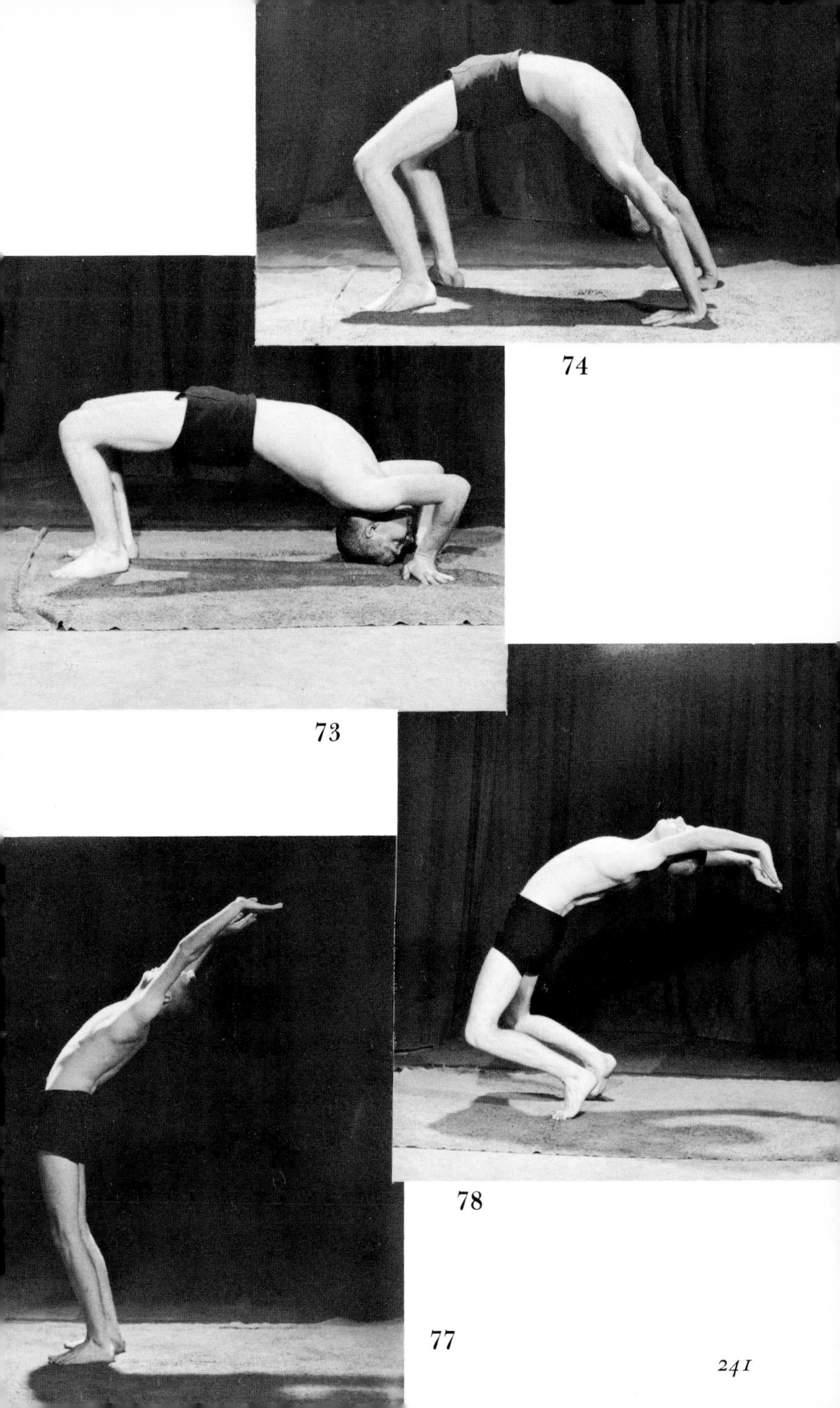

74

73

78

77

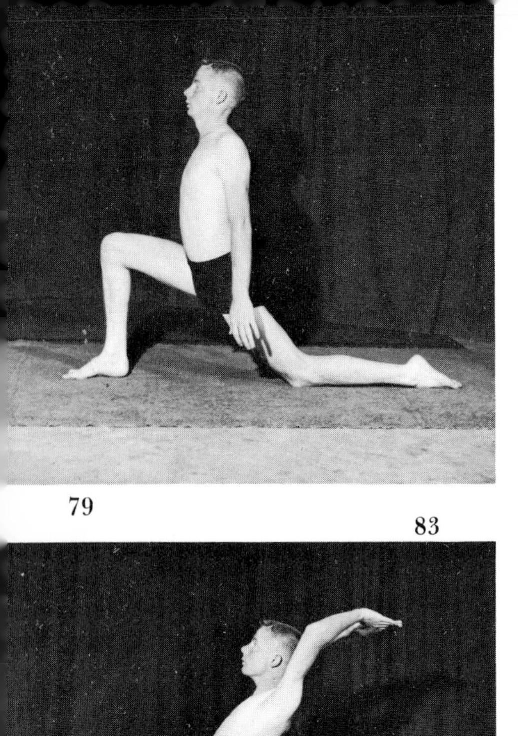

79

83

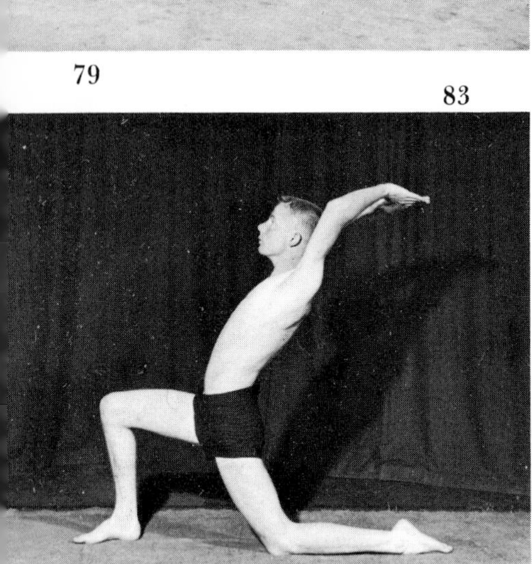

87

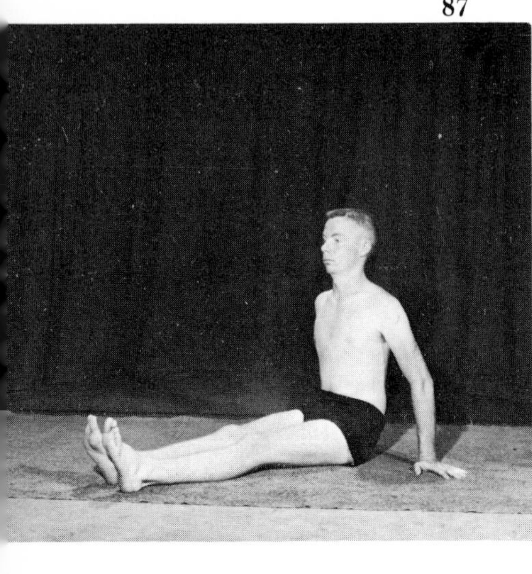

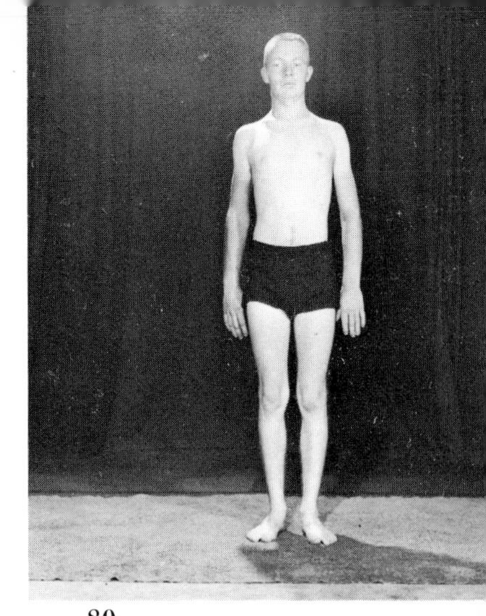

80

8

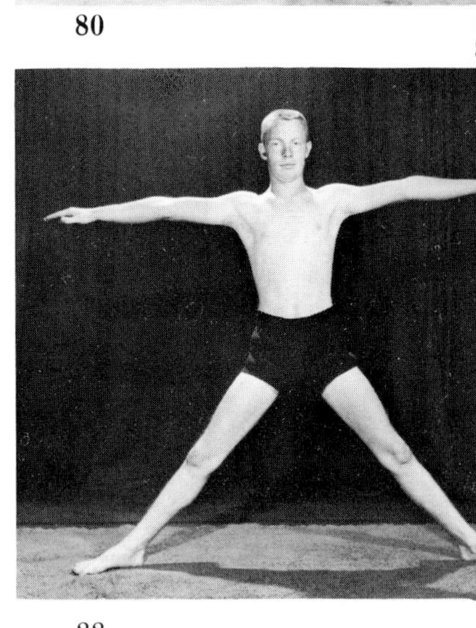

88

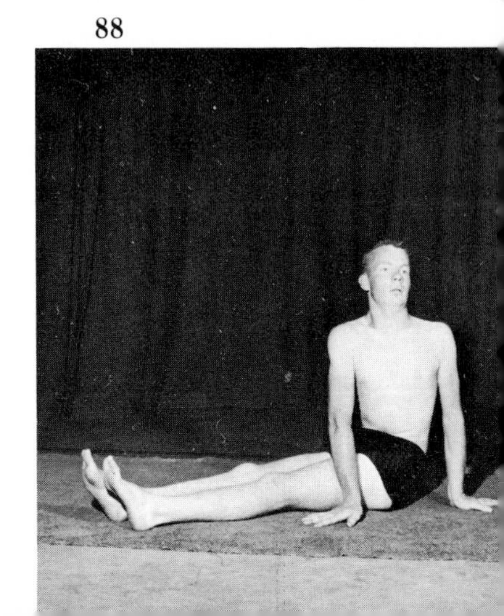

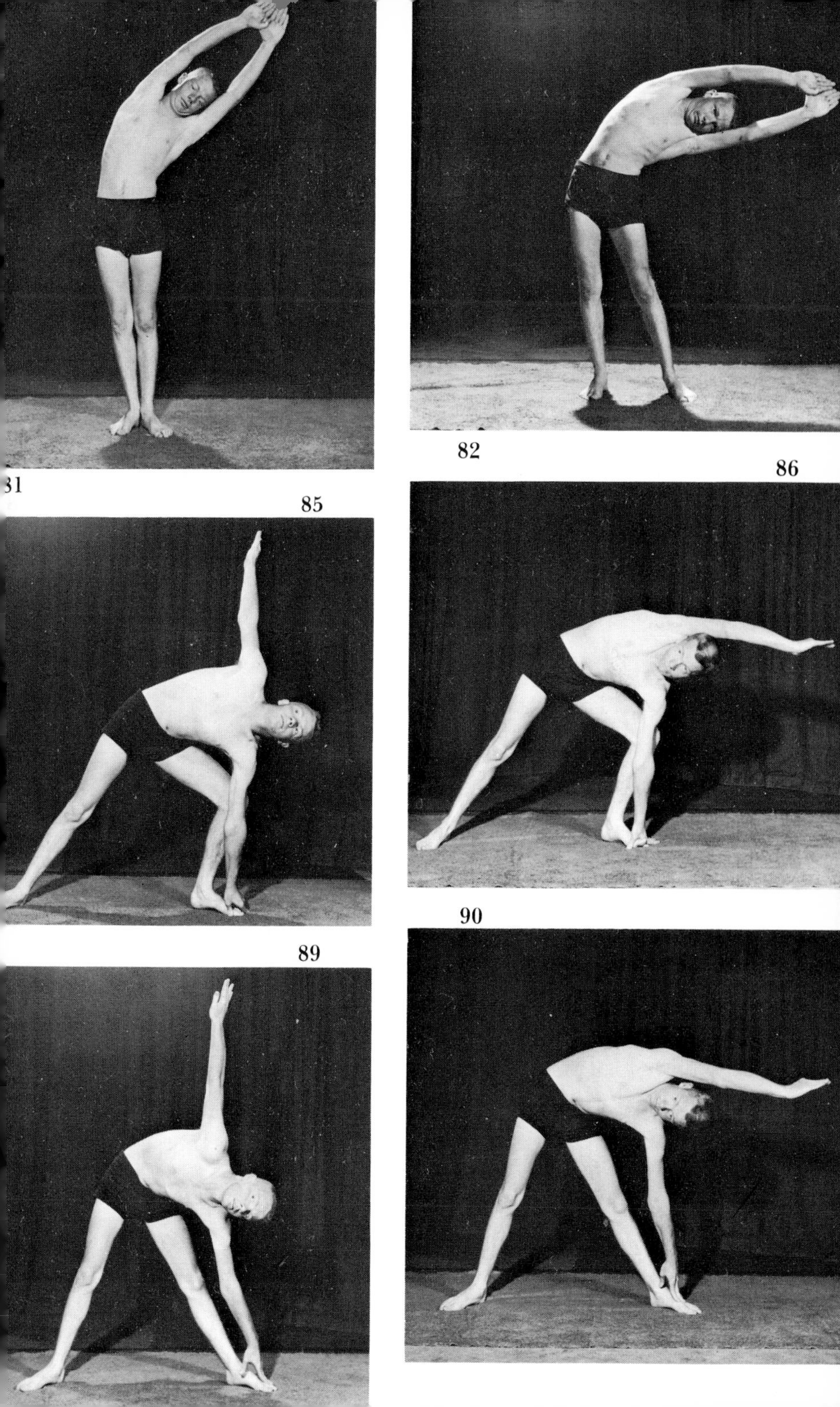

81

82

85

86

89

90

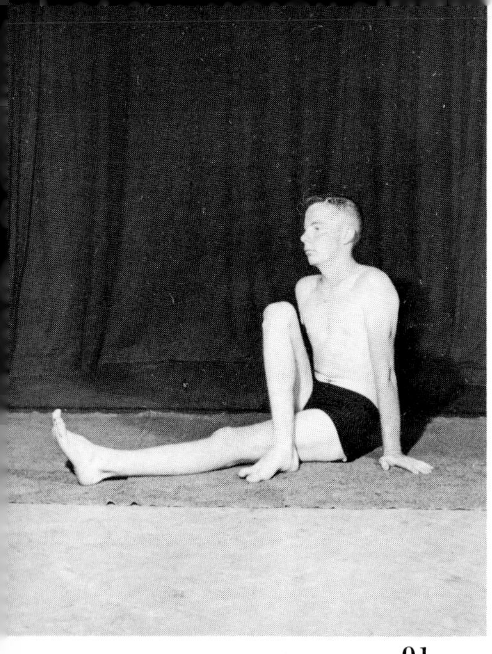

91

95

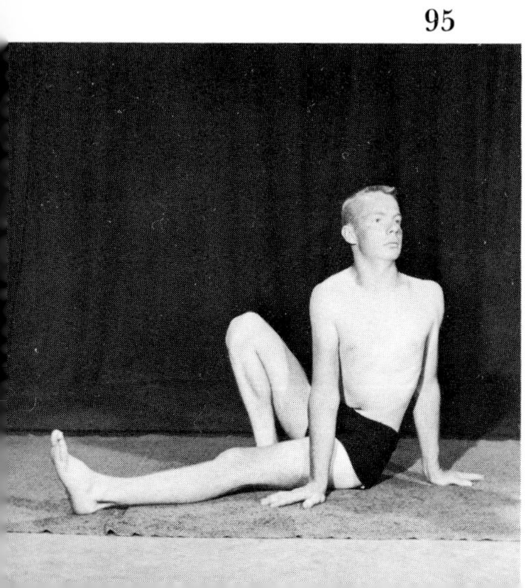

92

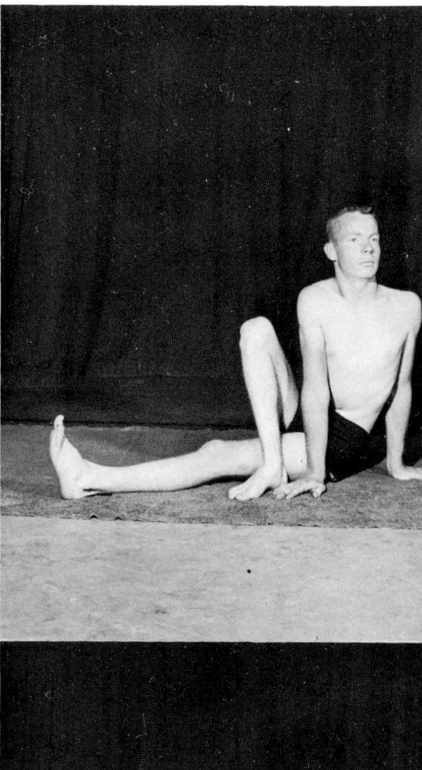

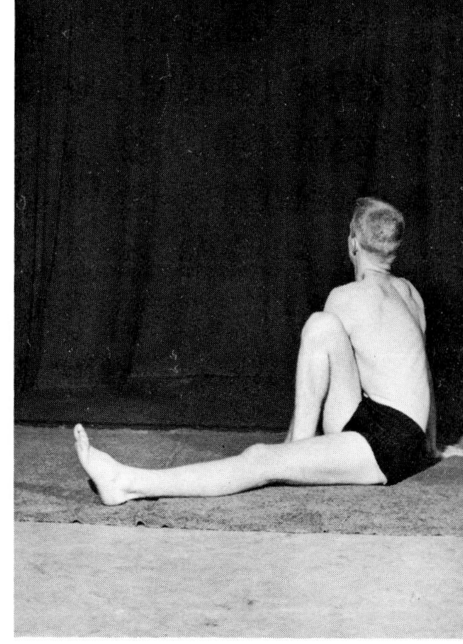

96

93

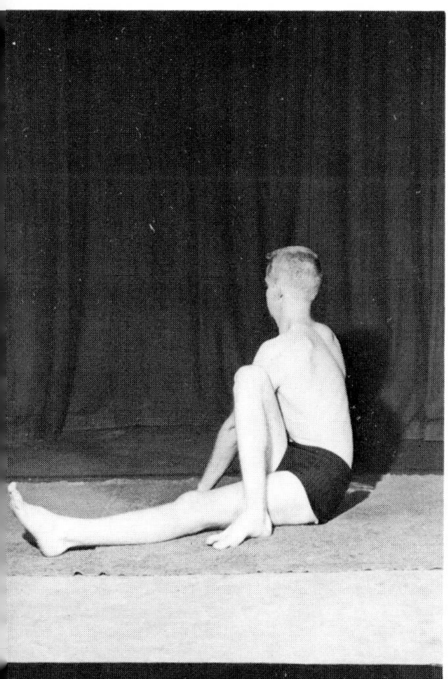

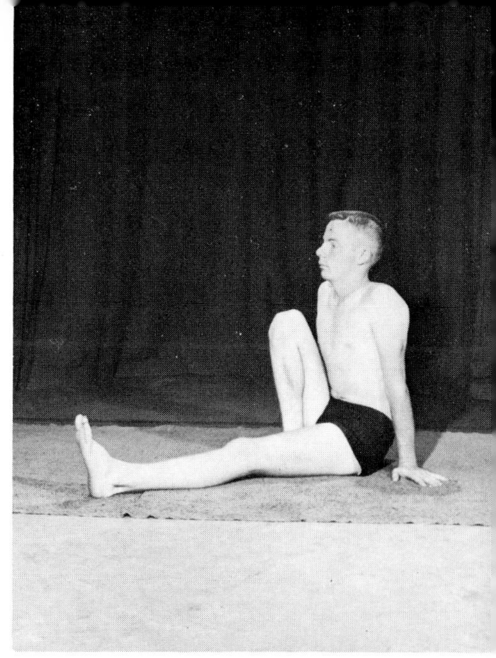

94

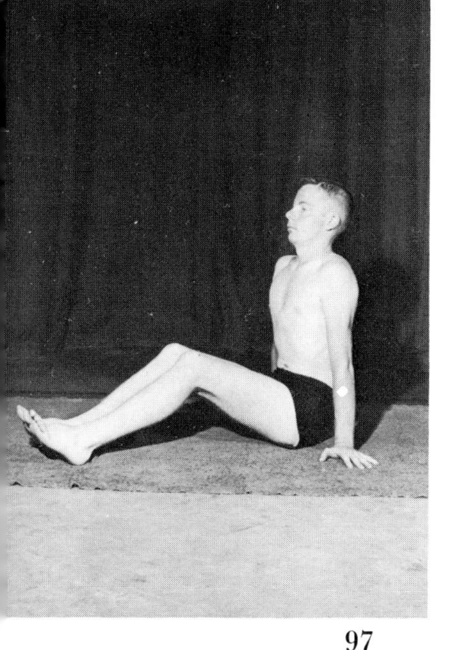

97

98

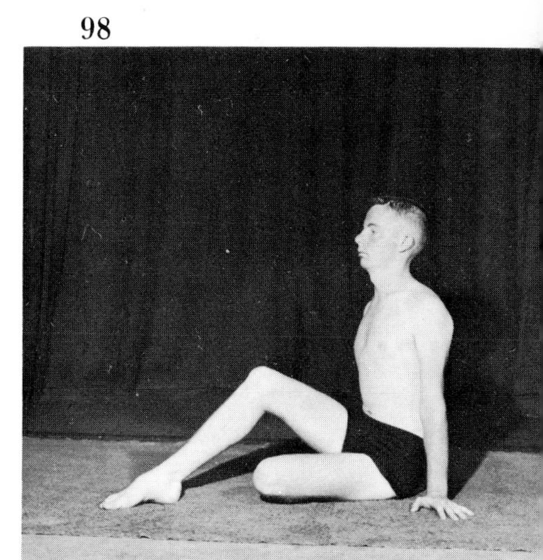

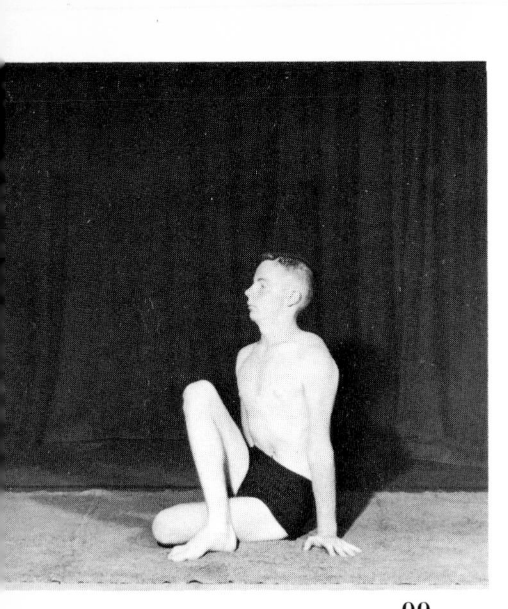

99

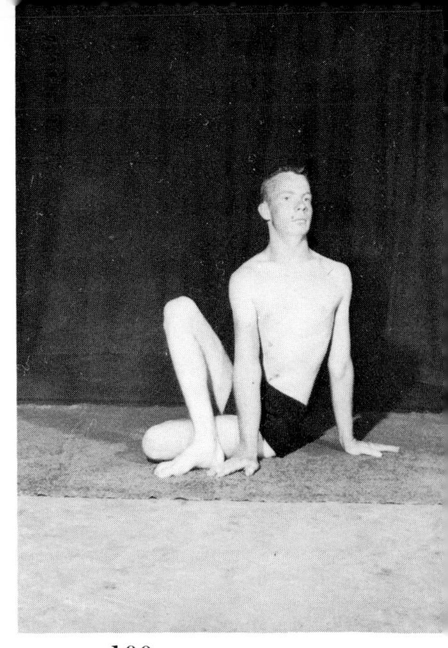

100

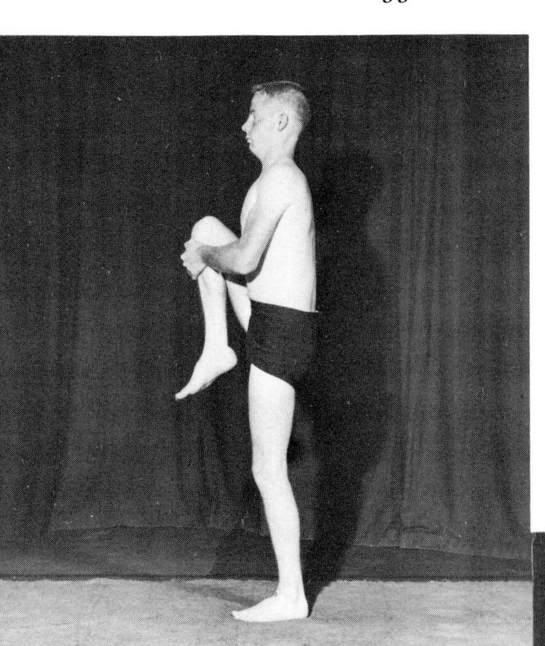

103

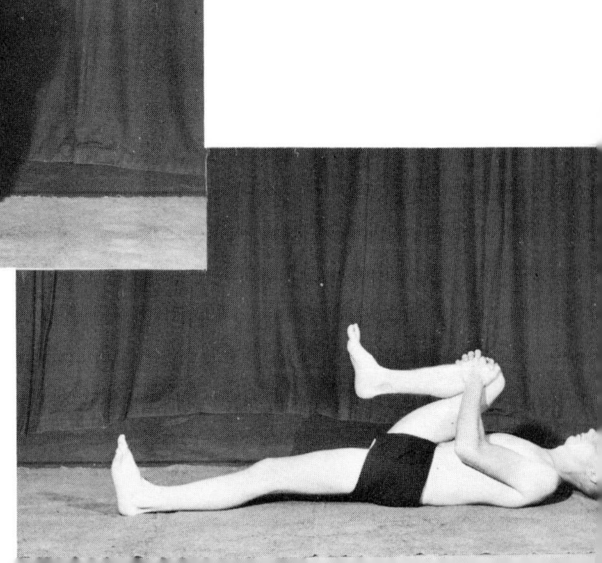

104

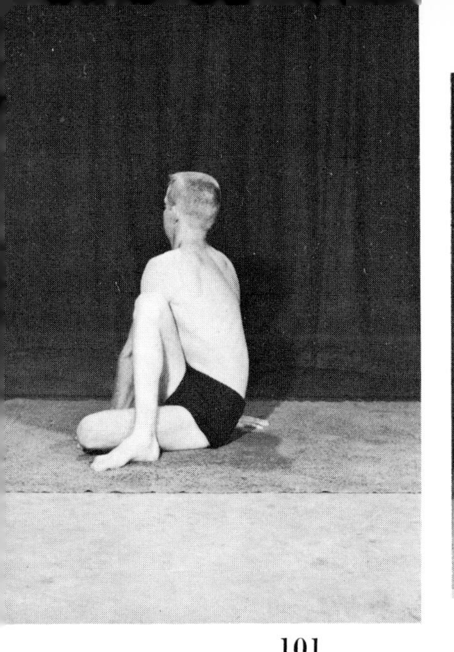

101

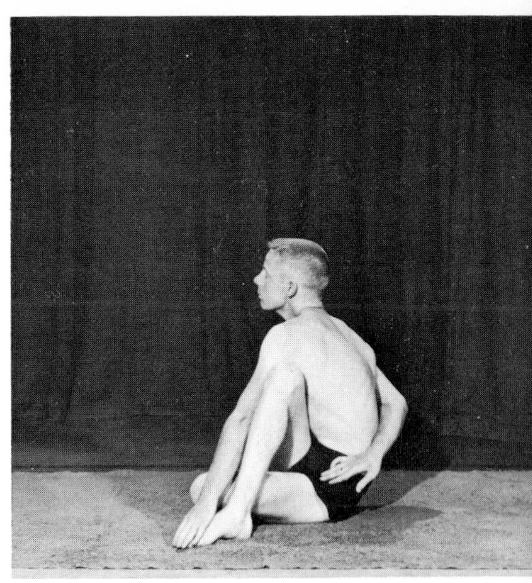

102

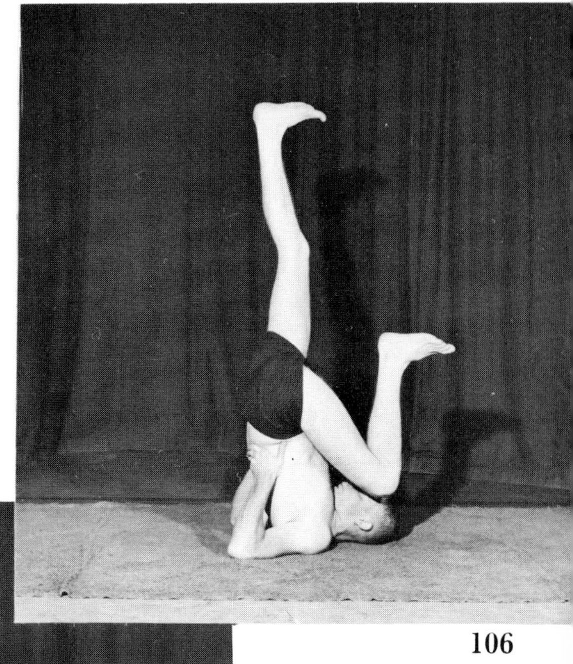

106

105

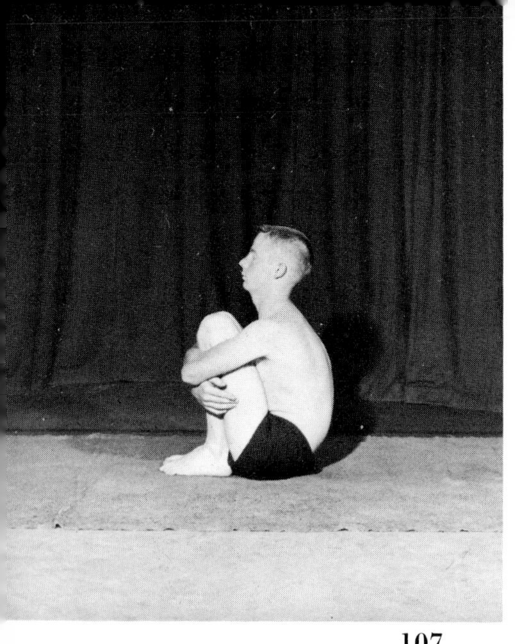

107

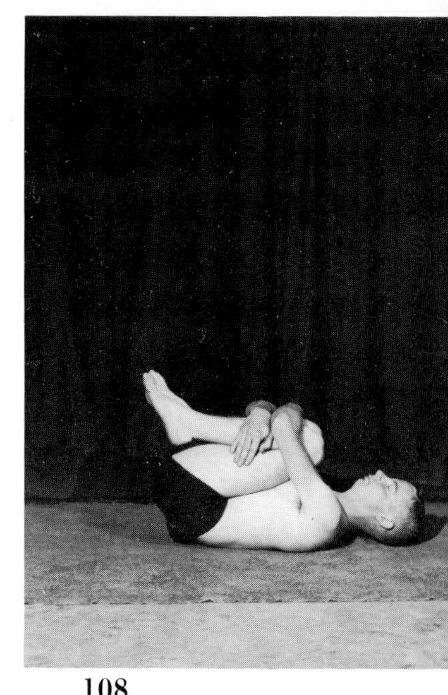

108

111

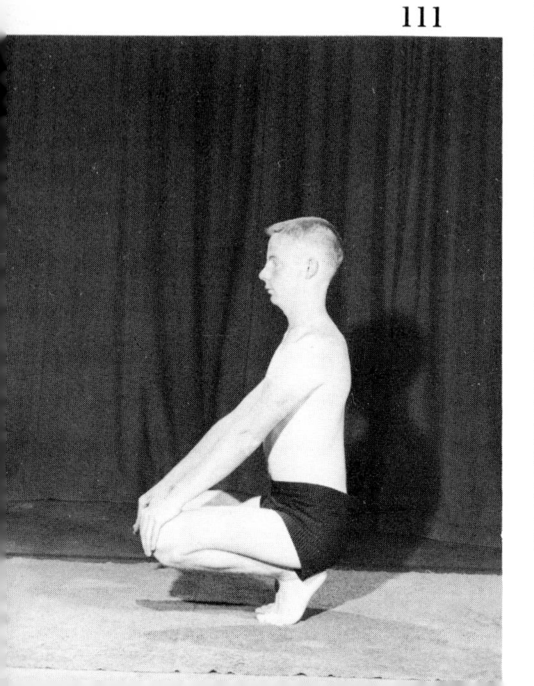

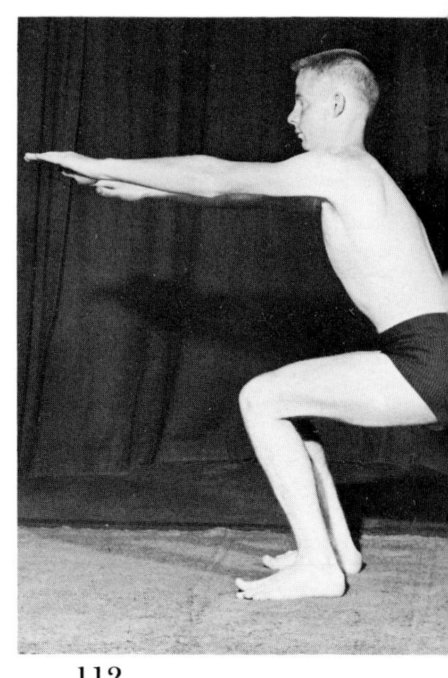

112

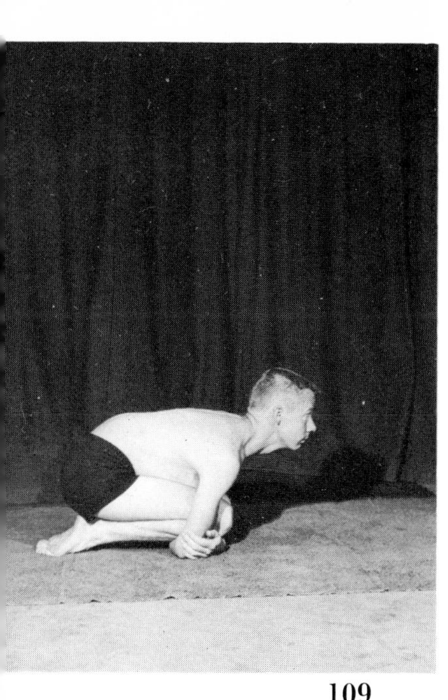

109

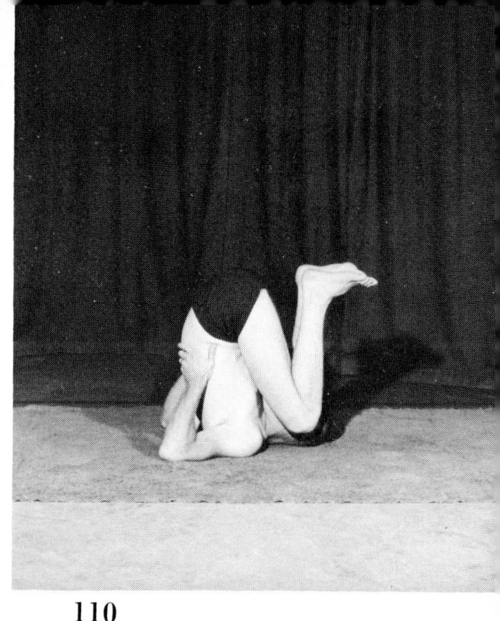

110

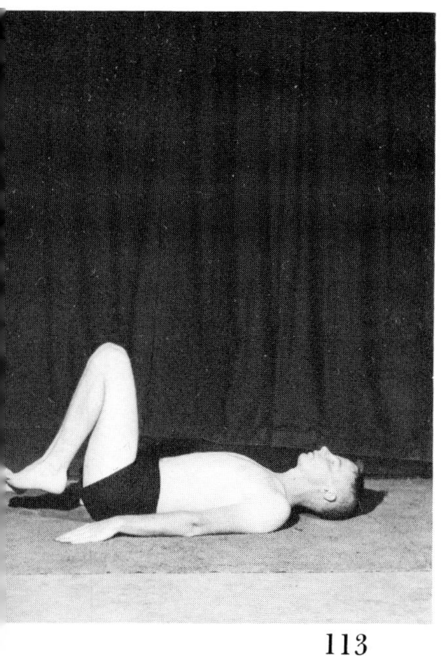

113

114

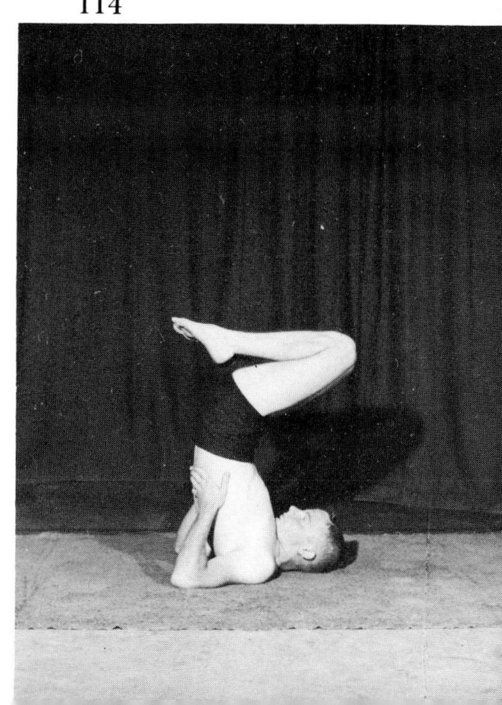

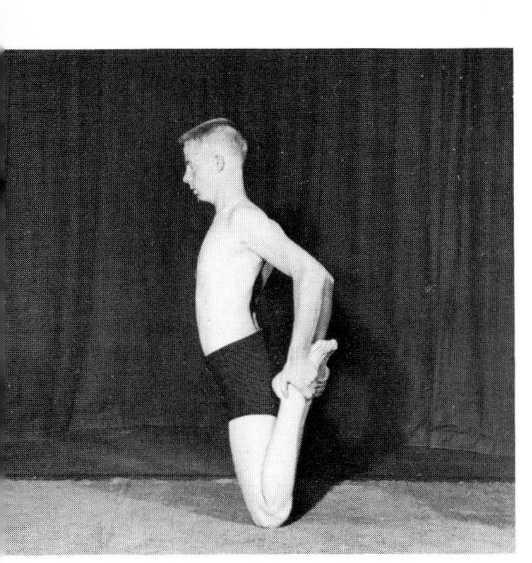

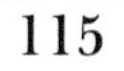

115

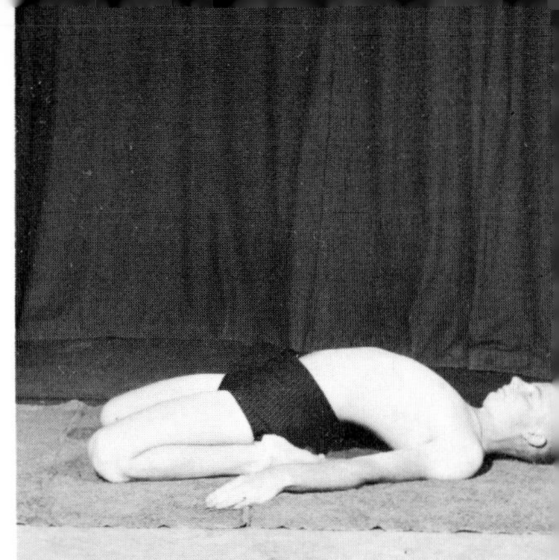

116

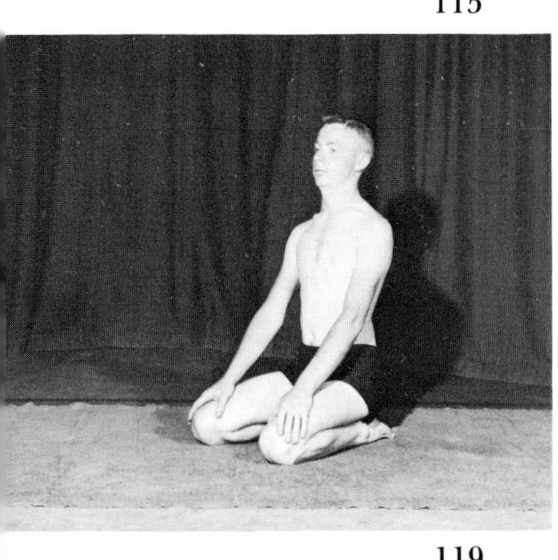

119

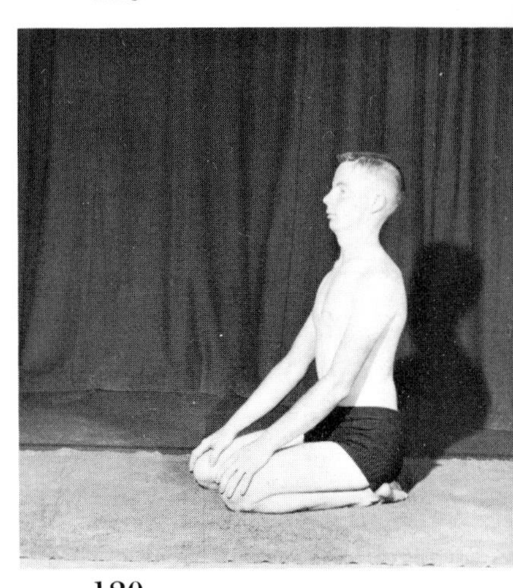

120

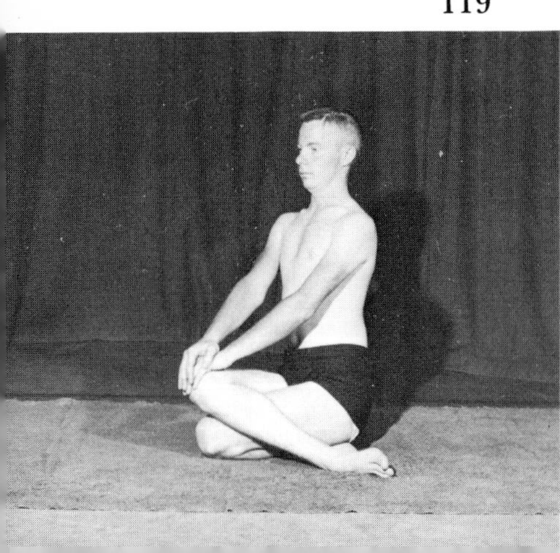

123

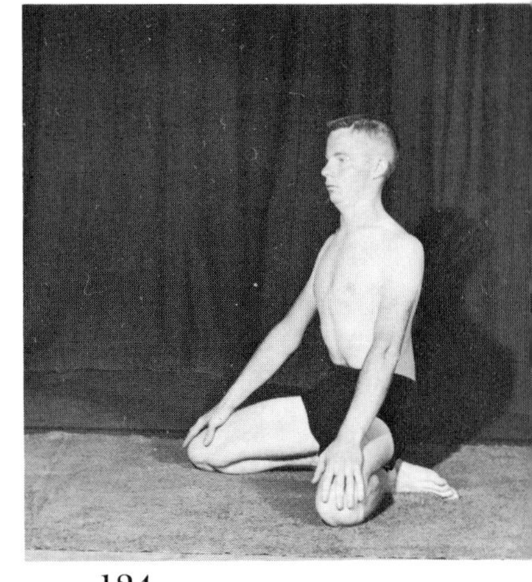

124

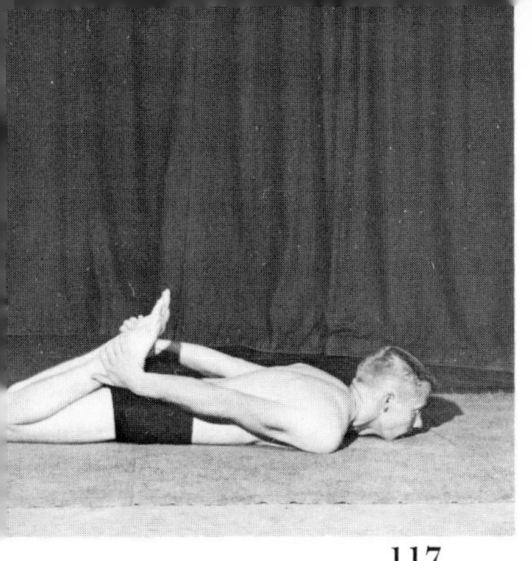
117

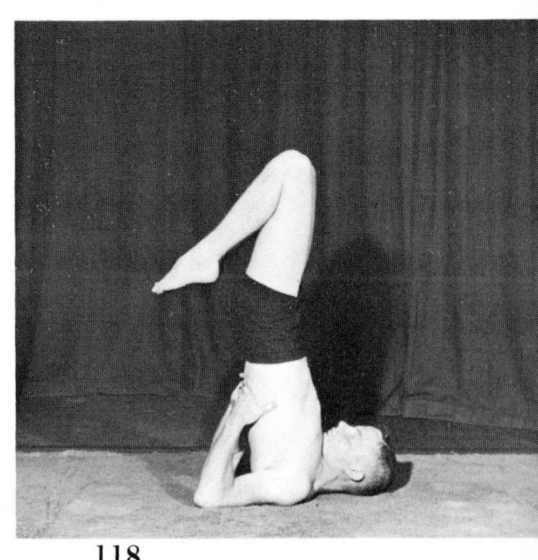
118

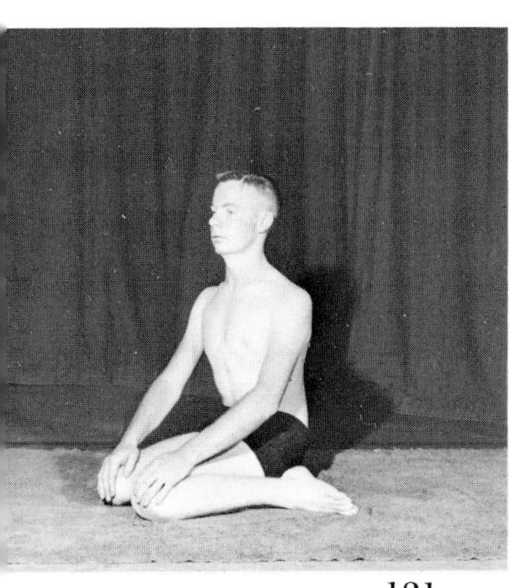
121

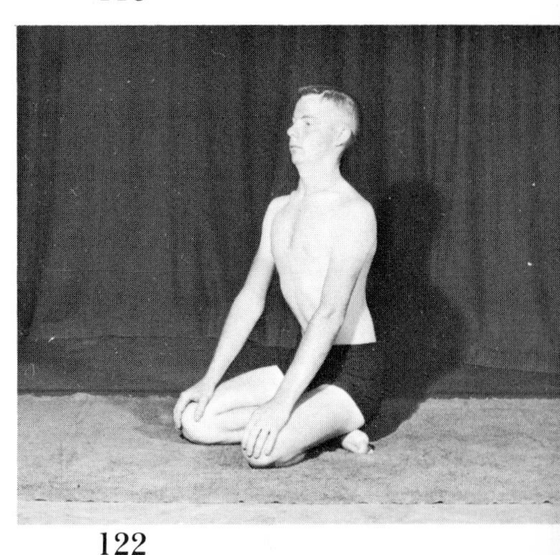
122

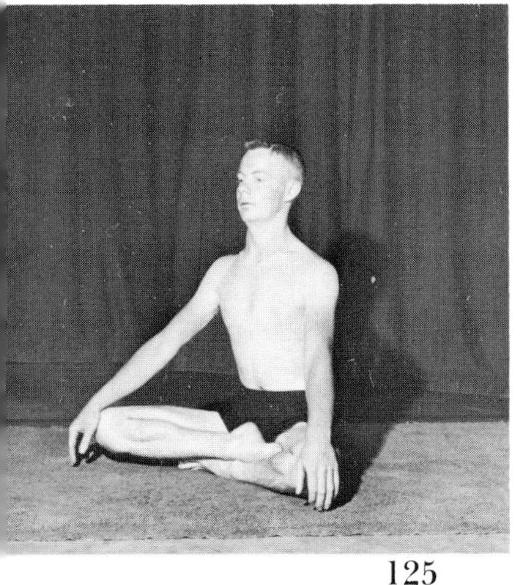
125

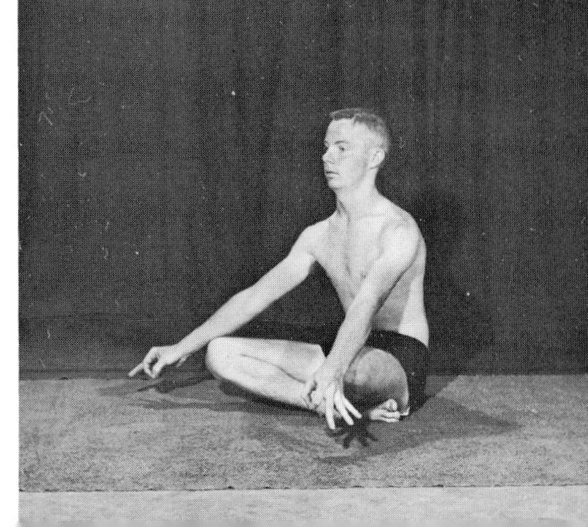
126

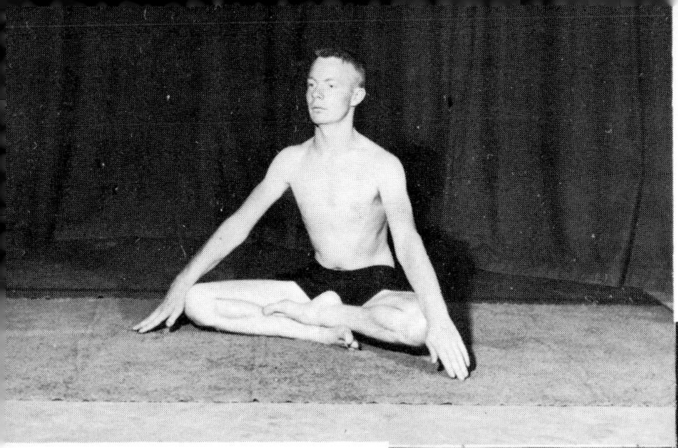

127

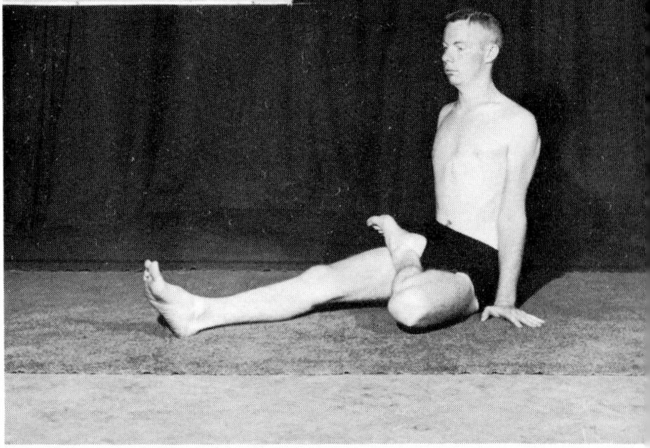

128

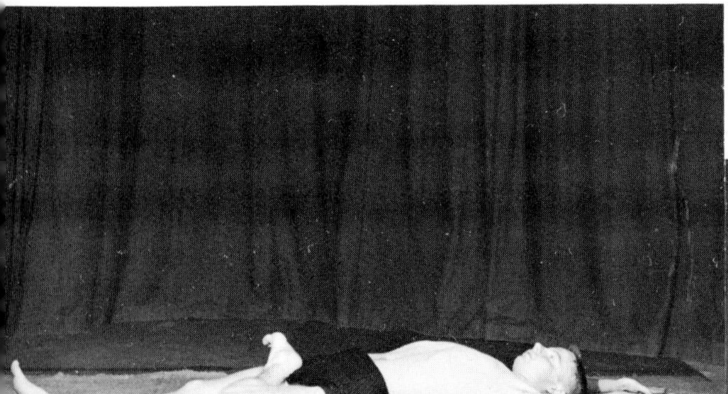

132

131

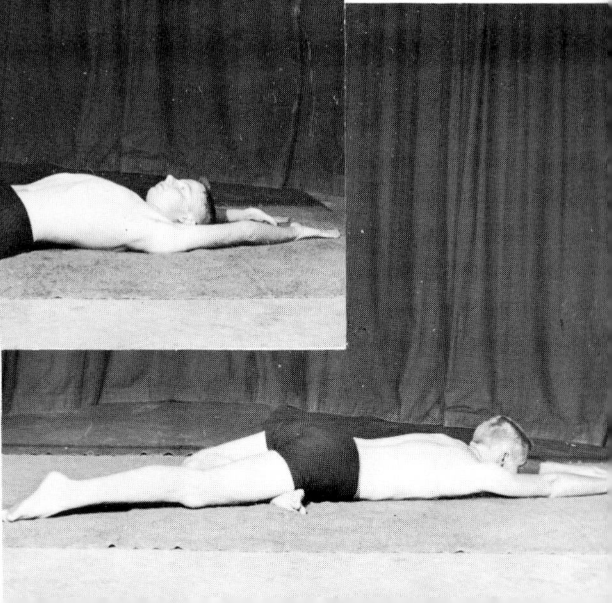

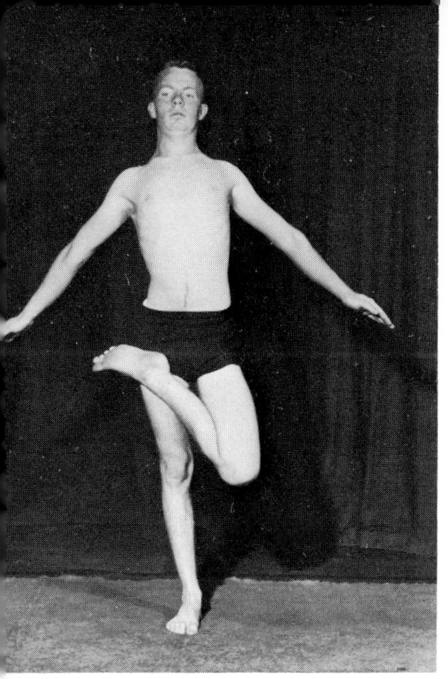

129

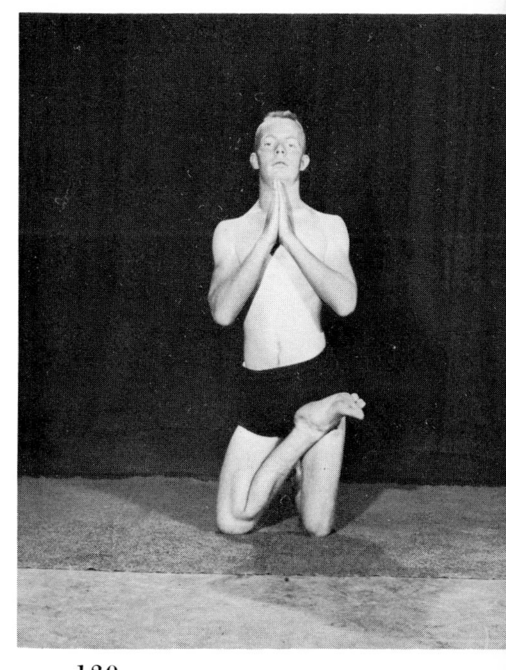

130

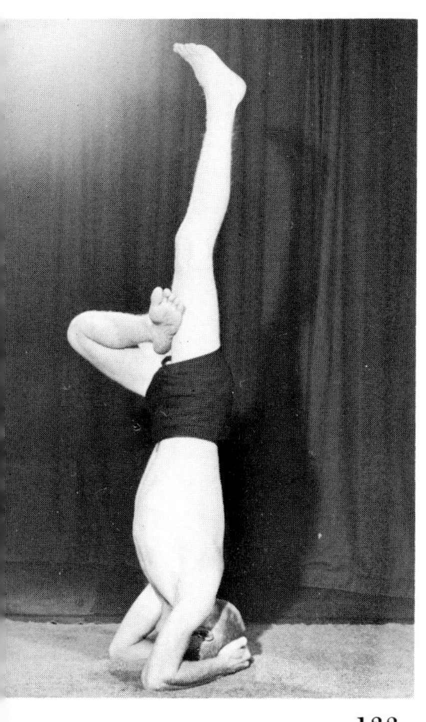

133

134

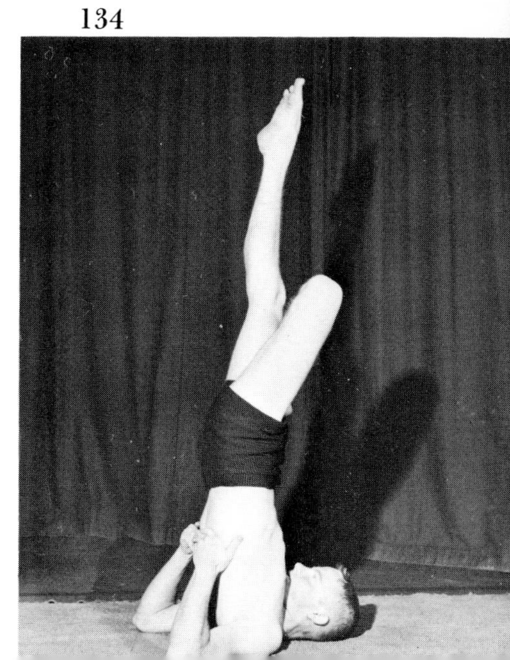

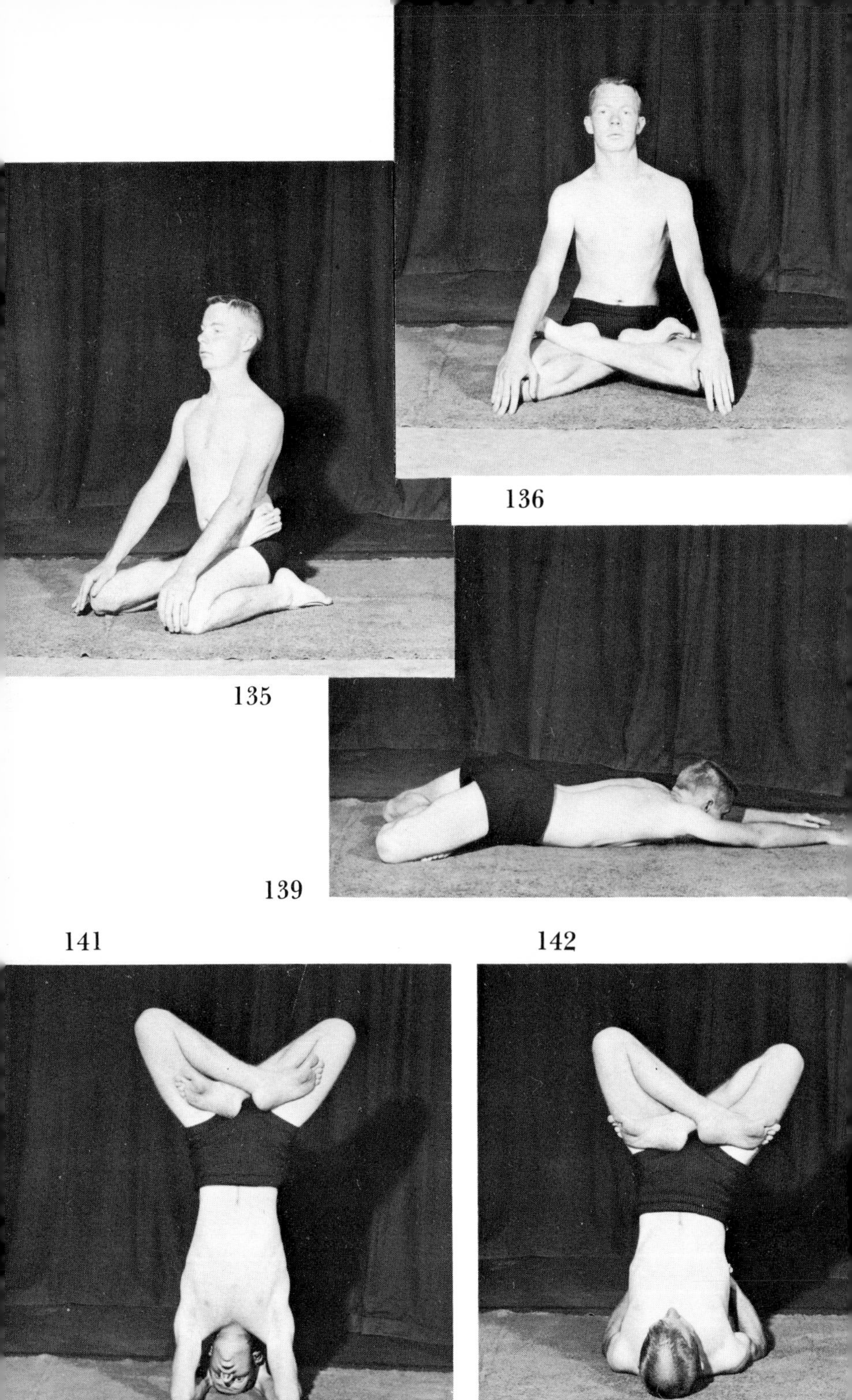

136

135

139

141

142

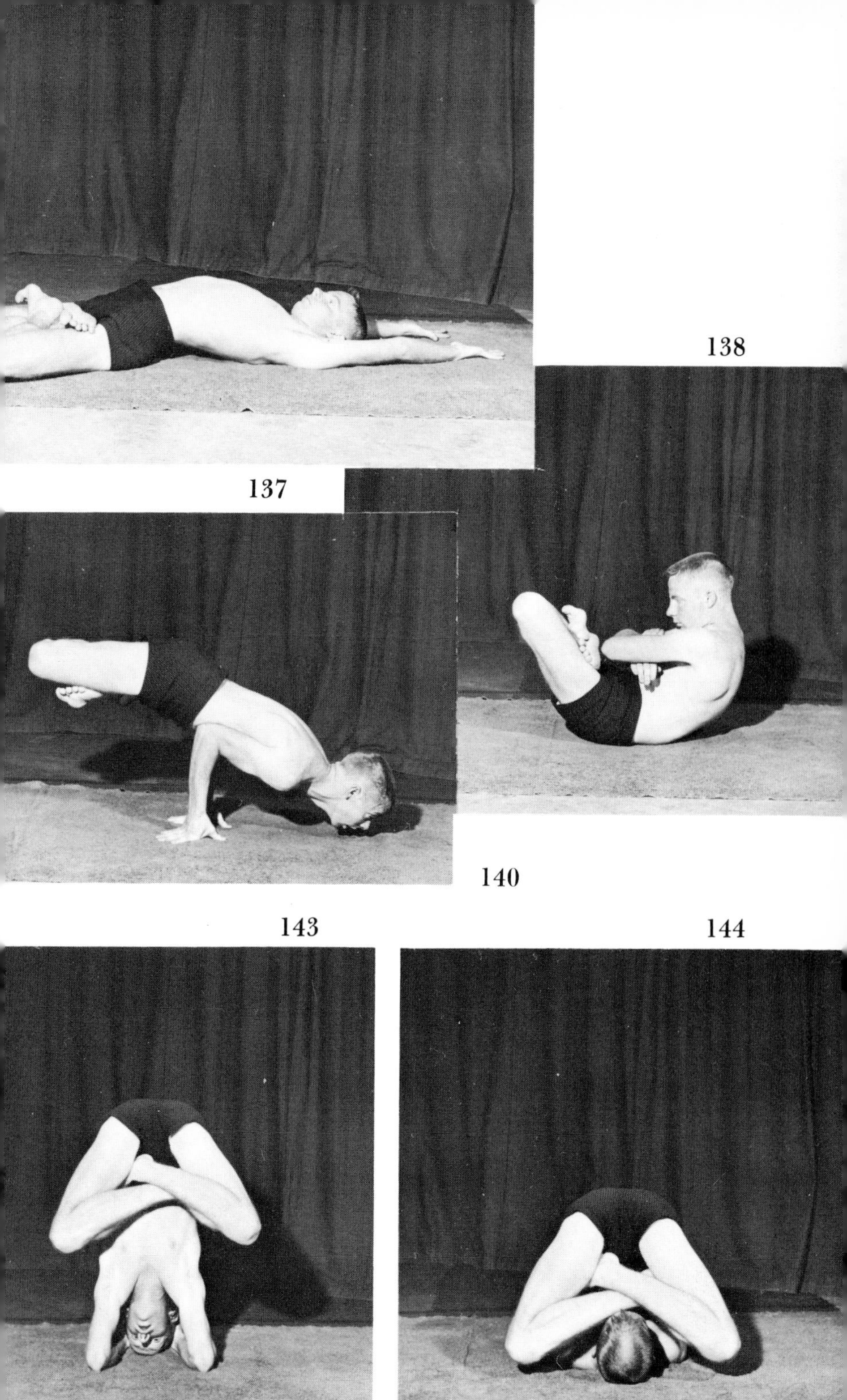

138

137

140

143

144

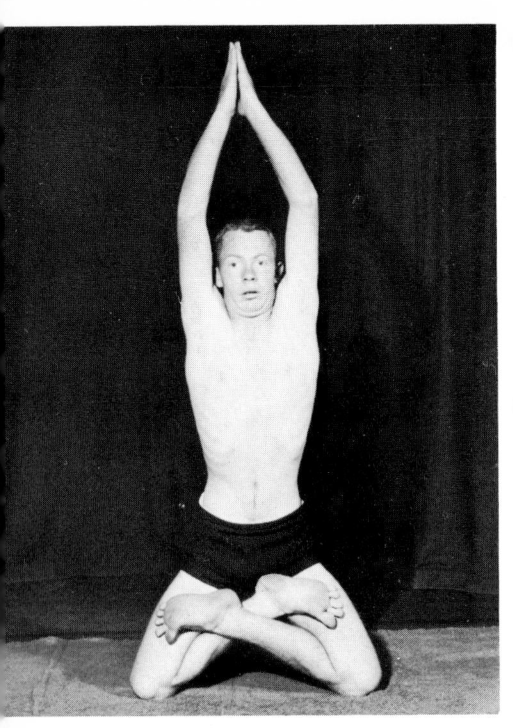

145

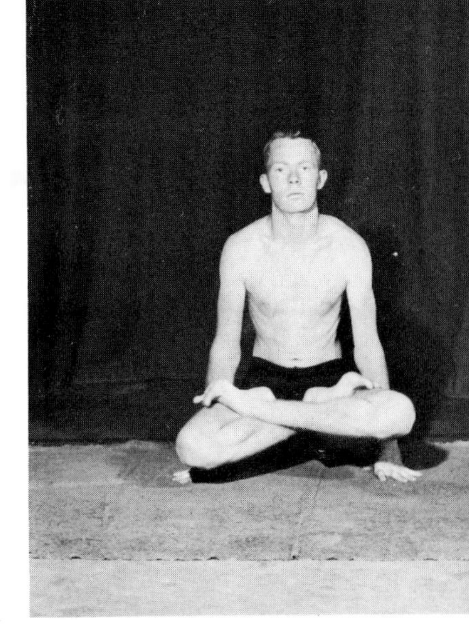

146

148

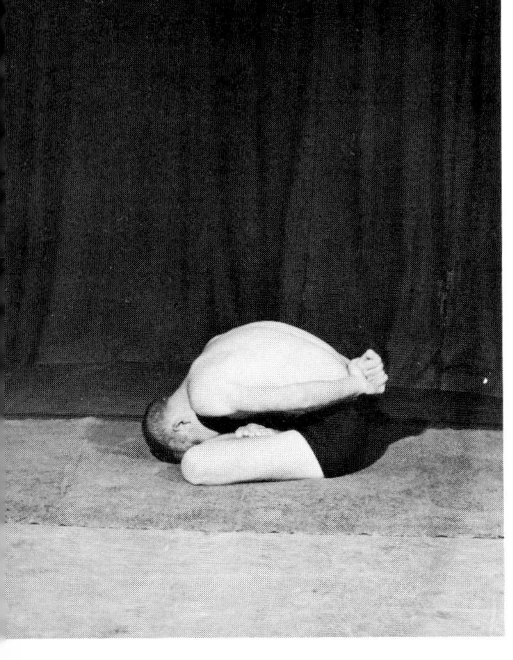

147

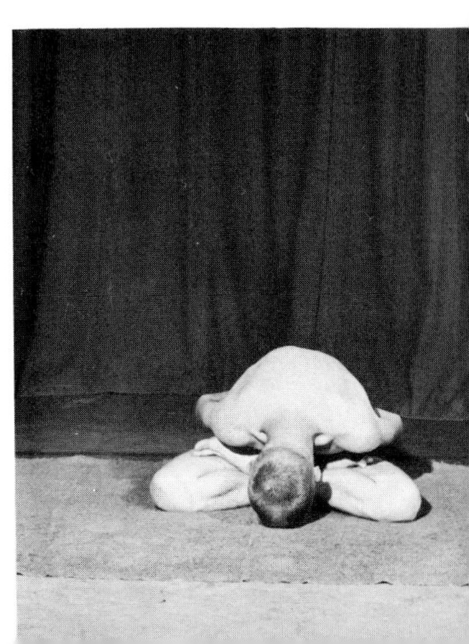

2. The Locust Series

The purpose of the Locust Series is partly the same as that of the Cobra Series, since one must bend his spine in the same direction, beginning from a prone position. As in the Cobra Series, the legs are kept straight. But the two series differ in that the head is raised during the Cobra Series while the feet and legs are raised in the Locust Series. By opposing each other in raising opposite ends of the body, these first two Prone-starting Series of the Front-stretching Postures function in much the same supplementary way as the first two Supine-starting Series of the Back-stretching Postures.

In the first stage of this series, one lies in a prone position (see Plate 5), just as in the preceding series. However, in his preparatory movements, one moves his hands to his sides and keeps his face to the floor. One may place his palms downward, keeping the fingers extended together on the floor, or one may place the backs of his hands on the floor, with his fingers doubled up in a fist. His head remains touching the floor, resting on either his chin or his forehead. Whichever option is adopted should be kept throughout the series.

Our second stage may be approached gradually through substages which everyone should be able to master in some degree. This stage is fully achieved when both legs, kept straight and together, are raised from the ground. No definite distance can be designated. We suggest that this posture has been formally achieved when the legs are held at about a forty-five-degree angle from the floor. (See Plate 75.) It will be noted that this posture is experienced more as a tightening of muscles of the buttocks and lower back than as a stretching of front muscles. Considerable pressure must be brought against the floor by the hands and arms, which are held straight, in order to raise and keep the legs in the air.

Substages consist, respectively, in raising first one leg alone and then the other, without twisting the spine. Considerable practice with these one-legged *(eka-pada)* stages may precede any attempt to raise both legs *(dwa-pada)* together. Since *Salabha,* the Sanskrit term for locust or grasshopper, provides the basis for this posture, *Salabhasana,* and posture series, the term *Ardha-Salabhasana,* or Half-Locust Posture, has come to be applied to the one-legged stages.

Few should expect to attain the final stage in which, ideally, the legs rise to a vertical position, bending the back much farther. Whereas in our second stage both chest and abdomen remain flat on the floor, now the abdomen begins to rise somewhat. Although even greater pressure and strain are needed on the hands, shoulders and back muscles in raising the legs higher, as they approach a vertical position, they tend toward a balanced condition in which some of the strain is relieved. Expert Vishnudevananda, raising even his chest off the floor and resting primarily on his shoulders and chin and arms, poses his legs at about a 135-degree angle from his arms still flat on the floor.

Lowering the legs to the floor again should be smooth and continuous. They ought not be dropped. If breathing has been stopped during the exercise, it should be resumed for a while before trying again. One should gradually coordinate exhaling and inhaling with movements into and out of postures, including this one.

3. The Bow Series

Some confusion, which quite often develops regarding the naming of different but related postures, seems to have become permanently embedded in teaching tradition. The Bow Series appears to us as combining the functions of the two preceding series. That is, it raises both ends of the body at once, rather than first the head and then the feet. In raising both head and feet at the same time, it performs a function of stretching the front even more than either the Cobra Series which raises only the head and trunk or the Locust Series which raises mainly the feet and legs. It does this in just about the same manner in which our Head-and-Feet Series involved more stretching than either the Head-first Series or the Feet-first Series of our Supine-starting Back-stretching Postures. A bow *(dhanura)*, one used for shooting arrows, is bent in a smoothly curved fashion. So *Dhanurasana* simulates this form as nearly as possible. Confusion seems to have arisen from the fact that a person, especially with heavy legs and light trunk, who tries to assume the Locust Posture, will find his head and shoulders forced off the ground somewhat. Hence what seems to us to be properly called the Bow Posture has sometimes been treated as a variety of the Locust Posture.

In our first, or prone relaxation stage (see Plate 6), one makes preparations for a second stage by extending his hands together on the floor in front of him and his legs together on the floor behind him. His body forms a straight line with all parts of the front of his body lying flat on the floor.

Our second stage, and the only one often confused with a variation of the Locust Posture Series, consists in raising both the extended arms and the extended legs up from the ground in a symmetrical manner. (See Plate 58. Also Plate 60.) That is, one tries to raise his arms, head and chest about as far from the floor as he raises his legs, lower and upper. The ideal is to form as smooth a curve as possible. One cannot always know whether his body does depict such a curve, unless he has someone tell him or observes himself in a mirror. But more important than seeing the curve is to feel one's body in such a backward-curved position. People with different weight distributions—heavier calves and feet or heavier busts and shoulders—should expect some problems in attaining evenness of curvature. However, the purpose of this posture is stretching front muscles and massaging the abdomen and spinal column more than attaining a perfect picture. One's weight will rest primarily on the abdomen, though beginners may have to leave much of their chest and hips on the floor in their first attempts.

Again, no definite distance from the floor for hands and feet can be specified for formal perfection. One will raise both as high as he can for purposes of exercise. One may set the angles depicted in the second stage of our Head-and-Feet Series for back stretching as his ideal goal for this front-stretching posture—the two angles together approximating forty-five degrees. One should, if possible, assume this position smoothly, not jerkily, and descend back to a prone position gradually.

Our third stage, which is unmistakably traditional, consists in attaining the bow position by means of bending the knees, raising the lower legs and grabbing hold of them with the hands extended behind the back. (See Plate 59.) One may do this either from a preparatory prone position or after he has raised both shoulders and knees from the floor. The hands are clasped around the ankles, arms are kept straight and knees remain together. The body from head to knees is then bent into a curved bow position, both by tightening the back muscles and by putting pressure on the lower legs as if he were tightening the string of a bow. As such pressure is exerted, the body tends to bend or bow more sharply and the weight of the body rests more fully on the center of the abdomen. If any particular position is held, the sharpness of the bend may be increased by inhaling. Caution again is needed for here one may employ well-developed muscles to force back bending more than is wise. Beginners who have difficulty with this posture may try grasping one leg at a time before attempting the more difficult posture. Extremely supple experts can draw their feet toward the head and place them upon it.

4. The Rocking Bow Series

Although few authors have mentioned rolling about while holding Bow Postures, we suggest that here is an unusually good opportunity for healthy exercise. Traditional yogic postures are essentially stationary positions held with firmness. Although movements are required for going from one posture to another, movements which should be slow as well as graceful, the focus of attention has been primarily upon the position to be held and only secondarily upon movements needed to get into or out of a position. Movement as movement, especially rapid movement, has been outside the concerns of yogic tradition. Efforts have tended more in the direction of slowing down movements rather than in that of rapid movement. Hence the present suggestions regarding a Rocking Bow Series or, perhaps preferably, merely a Rocker Series, may go counter to the main stream of yogic endeavors. Yet it is not without some antecedents, for Sivananda (in *Yoga Asanas,* pages 80, 81) not only suggests that one may move both forward and backward and from side to side but also admonishes us to "Swing, rock and rejoice."

Our Rocker Series, if such it may be called, presupposes attainment of our second stage of the Bow Posture. That is, one should raise both his arms, stretched out in front, and his legs, stretched out behind, at the same time, thus arching his back. (See Plate 60.) He should then move his weight a bit, forward and backward, keeping his back arched stiffly. Then his legs should rise a little higher and his arms descend a bit lower, or vice versa, for he may start his motion in either direction. Persons with different weight distribution may have personal preferences concerning which way to begin. As one rocks back and forth upon his abdomen, he will find he can raise his arms and legs farther from the floor than he can when he holds his body still in the Bow Posture. Neither his arms nor his feet should touch the floor during such rocking motions, although his arms and legs may do so when his rocking becomes extreme. When rocking backward, with his legs closer to the floor, he may raise not only his arms but also his chest and abdomen from the floor. (See Plate 61.) When rocking forward, with his arms closer to the floor, he may find that he can raise not only his hips and abdomen but perhaps even his chest from the floor. (See Plate 62.)

Caution about rocking too far and straining the back or neck may be needed. A person should practice with moderation and feel his way with regard to how much rocking he can do with safety and profit. Such rocking should be especially good for massaging the internal organs and for reducing the fat layer on the abdomen. One may also roll from side to side, and even rock forward and backward on one side and then on the other, if he can maintain his balance in such off-balanced positions.

5. The Peacock Series

With the Peacock Series we meet another dimension in yogic tradition. We come to postures which entail considerable muscular strain. Even though the aim here is not muscle building, it goes beyond the basic interest in stretching and limbering muscles. The spirit of gymnastic prowess begins to invade the scene and, although in line with the purpose of attaining complete self-control, the Peacock Series presents a challenge to muscular power which, though this may not be apparent to frustrated beginners, was not intentionally present in any marked degree in our previous series. We propose that the reader consider this and the following series too advanced for beginners, unless they already happen to have developed gymnastic abilities.

The arms, which have received little attention thus far, now become the most-exercised appendages because the whole weight of the body, as well as the strains involved in keeping the body balanced in all directions, fall upon them. The body is propped up and poised in the air, with the arms used as stilts. It remains in a much more precarious balance than in most postures. Although one may choose from among several options regarding the direction in which his fingers point when his hands are placed on the floor, the orthodox position calls for pointing them backward toward the feet. Whichever direction is chosen, the bent wrists must bear the entire body weight. Ability to bend the hands backward at more than a ninety-degree angle is needed.

We shall depict three preparatory stages in addition to the prone starting position. One may use any one of these, or all three of them, as he sees fit. Considerable initial experimentation may be needed, especially for people with imbalanced weight distribution (long and heavy legs or heavy head and chest).

Our first preparatory stage, and the most traditional, consists in kneeling on the ground with feet, close together, resting on toes, heels up, knees spread apart and hands, with palms flat on floor, between the knees with fingers pointing toward toes. (See Plate 67.) The little fingers should lie side by side and the elbows, held close together, are bent and placed against the abdomen which descends upon them. You are now ready to try to straighten your legs and hold them off the floor.

A second optional preparatory stage may begin from either the prone position or the position just described. Here one props up the middle of his body but leaves both his head and feet on the floor. The legs are extended. (See Plate 68.) If one begins from the prone position, he may first raise the middle part of his body, resting his weight upon forehead and toes, and then place his hands on the floor under him with elbows together touching the abdomen. One may well practice stretching his wrists in this position for some time before trying a more difficult stage. He can experiment with various locations of the elbows so as to attain both a most comfortable and a most closely balanced position.

A third optional preparatory stage or posture, which Sivananda calls *"Hamasana,"* is like the full *Mayurasana* (Peacock Posture) except that the feet remain on the floor, resting on the toes. (See Plate 71.) This too should be an excellent exercising position.

One attains the Peacock Posture itself when he balances his body on his elbows. (See Plate 72.) Although the elbows should be as close together as possible, in practice they tend to be forced apart as the weight of the body presses the chest and abdomen against the upper arms. Ideally, the body forms a horizontal line parallel to the floor. Perfection in this posture is difficult to attain. Legs should be kept straight, and the whole body should appear to approximate a straight line. We arbitrarily designate this as our fourth stage.

A fifth stage involves some genuine front stretching, for here the back is arched a bit and the legs form about a forty-five-degree angle above the horizontal line while the trunk remains relatively horizontal. (See Plate 75.) Although some more strain on the back muscles may be involved, one who can attain this position may find his weight even more balanced than it is in our fourth stage.

A sixth stage, which seems to me to go beyond what is usually meant by the Peacock Pose but which some include as a variation, consists in arching the back still more and extending the legs straight up in the air, in a vertical position, while lowering the head and resting the forehead on the floor. (See Plate 76.) Other variations may be found through bending or folding the legs and through changing the hand positions so that thumbs and fingers go in opposite directions or so that the weight rests entirely upon the knuckles of the hands made into fists.

6. The Crow Posture

Kakasana, the Crow Posture, is another balancing-the-body-on-the-hands exercise which is much easier than the better-known Peacock Posture. Here one puts his hands on the floor, palms downward with fingers forward, and places his knees on the backs of his upper arms and proceeds to balance his weight on his hands. The head faces the floor and the line of the lower legs, which is about level with the head, is horizontal. (See Plate 63.)

7. The Scorpion Series

Vrichikasana, the Scorpion Posture, is another upside-down pose in which the weight is placed upon the elbows, with the forearms and palms of the hands flat on the floor. One faces the floor and arches his back, and balances his legs straight up in the air. (See Plate 64.) Ideally, his legs will be kept straight. But one may arch his back in various ways and even bend his knees so as to touch his head with his toes. One may vary this also by standing on his hands, with arms straightened. This series is similar to the Headstand Series, except that one's head is raised from the floor and all weight is put on the elbows.

B. Supine-starting Series

We turn now to consider ways for stretching the muscles lining the front of the body by examining ways of bending backward beginning from the Most Relaxed Posture in which we lie comfortably on our backs. All of the postures considered here will be called Circle Postures or Wheel Postures *(Chakrasana)* or variations of them. Some of these variations will be related to postures in other series, as will be noted. Some of them will be only semicircular or Half-circle Postures. For convenience, we include here ways of getting into Circle Postures from other starting positions.

1. The Half-circle Series

From our supine position (see Plate 2) we move into a first or preparatory stage in which we bend our knees and draw our feet up close to our buttocks, and bend our elbows and place our hands beside our head, palms flat on the floor with fingers pointed toward our feet. (See Plate 69.) We can test our musculature and ability to begin to rise on all fours. The experience may be disappointing, but this is good exercise anyway. One who has not tried other forms of front-stretching exercises should try them first. The circle series is more acrobatic in spirit than most of the others. Since considerable back-bending is involved, one should try bending his back in easy stages. For example, he may experiment on the edge of his bed, first by letting his head drop over, then his shoulders, and then progressively additional portions of his spine. This should be a gradual adjustment process and not a speedy slide. Older persons will want to test the feelings involved in holding their heads down anyway. Another useful technique is to lie on a pillowed chair, back down, with feet and hands on the floor. One may put pressure against hands and feet and try to stand on all fours while in the chair-resting position. Experience here will enable him to estimate his ability to attain the Half-circle Posture *(Ardha-Chakrasana)* by other methods.

In a second stage, one may raise his hips off the floor and straighten the line of his body from knees to shoulders, leaving his shoulders and head on the floor. (See Plate 70.) In doing this, his lower legs will move from an almost vertical position toward a forty-five-degree angle from the floor, and the angle of his lower legs to his feet will sharpen. If one chooses to raise his heels from the floor and stand on his toes as he moves his knees, he may rest his buttocks on his heels, in this stage.

PICTOGRAPH CHART NO. 5

FRONT-STRETCHING POSTURES

B. Supine-starting Series

1. *The Half-circle Series*

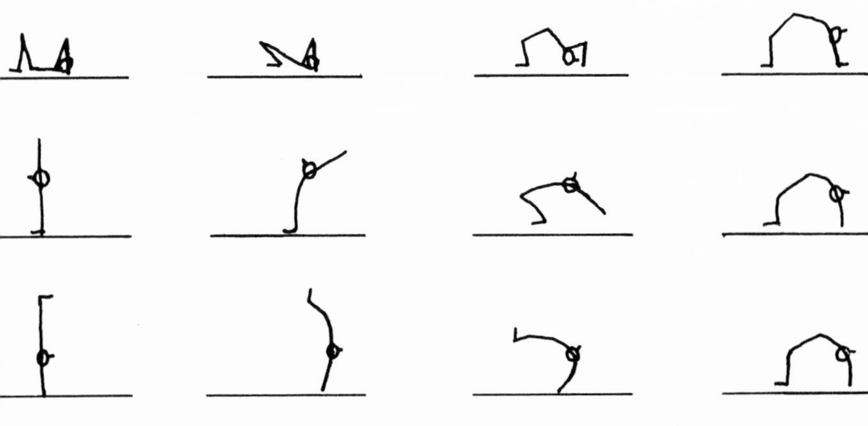

2. *The Full-circle Series*

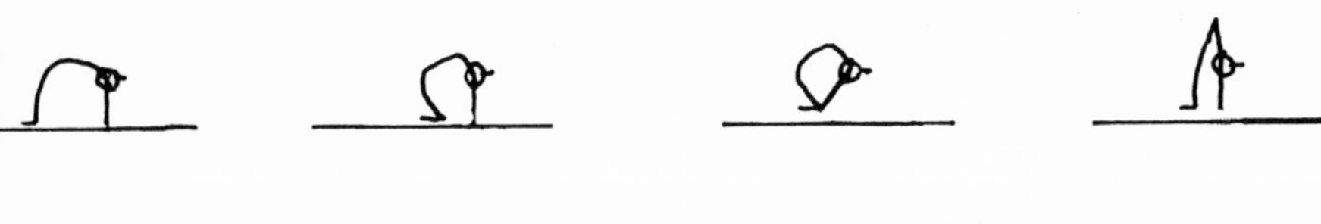

3. *Full-circle Variations*

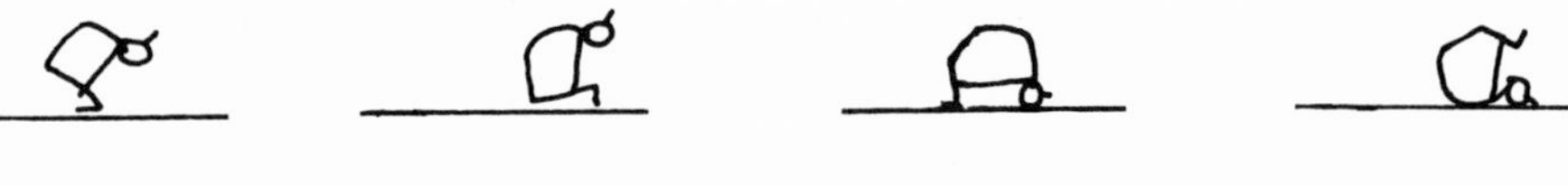

4. *The Kneeling Half-circle Series*

In a third stage, one raises his shoulders off the floor, but leaves his head on the floor. (See Plate 73.) The direction of his nose, which was vertical in the first two stages, begins to turn toward a horizontal direction, and he puts more weight on the top instead of the back of his head as his head turns during this movement. The angles of the legs at the knees are not so sharp and the angle of the body at the hips is sharper.

In a fourth and final stage, one then raises his head off the floor by pressing against the floor with his hands, until his arms become straight. (See Plate 74.) The knees still retain some bend in them but less than previously. One should not remain in this position long, unless he is fully acquainted with his abilities. He should descend gradually and reverse the stages through which he went in attaining the Half-circle Pose.

One may also attain the Half-circle Posture from a standing position. (See Plate 43.) Here one stands erect and then stretches his hands straight above his head in a preparatory gesture. He then bends backward as far as he can, keeping his legs straight, but shifting his weight as needed. (See Plate 77.) Then he bends his knees, bends his lower legs forward, and bends his back and arms as far as he can toward the floor, still holding his weight on his bent legs. (See Plate 78.) Then he drops his hands to the floor, palms down, and assumes the Half-circle Pose. (See Plate 74.) Persons interested in this technique of getting into the Half-circle Pose may experiment by placing their hands on a wall, fingers pointed toward the floor, as they begin their backward bending process. They may try "walking down the wall" on their hands. Done with moderation, this can provide excellent preparatory stretching exercise. As in all back-bending exercises, one should use extreme caution. One may use the above-noted way of getting out of this posture or, if he has the ability, he may rise again to a standing position by bending his legs far forward and placing more of his weight on his feet before he ascends.

Those who already have developed ability as tumblers or acrobats may also enter the Half-circle Posture from a headstand position. We have not previously mentioned the headstand position in which the body is held straight in a vertical position. Yogins have not favored this posture, but the possibility is mentioned here in order to note the formal symmetry in differing ways of bending the body. From the handstand position, one gradually bends his knees, legs and hips backward and lowers his feet to the floor, shifting his weight on his arms as he does so.

Those already skilled in attaining the Half-circle Posture may experiment further by lifting one leg, or one arm, or both one leg and one arm, and holding them in horizontal or vertical positions.

2. The Full-circle Series

Assuming the attainment of the Half-circle Posture, by whatever means, one then progressively bends his back and stretches his front more and more by moving his hands closer to his feet. In the first, or Half-circle, stage, one's lower legs and straightened arms approximate vertical directions. In a second stage, one halves the distance between his hands and his feet, usually by moving his hands closer to his feet. In a third and final stage, one moves his hands all the way to his feet so that they touch his feet. This represents the Full-circle Posture *(Purna-Chakrasana)* in its first form. However, a few extremely supple persons have been able to bend their spine near their hips so far that they approach a hairpin posture with legs straightened and head brought close to the back of the legs. No such position is recommended for business executives—or anyone, for that matter. But we may notice that this represents a formal reversal of the extreme positions observed as possible through the Back-stretching Series considered in Section V.

3. Full-circle Variations

The term *Chakrasana* or Circle Posture applies traditionally not only to what we have described as the Full-circle Posture in its first form—where the hands are kept on the floor, palms down and brought into contact with the feet—but also to modifications of this position. A first and most obvious is one in which the hands are raised from the floor and clasped around the ankles. Arms stay straight.

A second variation, which must be approached from a kneeling position, keeps the lower legs and tops of the feet flat on the floor. The hands clasp the ankles. The arms are held straight. When, from this position, one places his hands on the floor, fingers pointing away from his feet, and bends his feet so that his toes rest on the floor, he attains the Camel Posture *(Ustrasana)* which traditionally has been regarded as a distinct type of pose.

A third variation may be approached, through our third stage of the Half-circle Series, by keeping one's head on the floor and moving one's arms around and grasping the ankles while the feet remain flat on the floor.

A fourth variation has already been noted, and previously depicted, as the third stage of our Bow Series *(Dhanurasana);* and a fifth variation may be attained by moving from this Bow Posture in such a way that the weight is shifted from the abdomen to the chest and head.

4. Kneeling Half-circle Series

This series is usually classified elsewhere because it may be approached also from a sitting position; but since both the function of stretching the front by bending the back and the semicircular form are much the same as those of our Half-circle Series, we choose to emphasize this similarity by including it here. Traditionally, this pose has been called *Supta Vajrasana* or the Sleeping Thunderbolt Posture, and it will be mentioned again later. (See Section IX, A 1 D 2.) *Vajrasana* postures are those in which the lower legs are bent sharply against the upper buttocks, so that the heels are either against the buttocks or placed beside them. Although normally the knees stay together, they may be separated. Although this posture is usually introduced as a seated position, in which one either sits on his heels or sits on the floor with his heels beside his hips, one may also lie down backward from this seated position into a supine or sleeping pose, with the heels still under or beside the hips. One may approach his sleeping pose from either a kneeling, sitting or supine (legs stretched out) position, and we have chosen to call it the Kneeling Half-circle Series to indicate the fact that the lower legs remain on the floor and the knees stay bent throughout the series.

From a supine posture, with legs stretched out, as a first stage (see Plate 1), one may fold his legs under him or place his feet beside his hips on the floor, as a second stage. (See Plate 65.) He may rest in this position, placing his arms at his sides, folding them on the floor behind his back, folding them above his head, overlapping his hands on the floor behind his neck, or putting his palms together in a pointing prayer position on his chest.

The semicircular form appears as one arches his back as much as possible. His weight rests upon his head, with the crown down. (See Plate 66.) When this stage exhibits perfected form, the hands rest upon the front of the thighs and the arms are held straight. This is as far as most persons should expect to go, but for the athletically inclined, a still more extreme possibility is available.

One may place his hands upon his heels and lower his head

and rest it upon the upturned soles of his feet, by arching his back still more. This pose might also be obtained from our second Full-circle Variation or from the Camel Posture by bending the arms at the elbows until the elbows rest on the floor and the head is bent further to rest on the soles of the feet.

C. Standing Series

Arbitrarily we divide front-stretching exercises performed in a standing position into two groups: (1) Those in which one stands, and continues to stand, on two feet while bending backward, which we call Back-Bending Exercises; (2) those in which one stands on only one foot during all or most of the time while bending backward, which we call One-Leg Variations.

1. Back-bending Exercises

Every reader has already tried, and often, to bend backward, at least a little bit. Few escape physical education courses in which backward bends are included in their gymnasium exercises. We have already depicted a standing backward-bend series in illustrating ways to get into the Half-circle Posture and have depicted, at the end of our Full-circle Series, an extreme backward bend which very few will ever attain. We will refer to backward bending again when discussing the *Surya Namaskar* series in Section XII. Here we will mention only the obvious fact that one may use different arm positions—placing his hands on his hips, extending them out to his sides from his shoulders, holding them above his head or moving them in unison with forward and backward movements of his body. It is usual to combine a forward-bending exercise, such as touching the toes, with a backward-bending exercise for maximum benefit. Those who have forgotten how far they can bend or who have neglected backward bending for a long time should be cautioned against too vigorous or violent movements. Simple backward-bending exercises are obviously available for office use, as are the following one-leg variations.

2. ONE-LEG VARIATIONS

A person may stretch his front muscles one part at a time either by bending backward while one leg moves forward or by bending forward while one leg moves backward. In the pictographs depicting these variations, we have neglected to note the erect standing position which should precede each exercise. Restful stance and slow, steady and prolonged breathing promote healthy performance of these exercises. One who regards the depicted poses as a challenge to his ability faces trouble. He is bound to overexercise and is very likely to hurt his back. One who does only the first stage, or even only one of the first stages, in the following series may fully attain the purpose of front stretching, relaxing, and improved breathing and blood circulation. With considerable practice an exerciser may eventually attain the poses depicted in the second column. But those in the third column appear here only as possibilities to think about, perhaps aim at, but not poses which one can expect to achieve. We have omitted a fourth column which only ballet experts might achieve.

We believe that the pictographs will be sufficiently suggestive so that detailed comment seems unnecessary. The poses have been formalized and analogies among them and the other earlier posture series should be obvious. These one-leg variations should not be regarded as standard yogic poses. At least I have not seen them systematized in this way anywhere. But among the Bent-knee Variations (see Plates 79 and 83), which might be elaborated upon in great detail, our second pictograph is illustrated also by Vishnudevananda in his Plate 100, and called *Anjaneyasana* (Leg-split Posture). Our third

PICTOGRAPH CHART NO. 6

FRONT-STRETCHING SERIES
C. Standing Series

1. Back-bending Exercises

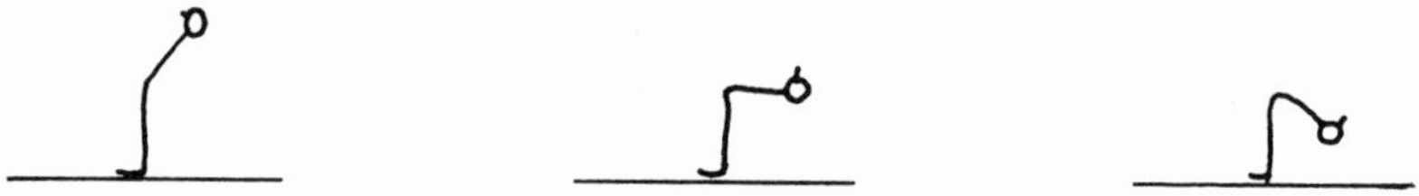

2. One-leg Variations / a. One-leg Forward

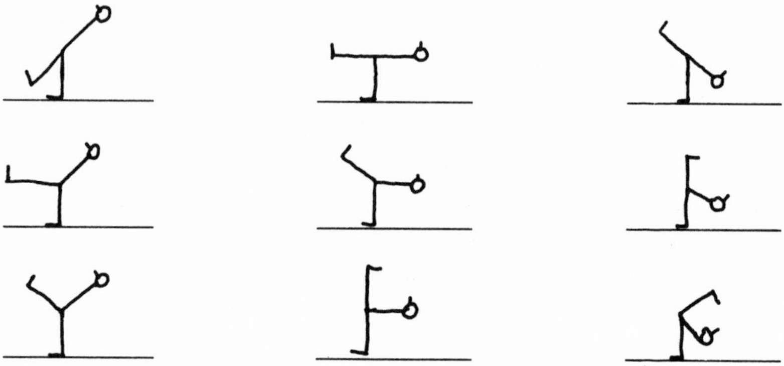

/ b. One-Leg Backward

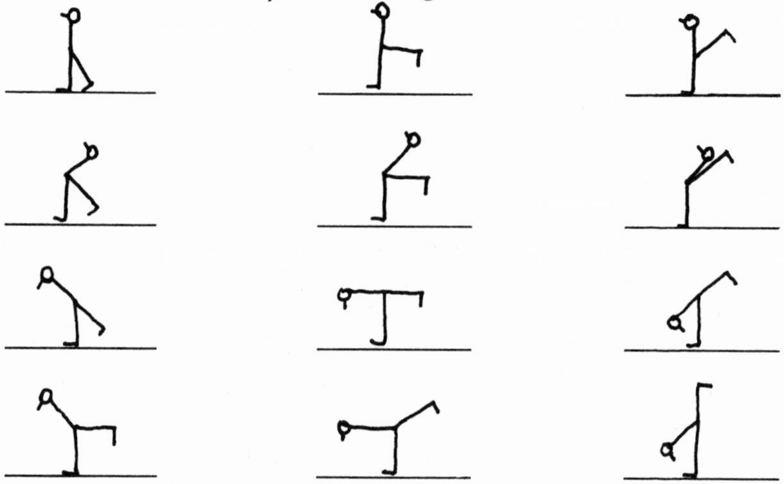

/ c. Bent-knee Variations

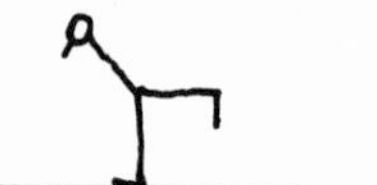

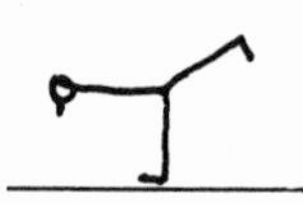

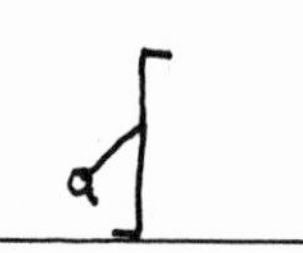

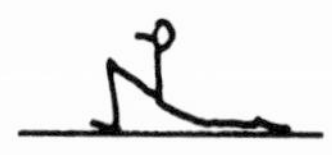

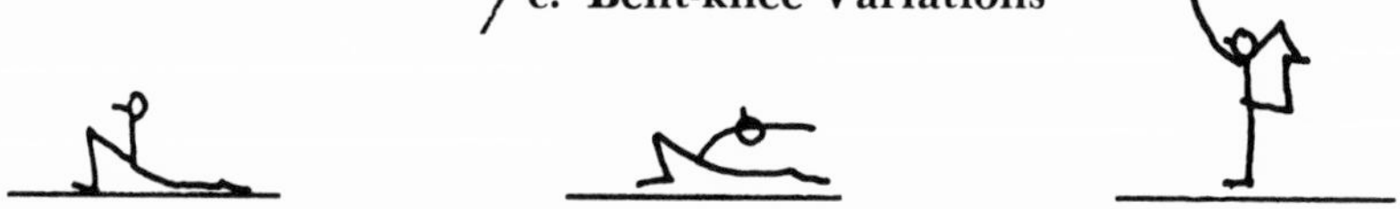

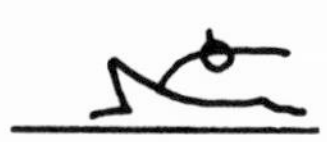

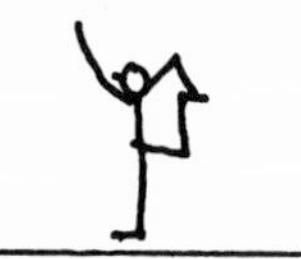

pictograph stylizes the famous traditional *Natarajasana,* or posture made famous by Lord Nataraja (illustrated by Vishnudevananda in his Plate 140); this, it may be observed, is much like a standing one-legged Bow Posture. By changing legs, one will note that he obtains another whole set of One-leg Variations series.

Many of our one-leg variations and one-leg-up series for both front and back stretching series could be duplicated in lying-down positions, either supine or prone. A reader with sufficient imagination can construct such a series for himself. Many of them may be easier and safer to practice, especially since the problems involved in balancing on one foot disappear. However, the standing exercises may be available for office use whereas those in prone or supine positions may work better at home.

VII. SIDE-STRETCHING POSTURES

The human body bends sideways, as well as forward and backward, and stretching the muscles on the sides of the body can be as relaxing as stretching those on the front or back. Of course, since our muscles consist not of single lines but often form broad bands of tissue, many of them spread from side to front and from back to side. Thus our artificial classification of postures must be recognized as one for conceptual convenience rather than one which presumes a knowledge of the multiplicities of muscular tissues in the body. The exercises already discussed have involved some side stretching, and the postures treated here as side stretching may have some forward and backward pulls also. When we bend to the left, the muscles on the right side stretch; when we bend to the right, those on the left stretch. When one moves from side to side in a slow rhythmical motion, breathing deeply as he does, he has more to gain than when he simply assumes a one-sided posture and stops.

Although a person may bend from side to side while lying down, on his side or in prone or supine positions, or even while standing on his head, we will limit our illustrations of postures here to two traditionally recognized types, called *Ardha-Chandrasana* or Half-moon Postures and *Trikonasana* or Triangle Postures. Postures may be held—and might be depicted as—bent in either direction, but depiction of one direction seems sufficient.

A. Half-moon Postures

Stand erect with heels together, arms at sides, abdomen in. (See Plate 80.) After a relaxed breathing period, raise hands above the head, keeping arms straight and close to the head, with thumbs interlocked and palms forward. Bend slowly to one side, keeping arms as straight as possible. Bend as far as you can, keeping heels together. (See Plate 81.) Some recommend also standing on your toes. After months of practice, the amount of bending possible may increase so that your body approaches a semicircle. As you bend farther, you may find it convenient to spread your legs a bit farther to aid in keeping your balance. (See Plate 82.) This posture is one of the most convenient for office use.

B. Triangle Postures

Two distinguishable types of triangle poses have gained traditional recognition. The first is easier and permits, or even requires, the bending of one knee. Yet in another sense it is harder, because here one tries to keep the bend of his body in a single plane and he is expected to reach down farther.

After a resting period, while standing in an erect posture, with feet together and hands at sides (see Plate 80), move one leg and place it on the floor so as to form a triangle with the two legs and the floor constituting its three sides.

PICTOGRAPH CHART NO. 7

SIDE-STRETCHING POSTURES

A. Half-moon Poses

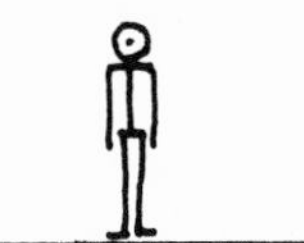

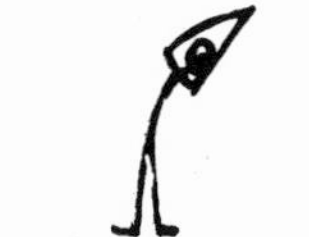

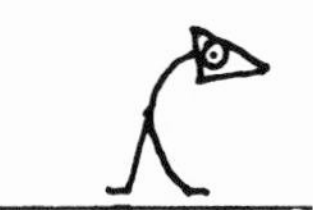

B. Triangle Poses

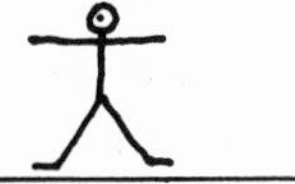

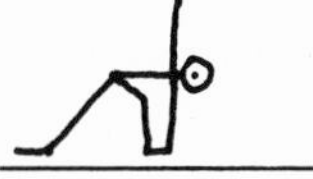

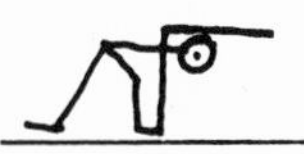

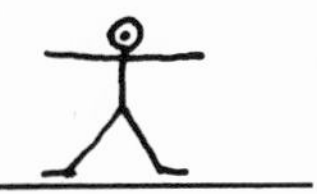

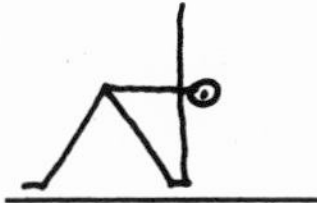

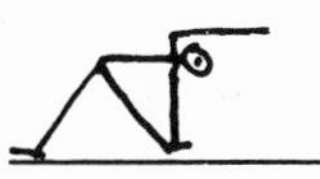

Although no definite angles can be specified, one's legs should be quite far apart and their form may approximate an equilateral triangle. Persons with different body builds and muscular capacities will make suitable adjustments here. The legs should be kept straight. The arms extend straight out from the shoulders. (See Plate 84.)

If one bends toward his right side, he should keep his left leg straight, both feet flat on floor, and bend his right knee enough so that he can touch his toes with his right hand. Arms continue to be held straight. Fingers point up and down. (See Plate 85.) In a final stage, the left side is stretched farther by bending the left arm down over the head into a horizontal position in line with the trunk, while the right fingers remain on the toes of the right foot. (See Plate 86.) Resume a standing position gradually and then repeat by bending toward the left side for symmetrical development.

The second type is exactly like the first except that here one keeps both legs straight throughout the exercise and it becomes necessary to shift the right hip, when bending to the right side, backward a bit. (See Plates 89, 90.) Although one may seek to place his right hand on his toes or even the floor, the formal posture requires only placing the palm on the ankle or the fingertips on the instep. One tries to keep his bent body confined as closely to a plane as possible; but the required shifting of the hip to permit lowering part of the abdomen in front of it makes this a slight forward bend also.

Persons especially interested in this type of exercise may experiment with placing their right hand on their left foot, and then their left hand on their right foot, in both of these types. Whereas in the standard types one's head continues to face forward, in the suggested experiments, it faces backward or toward what was the back of the body in its starting position.

VIII. SPINE-TWISTING POSTURES

Most of us fail to realize two things. The first is how far the spine can twist. It can twist as much as 150 degrees each way, if we include all the bending that can be done from the pelvis to the head, including the neck. The second is how much healthy exercise can come from twisting our spine regularly. We tend to sit, lie, stand and walk straight, as is natural, and the older we get the stiffer our spine twisting apparatus becomes. We even prefer to move our eyes right or left to moving our head right and left. The spine-twisting postures and exercises have been designed to massage and limber spinal muscles and to improve circulation of the blood in spinal areas. Other parts of our body become involved also, but here we have a primary focus of attention and effort.

One need not depend upon traditional yogic postures in order to keep his spine-twisting muscles supple. Yogic tradition emphasizes specific postures in a seated position on the floor, but one may also twist his spine while standing, sitting in a chair or lying down. One of the easiest and most effective ways is to stand erect and turn from side to side with a rhythmic movement. If one holds his arms out from his shoulder, they provide extra inertia which will carry the body around farther more easily than pushing. This exercise can be performed at almost any time when one has a bit of privacy and surely every business executive or professional person can spare a few moments for this exercise; if not in his office, then in the restroom. When sitting in a chair at a desk, or at dinner, or in conversation, one may deliberately turn his body and neck farther than usual and thus exercise himself while at work or otherwise in public. One may twist his body while lying in bed at night, slowly and persistently, and even lie in a twisted position for a while. Those who wish to try twisting exercises on the floor may lie on their backs, raise their legs in the air and wave them from side to side while trying to keep their backs flat on the floor. Since legs are heavy and cause the body to tip, one may bend his legs and roll his knees from side to side. One may precede and follow this exercise with rest in the Most Relaxed Posture.

Our attention will be directed here primarily toward some standardized yogic postures. We may well be amazed at our inability to perform simple turns, an inability we have acquired progressively as we have grown from infancy. Some reattainment of greater ability to turn is possible.

The postures to be considered here will be grouped into three related series, each with a Sanskrit name: (A) *Vakrasana* or Twisting Postures; (B) *Ardha-Matsyendrasana* or Half Spinal-twist Posture; (C) *Matsyendrasana* or (full) Spinal-twist Posture. Now *Matsyendra* does not mean "spinal twist," but happens to be the name of a famous yogin who supposedly originated the teaching of this posture. Most postures, we noted, have descriptive names, and early tradition assigned the names of animals ("cow," "lion," "crow," "peacock," "cobra") or other familiar objects, such as "moon" or "bow." But here we observe a rare exception in which the name of an originator has stuck and become orthodox.

A. Simple Twisting Series

We begin with a series which may be called *Vakrasana* or Twisting Postures. Of course, all of the postures considered in Section VIII are twisting postures, but since the names *Matsyendrasana* and *Ardha-Matsyendrasana* normally apply to the later series, it has become customary to call the simpler series *Vakrasana.*

The natural starting procedure for all of the following poses consists in sitting on the floor with legs stretched out together in front and arms on the floor at one's sides. It is better not to begin twisting immediately, except in minor ways, but to move backward and forward a bit, trying to touch your toes or to extend your fingers beyond them several times, breathing deeply and slowly and developing a relaxed attitude. Give attention to keeping the spine erect, legs flat on the floor, shoulders back, abdomen in, head back and face straight forward.

A first stage, and starting position, of this simple series involves placing the fingers of both hands on the floor at your sides. (See Plate 87.) Fingers should be pointed outward from the body in opposing directions. You may put the palms of your hands flat on the floor, if you can, but your arms should not be kept close to the body and no weight should be placed upon them. The arms should move freely at the shoulders and be bent as much as needed to keep them away from the body. You may discover some problems in trying to take and hold this very simple pose, and may need to practice it for some time before going on if you wish to avoid early frustration. You should reattend to your breathing and to your chest, abdominal and head positions after experimenting with hand and arm adjustments.

A second stage, also seemingly simple, consists in retaining the assumed position except for moving both of your hands from their positions on opposite sides of the body to a position on one side of the body. (See Plate 88.) Fingers should be kept pointing in opposite directions, as before, but now one set of fingers will be pointed in the direction which your legs take and the other set will be pointed rearward. In making this change, you must twist your spine, keeping it as straight as possible, with head and chest up and abdomen in. Do not bend forward to rest on your hands. Some compromises with the ideals expressed here must be made, but one should be able to feel when he is in both a suitably twisted and yet relatively erect position. If the palm of the

PICTOGRAPH CHART NO. 8

SPINE-TWISTING POSTURES

A. Simple Twisting Series

1 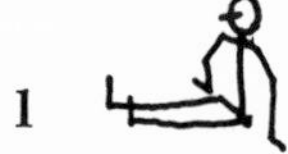

2 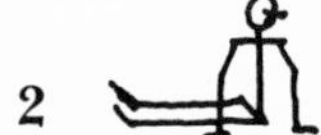

3 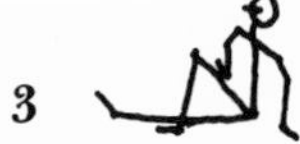

4 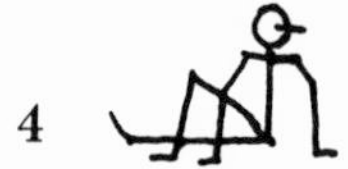

5 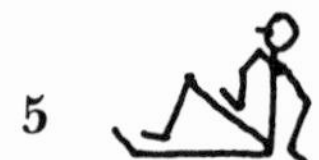

6 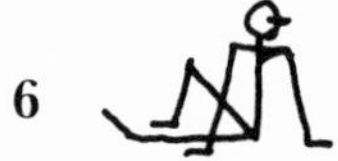

B. Half Spinal-twist Series

1 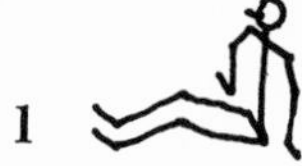

2 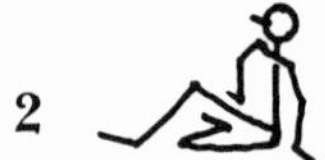

3 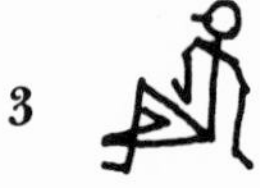

4 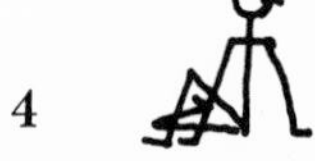

5 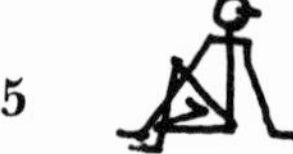

6 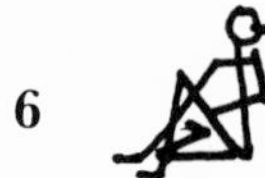

hand near your knee does not spread flat on the floor, or approach a comfortable finger-stretching position, twist your spine farther. After holding this position for a short while, move both hands to a corresponding position on the opposite side of the body, twisting the spine and moving the head accordingly. One's head naturally moves from facing forward to facing sideward in each of these and the following positions. But one should, while holding each twisted position, turn his head frontward again and then backward as far as he can.

After returning to the starting position, you are ready for a third stage. Raise one leg from the floor and move it across the other, bending it by drawing the knee and thigh up to the chest. (See Plate 91.) Place the sole of the foot of the bent leg flat on the floor by the thigh of the straight leg, near its knee.

Then, for a fourth stage, repeat everything in the second stage. If you bend your right leg first, twist your body first toward the left, since this is an easier adjustment to make. (See Plate 92.) Place your hands on the floor as before, palms down and fingers pointing in opposite—forward and backward—directions. (See Pictograph 4.) After bending your head backward as far as possible, then turn your trunk and head to your right side, keeping the right or bent leg in the same position. (See Plate 93.) Now a new problem arises. You will need to put your left arm outside of your right bent leg. Need for drawing in your abdomen and twisting your spine further may develop. You may need to work with this posture for some time before mastering it. But you must master this one if you are to proceed farther in these series. This simple posture provides a real challenge to many. Those with longer arms or shorter trunks may have some advantage here. A big stomach and thick legs are handicaps; facing a challenge here may provide additional incentive for abdomen reduction measures. This fourth stage is not finished until one has straightened his right leg and repeated the whole process again with his left leg bent.

A fifth stage in our simple series is exactly like the third stage except that this time, after returning to the starting position, one does not cross his legs as he bends one of them. Instead, he simply draws his leg up to his chest, keeping the foot of the bent leg on the same side of the other leg as when unbent. (See Plate 94.)

A sixth and final stage is like the fourth except for its foot location and some additional adjustment problems encountered as one swings his trunk and arms from the left side (see Plate 95) around to the right. (See Plate 96.) Before trying it, this may seem a simpler exercise, but it is really much more difficult, as experience will show. When finished with one leg bent, then straighten it and repeat the process with the other leg. Beginners may become so involved in making difficult adjustments that they need a reminder to restore as much as possible an erect, relaxed posture. One may be able to twist himself into some of these positions by bending forward, but for full benefit as a spine-twisting posture, the pose held here should keep the spine itself as straight as possible.

B. Half Spinal-twist Series

The first stage of our second series is like the first in our first series except that it terminates by bending both legs at the knees somewhat (see Plate 97) in preparation for crossing them in such a way that one leg (we begin with the left) may be bent under the right leg.

The second stage consists in bending this leg sharply in such a way that its heel touches the right thigh, hip or buttock, as the case may be with different body builds. (See Plate 98.) Although one may expect to keep both buttocks on the floor, some yogins advocate placing this heel in the perineal region and some sit on it with the right buttock. Individual experimentation to achieve maximum comfort in this posture seems in order. This bent leg remains flat on the floor throughout the series. One places his hands on the floor by his sides, with fingers pointing outward in opposite directions, just as in the first, third and fifth stages of our first series.

Our third stage consists merely in drawing the other, right, partly bent leg into a sharper bend so that its ankle touches the top of the knee of the left leg lying on the floor. The two legs are thus crossed in such a way that the ankle of the right leg crosses the left leg just above its knee. The sole of the right foot is kept flat on the floor throughout the series. Attention to erect posture, abdominal muscle control and breathing should continue.

Our fourth stage, like the second, fourth and sixth stages of preceding series, consists in turning the trunk to the left side and placing both hands on the floor with fingers pointing in opposite directions (forward and backward). (See Plate 100.) Then one turns directly to his right side so that his left arm is placed on the outside, or right side, of his right leg as he puts his hands on the floor. (See Plate 101.) Our pictographs for this series fail to indicate which way the body is turned, so one must take care to follow these directions as stated. One may expect to have to draw in his abdomen as his right leg presses against it, twisting his trunk further, using with caution, some pressure from his left shoulder against his right knee in promoting this twist. His left arm may now become straight; at least it will become and remain so during the next two stages. He may wish to stretch his spine further at his neck by turning his head backward as far as possible. One who has attained this stage may have gone far enough. But we will depict two more traditionally recognized stages and then discuss some variations.

Our fifth stage is like the fourth except that the left hand is moved from the floor beside his right leg to the toes of his right leg; or, if he cannot reach them immediately, first to the knee of his left leg, then to the ankle, and finally to the toes, of his right leg. (See Plate 102.) More Pressure from the right leg against the abdomen, more twisting of the spine and some adjustment of the hips may be expected. If the left knee tends to rise from the floor, especially as one grasps it during the first movement of his left hand, he must exert renewed effort to keep it on the floor. This effort should not consist in more willful strain but in a more willing resignation and relaxation of strained muscles. Again attention should be given to straightening the spine and neck, so far as is possible under the circumstances. The right hand remains on the floor during this stage, and its fingers and those of the left continue to point in opposing directions, except insofar as the fingers of the right hand become involved in grasping.

Our final stage is like the fifth except that here the right hand is raised from the floor and stretched behind the back as far as it can reach. (See Plate 102.) A slimmer person may reach farther than a fatter one. Formally one is expected to reach his left hip. Some reach far enough to grasp the top of the left thigh. Extreme contortionists can reach as far as the ankle of the right leg, which is drawn beside the left hip while the fingers of the left hand grasp the left knee. We will not depict these variations here. We should mention, of course, that the whole series should be repeated, beginning with the right leg which is then bent under the left.

C. Full Spinal-twist Posture

Without depicting or illustrating what is commonly regarded as the Full Spinal-twist Posture *(Matsyendrasana)*, which seems to go far beyond a full spinal twist by adding a leg-twisting feature, we merely note that this posture is like the last one except that the leg lying on the floor (the left one) should have its foot placed above the right thigh rather than on the floor next to or under the right buttock. In this case, the heel of the left foot is pressed deeply into the abdomen when the right leg presses against it and the abdomen as the posture develops. The variations previously noted are possible and one should also bend his head as far as possible, breathe as he can, relax as much as possible, hold the posture for a short while, and return gradually to his starting position and to a supine resting position if he is judicious. This posture series too should be repeated, reversing the positions of the two legs and the directions of spinal twisting.

IX. APPENDAGE-LIMBERING POSTURES

We turn now from exercises which aim at stretching the muscles of the full length of the body, whether of back or front or sides, or of those which control the turning of the trunk on its spinal axis, to exercises paying more specific attention to the appendages of the body. These include the legs, arms, neck and jaws, and additional portions of these such as toes and fingers, ankles and wrists, and even the tongue and eyes. We will not devote a separate section to each of these appendages and parts, but group them all together in a section entitled Appendage-limbering Postures. We arbitrarily divide the present section into four subsections entitled Leg Exercises, Arm Exercises, Jaw and Tongue Exercises, and Eye Exercises. The legs will receive the greatest amount of attention.

A. Leg Exercises

There are two basic ways in which legs can be stretched, in addition to trying to pull them lengthwise, a possibility which seems to have attained no traditional sanction. These two ways are: (1) by bending the legs at the knees (without twisting them); (2) by twisting them clockwise or counterclockwise (without bending them at the knees). Most traditional exercises both bend and twist at the same time. Twisting may be done with the legs straight, half bent or fully bent, either one leg at a time or both at the same time, and in standing, sitting, lying or upside-down positions.

When all of the possibilities of combinations and variations of these factors are considered, the number of distinguishable postures pertaining to leg bending and twisting alone is enormous. Only a few of these have retained prominence as types especially worthy of teaching. Some doubtless have gained continued attention because they exhibit striking attainments and may be held up as ideals toward which to strive. The emphasis among them upon floor-seated postures stems both from the fact that Indians traditionally did not, and today for the most part do not, sit in chairs and from the fact that traditional yogic posture exercises have aimed at preparation for meditation and thus attainment of formally approved and desirable meditation postures.

Our treatment of these postures will be somewhat schematic, systematized according to the possible ways of bending and twisting just mentioned. First we will consider some simple knee-bending postures and their simple variations and then some leg-twisting postures with their variations.

1. Knee-bending Postures

Six sets of postures will be depicted. More such postures exist, but only some of them will be mentioned. We will refer to them as set A, set B, etc., and to posture 1, posture 2, etc., in each set.

Set A consists of a very simple one-leg knee-bend exercise, known as *Pavanmuktasana* or Wind-freeing Posture because it may be used to release gas from the intestines. This posture

PICTOGRAPH CHART NO. 9

APPENDAGE-LIMBERING POSTURES

1. Knee-bending Postures

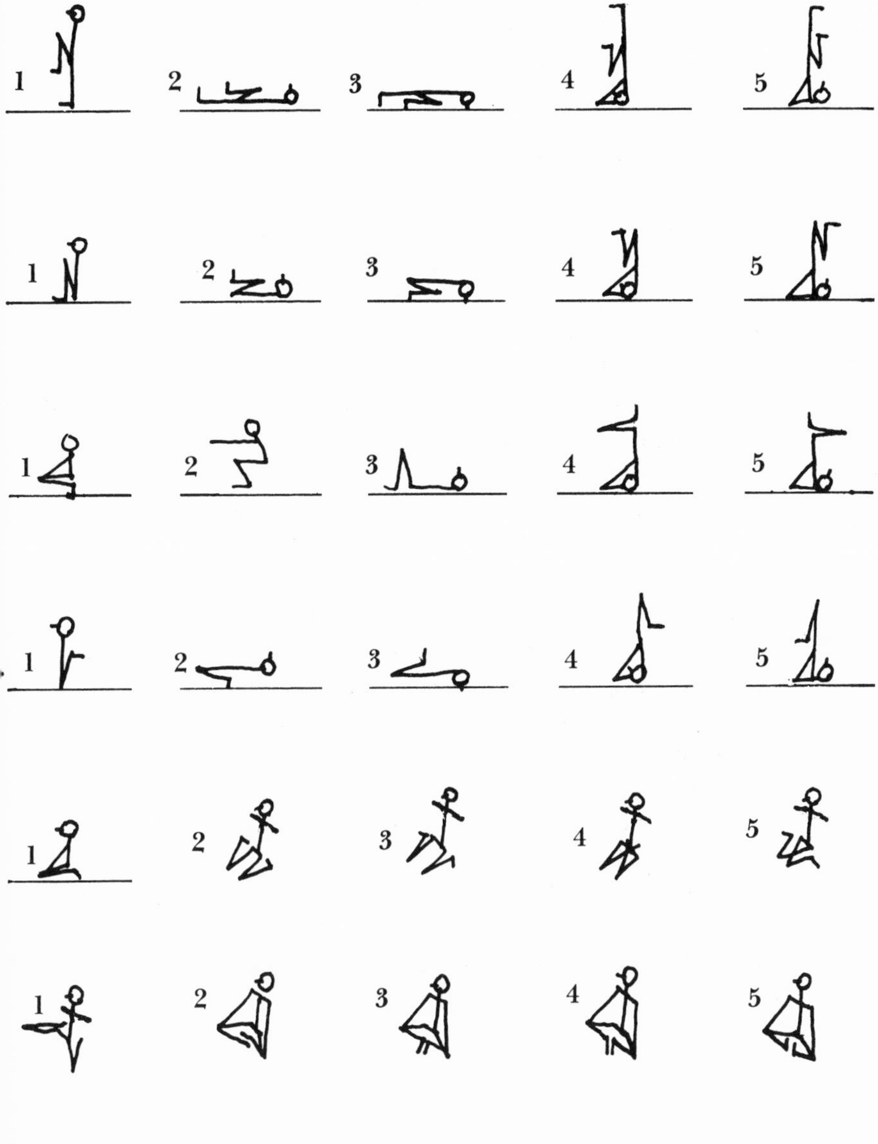

1 2 3 4 5

1 2 3 4 5

1 2 3 4 5

1 2 3 4 5

1 2 3 4 5

1 2 3 4 5

may take the form of standing on one leg *(eka-pada)* and drawing the other leg, bent at the knee, as tightly as possible against the body. (See Plate 103.) Traditionally this pose is free-standing, but one may put the foot of his bent leg upon a desk, table or windowsill to provide both pressure and stability.

More commonly, however, this posture is held in a supine position, in which one moves from the Most Relaxed Posture *(Savasana)* into this Wind-relieving Posture *(Eka-pada Pavan-mukta-asana).* One grasps his bent leg at the knee with both hands, which may be folded, and pulls it to and against his abdomen and chest. (See Plate 104.) He may exhale while increasing the pressure. He should then return the bent leg to a straight position and rest. Repeat the process with the other leg. Then bend and hug both legs. (See next set.) One author recommends that each pressure last from five to ten seconds, and that four repetitions of the three processes (one leg, the other leg, both legs) are sufficient. The reader will wish to experiment for himself.

One may, if he chooses, try this one-legged pose in a prone position (see Plate 105), though he can hardly do so comfortably unless he lies on a very soft bed. In this position, he can use the weight of his body for pressure, and he may use his arms to balance or adjust his weight. One may also assume a one-leg bent posture from either a headstand or a shoulder-stand position. (See Plate 106). Gravitational changes upon the intestines and colon and their contents may produce effects, however. In each of these one-knee bending postures, use of the other knee of course generates another such set.

Set B consists in postures in which both knees are bent as far as possible and drawn to the chest. The term *Pavanmuktasana* may apply here also, although some postures in this set may have other names also. Our first posture in this set depicts an upright position; but since one cannot stand upright with two bent legs, he must sit on the floor with his spine and neck straight and his feet flat on the floor. (See Plate 107.) He may hug both legs tightly to him, or he may tie a broad strip of cloth or a broad belt around his knees and back and free his hands and arms from pressure. This suggestion by Sivananda (*Yoga Asanas,* page 40) is the only exception which I can recall of using an instrument of any sort in aiding the holding of a posture. When the lower legs are crossed, with feet facing in opposite directions rather than forward, parallel and together, this becomes a form of *Sukhasana* or the Easy Pose, which we have yet to discuss.

One may vary this both-legs-pressed-to-the-chest form by holding it in a supine position (also called *Pavanmuktasana*) (see Plate 108), in a prone position (which some mistakenly consider a variation of *Yoga Mudra*) (see Plate 109, in a headstand position, or in a shoulderstand position. (See Plate 110.) When posture 3 is modified so that the arms, which may be hugging the knees or clasped behind the back or resting on the floor at one's sides, are stretched out on the floor in front with hands together and palms down, it becomes *Ardha-Kurmasana* or the Half-Tortoise Posture. If one elevates his bent legs by putting his hands flat on the floor, his lower arms in a vertical position, and his knees on the backs of his upper arms near the armpits, keeping his lower legs, shoulders and head in a straight horizontal line, he attains *Kakasana,* the Crow Posture. These variations of posture 3 are not depicted here. For depictions of the latter see Section VI, A, 6.

Set C is like set B except that here the sharply bent legs are held at ninety-degree angles from the trunk instead of being drawn tightly to and parallel with the trunk. If one begins this set with an upright position, he finds himself either standing on his toes (see Plate 111) or squatting on his heels. When standing on his toes (and here is a posture in which the toes are appendages receiving much stretching), one may find himself excessively devoted to keeping himself balanced. This posture has been called *Utkatasana* or the Difficult (or Hazardous) Posture. The hands rest on the knees in this seated position. Approaching it, as depicted in our posture 2, by lowering the body into it gradually from a standing position, keeping the spine and neck straight and the feet flat on the floor as long as possible, will also be found difficult. (See Plate 112.) This approach may also be called *Utkatasana.* The feet are kept together in both of these postures. One may keep his hands on his hips or extend them in front of him to aid in balancing when descending.

When one squats on his heels, with his heels on the floor, this posture is much easier, at least for most Orientals. I was surprised, early in my stay in Burma, to find Saw Tha U, our cook, sitting on the kitchen stool by squatting on his heels. He explained apologetically that he was more comfortable that way. Without chairs from time immemorial, most Orientals have adjusted themselves to sitting on their feet flat on the floor. This position is both very comfortable and very stable, once you get used to it, and very convenient since you carry your seat with you wherever you go. But when I tried it, I could not do it. When my heels reach the floor, I tip over backward. Western culture has made me incompetent at this point. Yogic efforts may make possible regaining a lost advantage But yogic tradition tends to assume Oriental abilities in this respect and hence no special foot-stretching exercises for this purpose have become traditional.

Set C, as we depict it, includes a very easy supine posture, in which one draws his heels to his buttocks (see Plate 113), a headstand posture and a shoulderstand posture. (See Plate 114.) No prone pose seems possible. One may also hold all of these postures with only one leg bent and the other straight, and of course change legs. Approaching the squatting position from a standing position, keeping one leg straight in front of him, is an excellent knee-bending exercise. One may vary *Utkatasana,* the Difficult Pose, involving balancing himself on the toes of both feet, by assuming a still more difficult balancing pose, called *Padangushtanasana,* in which he balances himself on the toes of only one leg while the other foot rests upon the knee of that same leg. This involves a twisting of the other leg, so perhaps we are getting ahead of our story.

Set D consists of postures in which the upper legs remain in a straight line with the trunk and head while the lower legs are so sharply bent that the heels press against the buttocks. Our upright posture 1 is normally preceded by posture 1 of set E (see Plate 119), which is called *Vajrasana,* "a high and mighty" pose, and translated either as the Thunderbolt Posture or the Adamantine Posture. *Vajrasana* has many variations which will be noted. In a simple *Vajrasana,* one sits on his heels, as in *Utkatasana* or posture 1 of set C, except that now his lower legs are flat on the floor as are the tops of his insteps and toes. In order to attain posture 1 of our present set D, one needs to raise himself up on his knees by bringing his upper legs into a straight line with his trunk which continues to be held in an upright or perpendicular position. (See Plate 115.) One should be sure that his rug or pad is sufficiently soft to prevent injury to the knees in this movement. One may practice by holding onto a table or desk at first, but ordinarily this posture should be attained without instrumental assistance. Although one may use his arms in any way he chooses to attain and maintain balance, formally in this posture the arms are extended directly above the head, also in a straight line with the trunk and upper legs. This is like, and may be considered a variation of, *Parvatasana,* the Mountain Posture, yet to be considered. (See Plate 145.)

Posture 2 of set D, *Supta Vajrasana* or the Sleeping (or

Supine) Thunderbolt Posture, consists in lying on one's back in a supine position with his legs bent under him. His feet then lie, soles upward, beside his hips. (See Plate 116.) Variations in foot positions and their relations to the hips are possible. Normally one enters this position from an upright or seated *Vajrasana* by bending backward. He may use his elbows to ease his descent. The back may be highly arched at first, though less highly as one becomes accustomed to the position. Various arm positions may accompany this pose. One may rest his head on his arms crossed at the wrists. One may straighten his arms and place his hands on his thighs. One may fold his arms on the floor behind his back. Or one may place his palms together on his chest in a prayer position. (See previous reference to this posture in Section VI, B, 4, posture 2 of our Kneeling Half-circle Series.) Because of its relation to *Savasana,* the Most Relaxed Posture, this posture is sometimes called *Ardha-Savasana* or the Half- (or Semi-) Supine Posture.

Postures 3, 4 and 5 of set D are depicted as holding a similar bent-leg form. Posture 3 involves a prone position in which the hands may be used to press the heels against the buttocks (see Plate 117) or against the floor beside the hips. Some consider this a variation of *Dhanurasana,* the Bow Posture. Posture 4 consists in a headstand position (noted previously in our Bent-leg Headstand Series) which may be called *Sirsha-Vajrasana* or the Headstand-Thunderbolt Posture. Posture 5 consists in a shoulderstand position (see Plate 118) which may be called *Sarvanga-Vajrasana* or the Shoulderstand-Thunderbolt Posture, though these names have not become popular. We will not depict or discuss another similar set of postures in which only one leg is bent while the other is kept straight. Ways of getting into some of these will be different.

Set E begins with the Thunderbolt Posture *(Vajrasana)*

which we have already started to discuss. In it one sits on his ankles which rest on the floor, as do the tops of his instep and toes. (See Plate 119.) Knees are kept together. Spine and head should be held erect and arms kept straight with hands resting on the knees. This is a simple position which most persons can hold, even if not for very long. However, yogins hold this position for a long time comfortably. Like the Easiest Posture and the Prone Posture, it serves as a starting point for several other postures, some of which we have just examined above and some of which will be considered immediately. A person may vary the position of his feet in this posture by twisting them so that both lie on the floor with their toes pointed out toward the sides of the body or with their toes pointed toward each other (see Plate 120) ; one's weight pressing against the ankles or heels promotes such twisting. Or one may spread his feet apart and sit on the floor with his feet, insteps down, beside his hips.

Two other prominent variations of *Vajrasana* constitute our postures 2 and 3 of set E. In each, one spreads his feet apart and sits on the floor, keeping his hands on his knees and his arms straight. In the first of these two, his ankles twist so the toes of the feet turn toward each other behind the buttocks. In the second, the ankles twist in the opposite direction and point away from each other. (See Plate 121.) Beginners should not hold these positions long. Variations include sitting on one leg only, while the other buttock rests on the floor with the other leg beside it.

We now turn to two somewhat different but related postures. The first of these, posture 4, is like *Vajrasana* except that the legs cross at the ankles and the top heel presses into the perineum. (See Plate 122.) I find no commonly accepted Sanskrit name for this pose, but one author calls it a "Crossed Posture" and suggests also crossing the wrists behind the hips so that the fingertips of the right hand touch the toes of the right foot and the tops of the left fingers touch the toes of the left foot; with chest out and shoulders back. Those having long arms may place the palm of the right hand on the sole of the right foot, and the left palm on the left sole. Other hand positions apparently are optional. One may vary this posture also by turning his feet on their sides while the ankles remain crossed.

The second of these, posture 5, involves crossing the legs at the knees instead of the ankles. (Plate 123.) In order to do this, a person will first sit on the floor and then proceed, in either of two ways, to cross his legs in such a way that one knee will be directly above the other and the right foot will lie, sole up, beside his left hip, and his left foot, sole up, beside his right hip. In one manner of proceeding, as in our Simple Spine-twisting Series, stages 1 and 3, both legs stretch in front, flat on the floor, and then one leg is bent and placed over the other; instead of placing it flat on the floor, however, it is drawn toward the hip, assisted, if necessary, by both hands which in this posture are placed, palms downward, on the knees. Then the other leg is bent and drawn toward the other hip. In the other method of proceeding, as in our Half Spinal-twist Series, stages 1, 2 and 3, both legs are bent slightly at the knees so that one leg may be slipped under the other and its foot drawn to the hip while the other leg is moved over the first and its foot is drawn to the hip.

No matter which way one proceeds, he attains a posture in which he sits erect, head up, arms straight, with hands folded above or in front of the top knee, with one knee on the floor and the other knee directly above it, and with both heels pressed against the sides of the legs. Persons with broad hips and thin legs may even be able to sit on their heels, as a variation of this posture. One will try this pose twice, starting with a different leg each time. The name of the posture seems somewhat uncertain. Some call it *Samkatasana,* meaning the Contracted Posture, indicating, I suspect, that the legs and knees are snuggled or pressed closely together rather than being parallel or, as in the following set, spread out. But since so many postures involve contractions, this hardly seems specifically descriptive. Some have preferred another possible translation of *Samkata* as "dangerous" and have called this the Dangerous Posture, although it seems no more so than many others.

The postures of this set may be combined with the arm exercises we have yet to discuss for producing variations of *Gomukhasana,* the Cow-faced Posture.

Set F consists also of seated postures in which the legs are bent at the knees as sharply as possible, but here in all cases the knees become spread apart as far as possible (see Plate 124) rather than kept close together as in the four preceding sets.

Posture 1, *Mandukasana* (The Frog Posture), is like a variation of *Vajrasana,* the Thunderbolt Posture, in which one sits with his buttocks on the floor and his feet beside his hips with his heels up. However, he spreads his legs as far as possible, so that the knees point in opposite directions. The form of the opposing legs and hips may approach a straight line and one can even try to sit on his heels in this position. Arms should be held straight, with one hand clasping or hooked over each knee.

Posture 2 is like posture 1 except that now the feet lie on the floor in front of the trunk instead of behind it. (See Plate 125.) It is also like *Samasana,* the Symmetrical Pose (see Section IX, A, 2, 2), except that here both feet lie on their sides on the floor rather than one above the other or with ankles crossed, and the hands stay on the knees with fingers folded over them. It may appear to be like *Siddhasana,* the Adept's Pose (see *ibid.*), but in *Siddhasana* one heel is pressed against the perineum whereas here the heels remain free from pressure.

Posture 3 is like posture 2 except that now the soles of the feet are placed together, touching each other from heels to toes. If the knees do not touch the floor, one may need to put some pressure upon them with the palms of his hands or readjust the position of his pelvis and abdomen. If one draws his heels close to the body so that they touch the groin, this posture is then called *Bhadrasana* (the Gentle [or Auspicious] Posture). If one then moves his body forward and sits on his heels, the posture is called *Gorakshasana,* the Cowherd (or Goatherd) Posture.

Posture 4 presupposes posture 3 and is too difficult for most persons to try. It consists in keeping the soles of the feet together while the heels are raised into a vertical position with the toes on the floor. One will need to grasp his ankles and draw his heels toward his abdomen and twist his ankles. This posture goes beyond mere leg bending and involves both leg and ankle twisting. Posture 5, *Khandapitasana,* or the Crippled (or Clubfoot) Posture, continues the ankle-twisting process in the same direction by raising the body and moving it forward so as to sit above the feet; the toes remain fixed on the floor while the heels bend forward. These postures can hardly be of any significant use to business executives that I can see, but they do illustrate the extent to which knee-bending and ankle-twisting exercises can go. (See Vishnudevananda, Plates 118 and 119.) Those zealous enough to try these postures may experiment first with one foot at a time.

2. Leg-twisting Postures

Although some leg twisting has been involved already in the preceding sets of postures, the primary emphasis has been upon knee bending. Now we come to some sets where leg twisting is primary and knee bending secondary, even though the knees may be bent also. By leg twisting we mean turning the legs clockwise or counterclockwise. Such turning may occur when the legs remain straight, but little attention seems to have been given traditionally to twisting straight legs. One can twist both legs in the same direction and then both in the opposite direction, or he can twist them in opposite directions so that the toes of the feet both turn toward each other and then away from each other. Children often play at walking sideways, either by standing alternately on both sets of toes and both heels and moving the heels and toes alternately in the same direction, or by standing on the toes of one foot and the heel of the other and moving the heel of the first foot and the toes of the other foot in the same direction. This little game can be played in the office, if anyone happens to care to do it, and it may serve as a little yoga.

Ankle twisting has already received some attention, even if incidentally, in the two preceding sets and some extreme emphasis in the last two postures. In the following sets we will be concerned with twisting both the upper and lower legs.

Twisting of an upper leg may best be visualized and experienced when the knee bends at a right angle and then the lower leg turns ninety degrees. One might do this in either direction, but counterclockwise movements of the right leg and clockwise movements of the left leg appear to have been largely neglected. Some leg twisting occurred in posture E, 3 above, but mainly in the lower legs and ankles. Most traditional postures—and all of our immediately following descriptions and pictographs—pertain to twisting the upper legs in such a way that the lower legs turn toward each other or in such a way that the upper right leg turns clockwise and the upper left leg turns counterclockwise.

Twisting the lower legs may also take both clockwise and counterclockwise directions, and they may be turned in both the same or different directions at one time. The lower part of a leg may be twisted in a direction opposite to the twist in the upper part of that same leg. However, traditional composite postures tend to twist upper and lower parts of each leg in the same direction. *Virasana,* the Hero Posture, may be an exception.

We have selected and arranged twenty-five postures, many of which have variations, in a somewhat systematic order for serial treatment. Although we cannot say that these postures constitute a single series, some serial development will be noted. All of them either lead up to or derive from *Padmasana,* the Lotus Posture, which plays a central role in yogic tradition. The attempt to organize these postures into four sets of five each results in somewhat arbitrary groupings, though it serves the purpose of pictorial convenience. Decision to treat some postures as distinct and others as variations is partly arbitrary and partly a product of differing interpretations which have developed among hatha yoga teachers. We shall designate our twenty-five pictographs by number. Our first ten postures may all be regarded as preparatory to the Lotus Posture, though each may have its own independent merits and variations also.

Posture 1. We begin this set with *Sukhasana,* the Easy Posture, one so easy that everyone can do it without practice. This traditionally recognized seated posture should not be confused with the Supine Posture *(Savasana)* which we have called the Easiest Posture. Yogins who adopt other seated positions do not often return to this posture for rest. Yogins usually regard this posture as too easy and recommend it only for beginners or old people. Perhaps the most striking characteristic of this posture, when compared with other seated postures, is that the knees remain off the floor. (See Plate 126.) Most seated postures require that the knees be kept on the floor. The reasons for this requirement are at least twofold: One can attain a more stable position when his knees stay down, a virtue needed for success in meditation. One's abdomen more naturally remains in and under mus-

APPENDAGE-LIMBERING POSTURES

2. *Leg-twisting Postures*

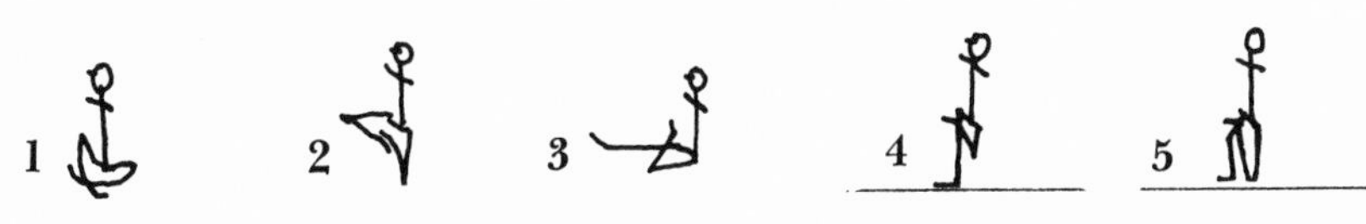

6 7 8 9 10

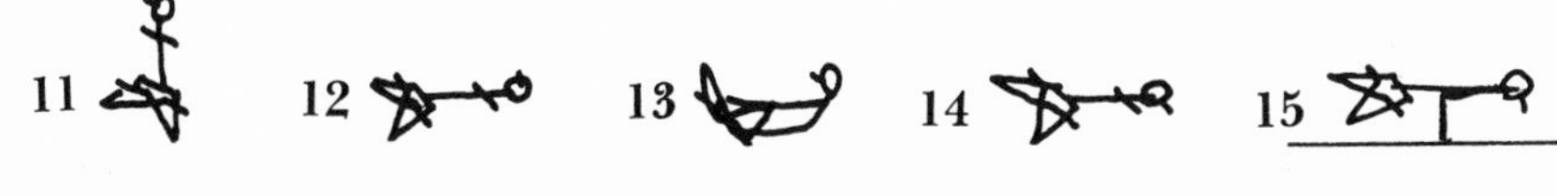

16 17 18 19 20

21 22 23 24 25

cular pressure when the knees stretch down. Also, more stretching takes place when the knees are down. So *Sukhasana,* while easy in the sense that it requires a minimum of effort and bending, may provide few of the effects desired from yogic postures.

Sukhasana consists in sitting comfortably on the floor (traditionally Hindus did not use chairs), with legs bent, drawn up toward the body and crossed at the ankles. The feet then rest on the floor with their outer sides down and with the calves resting on their upper sides. Almost no twisting of the legs is felt. The feet may be moved farther apart or closer together, or farther from or closer to the seat, in order to attain a most comfortable position. Different leg and body proportions will cause some variety of form in different people. The back and neck should be erect. Many options regarding hand positions exist, and these will be considered more fully in connection with meditation postures.

Sivananda suggests one variation of *Sukhasana* for older people or those who, for any reason, have difficulty in holding themselves together stably without assistance. As already mentioned, one may use a broad band or belt, tied around his knees and back, to bind himself together. In this case, the knees will be raised higher and press against the abdomen and the feet will tend to rest on their heels or soles and point in opposite directions. One may then sit in this condition for long periods of meditation.

Posture 2. For pictographic convenience we here group together traditional postures having five distinct names. Sometimes they are regarded as distinct postures and sometimes as identical. They are: *Samasana, Siddhasana, Muktasana, Guptasana* and *Svastikasana.*

Samasana, the Symmetrical (or Equal) Posture, appears to be the next easiest of leg-twisting postures. One lower leg, usually the left, lies flat on the floor, instep down, with its heel placed at the beginning of the right thigh near the crotch, while the other or right lower leg rests on the first, instep down, with its heel near the beginning of the left thigh. Difficulties which a novice should expect here will be those involved in getting and keeping his knees on the floor, maintaining his balance (since he may encounter a tendency to tip in the direction of his right knee) and relaxing. So long as one remains tense, not merely nervously but muscularly, he can hardly expect to succeed. Attention to drawing in his abdomen and straightening his spine may be needed and should prove helpful in adjusting leg positions.

Siddhasana, the Adept's Posture, was so called because *Siddhas,* or ancient yogins who had attained mastery over their bodies, commonly used this position, apparently. Since they had completed attainment, they came to be called "perfected yogins," and hence this is sometimes called the Perfect (or Perfected) Posture. It is like *Samasana* except that one heel is placed at the anus instead of being closer to the thigh. The other heel lies in front of it, touching the pubic bone. This has also been called *Muktasana,* the Free (or Freed) Posture, again presumably a name indicating the attainment of freedom from bodily disturbances by successful yogins.

Guptasana, the Hidden Posture, is like *Siddhasana* except that one heel is placed in front of the pubic bone and the other directly above it, with the toes of the top foot inserted between the calf and thigh of the other leg.

Svastikasana, the Prosperous Posture, is like *Siddhasana* and *Guptasana* except that the toes of both feet are inserted between calves and thighs. This involves stretching and bending the toes of the lower foot so that they will reach upward and lie partly on top of the other calf.

Posture 3. *Ardha-Padmasana,* the Half-Lotus Posture, is a general name for some partial approaches to the Lotus Posture. The Lotus Posture is the best known of all yogic postures to people otherwise unfamiliar with yoga, partly because so many Buddhist, Jain and Hindu statues depict figures seated in it. However, an important ambiguity in the use of the term *Padmasana* or Lotus Posture needs to be made clear. Although, on the one hand, it applies primarily to a single, definite, seated posture especially recommended for meditation, it also serves as a general name for all postures with similar leg positions—whether seated or not. The most obvious general characteristic of Lotus Postures consists in placing the left foot upside down on the right thigh and the right foot upsidedown on the left thigh. Since this characteristic occurs in all of our postures 11–25, all of them may thus be called "Lotus Postures" in the general sense of this term.

Since attainment of any Lotus position may be very difficult for beginners, most will approach it by means of Half-Lotus Postures in which the foot of only one leg rests on the thigh of the other. (See Plate 128.) Since all of our postures 3–10 exhibit this characteristic, they may all be regarded as *Ardha-Padmasanas* or Half-Lotus Postures. Nevertheless, this term also is used primarily to designate a seated posture, with the others regarded as variations of it. Even so, some uncertainty exists concerning whether such primary usage pertains to the postures we have depicted and described as follows or to either of the two varieties of *Virasana* as explained in posture 10.

Posture 4. *Vrikshasana,* the Tree Posture, consists in standing on one leg, bending the other leg sharply and placing the instep of the foot of the other leg in front of the thigh or, if possible, in the groin, of the first leg, and then placing the arms and hands in a position which somewhat resembles the branches of a tree. (See Plate 129.) Some hold their arms above their head with palms together and forearms creating a ninety-degree angle, presumably to represent the slope of a pine tree. Others drop their arms from their shoulders, keeping them straight and holding them out from the sides at symmetrical angles which again simulate the sloping form caused by the branches of a pine tree.

Posture 5. *Vatyasana* consists in standing on one leg and one knee with the instep of the foot of the bent leg resting on the thigh or in the groin of the first leg which must be partly bent. (See Plate 130.) Directions call for starting from *Vrikshasana,* the Tree Posture, and then slowly bending the straight leg until the knee of the bent leg touches the floor. I have been unable to find a reliable translation of this Sanskrit name. Danielou calls it "The Horse Posture." But I suspect that it refers to a banyan or Indian fig tree. The banyan tree drops limbs which take root and become additional supporting trunks. So I suggest that this be called the Banyan Tree Posture. One may try various optional arm and hand positions, but a formal pose has the palms of the hands put together in a prayer position and held in front of the chest.

Postures 6–9. The form of the body held in the Tree Posture, a standing position, may be repeated in a supine position (and called *Supta-Ardha-Padmasana* or the Supine Half-lotus Posture) (see Plate 131), in a prone position (and called *Adva-Ardha-Padmasana* or the Prone Half-lotus Posture) (see Plate 132), in a headstand position (and called *Sirsha-Ardha-Padmasana* or the Headstand Half-lotus Posture) (see Plate 133), and in a shoulderstand position (and called *Sarvanga-Ardha-Padmasana* or the Shoulderstand Half-lotus Posture). (See Plate 134.) In all of these postures the spine and one leg form a straight line while the other leg is bent with its instep touching the thigh or groin of the straight leg. Numerous other variations of Half-lotus positions may be explored. The form exhibited in our posture 3, a seated position in which the straight leg and the trunk form a right angle, may be repeated in supine, prone, headstand and shoulderstand positions, and all of the typical angles illustrated repeatedly in our Section V may be deliberately held. These have not become popular exercises with yogins who have selected from the maze of possibilities only a few of the most effective postures for their purposes.

Posture 10. *Virasana,* the Hero Posture, is a name unfortunately applied to different positions by different yogins. We choose to apply it here primarily to that Half-lotus Posture which is also a Half-thunderbolt Posture—a seated position in which the foot of one leg rests on the thigh or in the groin of the other leg while the foot of the other leg is placed flat on the floor, instep down, beside its own hip. (See Plate 135.) That is, both legs are sharply bent, but only one receives much twisting. This combines some advantages of the Thunderbolt and Lotus postures. Since many persons will be unable to attain the full Lotus Posture, they may find this posture—in which first one leg is twisted and then later the other—to be the limit of their capacity and thus fully sufficient for them.

Perhaps we should mention the fact that the term *Virasana,* the Hero Posture, may apply also to a simpler position closer in form to those included in the group represented by our posture 2. Sivananda, in *Yoga Asanas,* page 32, describes this posture as consisting in putting the foot of one leg on the thigh of the other and the foot of the other under the thigh of the first. This should be a relatively comfortable position for some beginners and a limit of achievement for others. One who cannot attain this position can hardly expect to achieve the Lotus Posture or any of its more advanced variations.

Posture 11. *Padmasana,* the Lotus Posture, stands out among all yogic postures as most typical and representative. (See Plate 136.) It has become symbolic of yoga or, indeed, of Hindu cultural ideals. The reason why the term "lotus" was chosen for this posture, when the posture in no significant way resembles a lotus, should be made clear. The lotus flower itself may be seen to symbolize the quiet, peaceful isolated, undisturbed goal of yoga. A lotus blossom floats serenely in a quiet pool, having no apparent connection with other flowers or with the shore. It blooms in all its beauty in a perfectly quiet, unentangled, pure, symmetrical, circular (hence unified) self-sufficiency. Thus the lotus blossom, which had become a sacred symbol for those seeking spiritual peace, was a natural symbol for signifying the spiritual goal sought and commonly found in this particular posture. As should be expected of a symbol surviving through such a long history, fantastic varieties of interpretations, both in story and sculpture, have developed around it. To emphasize the sacred symbolism, yogins, Buddhas and respected deities of every sort are carved as seated on or in a huge stylized lotus blossom, often having dozens of petals. Superficial observers of Hindu statuary may conclude that monstrous lotus blossoms, rather than kusha grass and animal skins, were the original foundations for yogic exercises. But anyone induced into, and sympathetic with, belief in the worthiness and sacredness of perfect quiescence can hardly fail to appreciate the aptness of choosing the name Lotus Posture for this most representative position.

The Lotus Posture consists essentially in a seated position with the insteps of both feet placed high on the thighs or in the groins of their opposite legs. The knees should be kept on the floor to maintain stability. The spine should be straight, the head erect, the abdomen in and chest out. Above all the position should be comfortable, since it is designed primarily for meditation during long periods. Various hand positions are possible and these will be surveyed in Section XI. Often the arms stay straight while the hands rest on the knees, either the palms down in a knee-clasping position, or with the palms up and thumb and index finger in a symbolic gesture. Often the arms relax at the sides with the hands, palms up, dropping separately on the thighs. Sometimes the elbows bend slightly while the hands rest together, the palm of one against the back of the other, in a formal fashion in front of the abdomen.

Bandha Padmasana, or *Baddha Padmasana,* the Bound Lotus Posture, is a variation not depicted here. It consists in the Lotus Posture with the knees drawn together somewhat, the feet extended farther over the thighs and twisted farther so that their heels become pressed into the sides of the abdomen, while the arms are crossed behind the back and the fingers of the right hand grasp the toes, or big toe, of the right foot while the fingers of the left hand grasp the toes of the left foot. Not only may a practitioner perform this exercise one leg and hand at a time, but he may need to practice it in this way for a long while before trying and succeeding with two. When only one leg is bound, this may be called an *Ardha-Bandha-Padmasana,* or Modified (or Half) Bound Lotus Posture. This Bound (or Locked) Lotus Posture is not designed for meditation but as an additional massaging, stretching and twisting exercise. When one returns from a Bound Lotus Posture to a regular or full *(Purna)* Lotus Posture, he may find himself becoming more comfortable than if he neglects to do the extra stretching first.

Posture 12. *Matsyasana,* the Fish Posture, consists in first assuming the Lotus Posture and then lying down backward until you become flat on your back. The hands may then be folded above your head on the floor, used to prop up your head or stretched on the floor above your head. (See Plate 133.) One may get into this position directly from a supine position also, and those frustrated in their initial attempts to attain the seated Lotus Posture may practice in bed over a long period to attain the Fish Posture first. It will be natural to try this one leg at a time. Another variation of the Fish Posture retains an arched back and neck with weight resting on the crown of the head and the hands resting on the thighs, clasping the feet, or locked around the big toes. Or one may fold his arms behind his arched back. Since this is primarily a supine posture, it may also be called *Supta Padmasana* or the Supine Lotus Posture. It is similar to *Supta Vajrasana*, the Supine Thunderbolt Posture, except that the feet lie crossed on top of the thighs instead of below or beside their respective hips. I suspect that this is called the Fish Posture because the pattern formed by the bent knees resembles the tail fins of a fish. One may wave his fishtail up from this supine position, thus attaining a form similar to that in his sitting position except that the whole form has been turned a ninety-degree angle. But he will have to wait for postures 14, 15, 17 or 19 to wave it in the opposite direction.

Posture 13. *Tulasana, Tulitasana* or *Tolangulasana*, the Balanced Posture, begins as a Fish Posture. Then one places both hands under his buttocks, supporting and balancing his entire body on his elbow and hands. The head and upper part of the body are raised and bent forward and the knees are raised or bent forward also. The posture is so named, doubtless, because the two ends of his body balance each other and may move up and down slightly in a way resembling the action of a balancing or weight scale. As one raises his head and knees as far as possible, his form becomes somewhat analogous to a reversed Bow Posture in which his abdomen faces up and away from the floor rather than down on the floor. One may perform a similar exercise by folding his arms above his chest and then drawing his folded arms and folded legs together as close as he can. (See Plate 138.)

Posture 14. The Prone Fish Posture appears to have no special Sanskrit name, unless it be *Adva-Matsyasana*. It consists in holding a Lotus position while lying face down. (See Plate 139.) It may be approached from a Prone Posture, *Advasana,* or from a Mountain Posture, *Parvatasana* (see our posture 16). One may rest his head on his chin or forehead or on his hands or arms folded under his head. It is possible also to vary this position by raising the body up into an inverted bow form by bending his fishtail forward and under, bending his head and neck forward and under, and arching his back with the aid of the hands placed under his abdomen. This modification may serve as an approach to postures 15, 17 and 18.

Posture 15. *Lolasana,* the Swinging Posture, may be thought of as a combination of the Peacock Posture, *Mayurasana,* and the Prone Fish Posture. It consists in holding a Prone Fish Posture while raising the whole body up in the air and balancing it on the elbows with the forearms being held in a vertical position. (See Plate 140.) It may be approached from a Prone Fish Posture, as just described under posture 14, by bending the knees and head under the body and toward each other and by raising the body up on the elbows after placing the arms under the abdomen. Then, after a balanced condition is attained, the head and knees may be raised gradually into a modified Peacock Posture. One may approach it from the Mountain Posture, *Parvatasana,* by then putting his hands on the floor in front of him and proceeding as in approaching the Peacock Posture. Or, if he has advanced sufficiently in suppleness and self-control, one may even first assume a Peacock Posture and then proceed to fold his legs in the Lotus Posture or fishtail fashion. Once in position, one may vary the horizontal line of his body by tipping it, lowering his head or knees or both successively to simulate a modest seesaw motion, or he may move his body forward and backward on his hands in a slightly swaying motion. This posture could be called a Peacock-Lotus Posture *(Mayura-Padmasana).*

Posture 16. *Parvatasana,* the Mountain Posture, consists in assuming a seated Lotus Posture, *Padmasana,* and then raising the body straight up in the air by standing on the knees while retaining the folded-legs form. The arms are extended, held straight and used for balancing and steadying the pose. When in final form, the arms extend above the head so that either the arms, trunk and upper legs form a straight line or the arms meet the hands in forming a peak resembling a mountain peak. (See Plate 145.) Be sure that padding under the knees is sufficient to prevent injury or discomfort. This posture is related to posture 1 of set D of our Knee-bending Postures (see Plate 115) but differs from it by holding the feet in front of the thighs or groin instead of behind the buttocks or by holding the legs in a Lotus rather than in a Thunderbolt position.

Posture 17. *Sirsha-Padmasana,* the Headstand Lotus Posture, combines holding the legs in a Lotus position while the remainder of the body attains a Headstand position. (See Plate 141.) This and the following three postures may also be called *Urdhva-Padmasana* or the Aloft Lotus Posture. (*Urdhva* means elevated, raised, high, above or aloft.) One may get into this position either by first attaining a headstand and then folding his legs in a Lotus position or by arising out of a Prone Fish Posture, as suggested in our discussion of posture 14. In this latter case he will first assume our posture 18. Once in a full Headstand Lotus Posture, one may exercise further by waving his fishtail not only forward and backward but also by twisting it and his spine clockwise and counterclockwise.

Posture 18. *Sirsha-Padmasana,* the Headstand Lotus Posture, also names the position in which the Lotus-folded legs are lowered from the full *(Purna) Sirsha-Padmasana* until the calves or knees touch the chest. (See Plate 143.) If one uses the conventional Western headstand position in which he balances on his head and hands, with elbows raised in the air—rather than the traditional Yogic headstand in which his hands are folded around his head and he balances on his head and elbows, then when he lowers his folded legs he may rest his knees on his raised elbows. We might call these postures (and posture 20) *Ardha-Urdhva-Padmasana,* the Half-aloft Lotus Postures.

Postures 19 and 20. *Sarvanga-Padmasana,* the Shoulderstand Lotus Posture, seems to have received little attention in yogic practice. It consists in combining a Shoulderstand Posture with a Lotus position for the legs. (See Plate 142.) One may first attain a Shoulderstand Posture and then fold his legs, or he may first attain a Supine Lotus Posture (which may be preceded by a seated Lotus Posture) and then raise his legs in the normal manner for rising into a Shoulderstand Posture. One may, after attaining this position, also wave his fishtail forward and backward and twist it and his trunk clockwise and counterclockwise. If he lowers his legs in the direction of his head and touches his chest with them, he attains our posture 20. (See Plate 144.) (Illustrated, with further advanced modifications, in *Self-Realization Magazine,* July-August, 1961, page 7.)

Posture 21. *Utthita Padmasana,* the Aloft (Elevated) Lotus Posture, consists in a seated Lotus Posture retained while raised in the air by placing the hands beside the hips and pushing the whole body upward. (See Plate 146.) All weight rests on the hands. One may need to adjust his hand positions several times before he attains a balanced condition which can be held with relative comfort for a short time.

Posture 22. *Kukkutasana,* the Cock Posture, is also an elevated posture and is exactly like the Aloft Lotus Posture, *Utthita Padmasana,* except that the arms are placed inside rather than outside the thighs before raising the body. That is, the arms must be placed between the thighs and calves before and during holding this position. If one spreads his fingers out on the floor, his hands will look more like rooster's feet. Some prefer to double up their fingers into a fist before trying this one. Although presumably the name Cock Posture applies to this position regardless of the distance which the body is raised from the floor, full achievement of the posture has not been attained until the legs rise above the elbows and become supported thereon.

Posture 23. *Garbhasana,* the Foetus Posture, is like the Cock Posture except that one rests on his buttocks and balances himself thereon while retaining the lotus-leg position with his arms thrust through between the thighs and calves up to the elbows and then bent up so that the hands touch the cheeks. This posture is supposed to resemble the form which an unborn child takes while in the womb. It may be regarded as a variation of *Kukkutasana* if one first assumes the Cock Posture and then sits down and balances himself in an upright position while resting on his buttocks. Formal directions call for touching or grasping the ears with the fingers.

Posture 24. *Uttana-Kurmasana,* the Upside-down Tortoise Posture, appears to be a most difficult one and I have seen no illustrations of it. It was described in the ancient *Gheranda Samhita,* Part II, Sutra 33, as follows: "Assume a Cock Posture, catch hold of the neck with the hands, and stand stretched out like a tortoise." *Uttana* means "stretched out" and "lying on the back" or "with face upward." Thus, this posture appears to be one in which the Lotus position of the feet is retained while rolling out of a Cock position onto one's back. How one can cross his hands behind his back and grasp his neck seems uncertain to me, but slimmer and more supple persons may be able to do so. An upside-down turtle does stretch his neck backward and such backward stretching of the head may make reaching it with the hands easier. This position might also, I suspect, be approached from the Fish Posture, *Matsyasana,* or, better, from the Balance Posture, *Tulasana.*

Posture 25. *Yogasana,* the Yoga Posture, is a term with a confused history. The *Gheranda Samhita,* Part II, Sutra 45, says, "This is called the Yoga Posture assumed by the yogins when practicing Yoga." Now, in a sense, all of the postures used by yogins are properly called yoga asana or *yogasana,* "yogic postures." However, if we read the description given, preceding the above-quoted sutra, we notice that it describes a very simple *Padmasana* or Lotus Posture with a hand position which appears to have been modified or abandoned by later usage. "Turn the feet upward, place them on the knees; then place the hands on the ground with the palms turned upward; inspire, and fix the gaze on the tip of the nose." Notice here that the hands appear to drop on the floor beside the hips or legs, whereas resting the hands in front of the body above the legs has become traditional.

However, we choose to identify *yogasana* with yoga mudra. Mudra means "form" or "shape." Although asana means "posture" or "position," and originally a "seated position," the elaboration of varieties of postures having different forms make it possible to regard each posture as a form or mudra; and each position designated as a mudra is, in effect, a variation of the form of some prior, or previously recognized and designated, posture or asana. Thus, so far as practice is concerned, the name mudra amounts to an alternative name for asana, though the use of the term mudra to name some asanas has become traditional. Since the term *Padmasana* or Lotus Posture has now become the dominant name for the position earlier called *Yogasana* and since the term yoga mudra designates a different, well-defined, specific posture, we choose to treat it here as *Yogasana.* This posture consists in taking a Lotus Posture and then bending the trunk forward until the forehead rests upon the floor. (See Plates 147 and 148.) Various hand positions are optional. One may place his palms on his heels, thus increasing the pressure in the abdomen. One may keep his arms as straight as he can and clasp the wrist of one hand with his other hand behind his back. One may place his hands with palms together in a prayer position pointing upward behind his back. This position should not be confused with a similar position in which the feet are under rather than on top of the thighs, as in the prone variation of *Pavanmuktasana* (set B, posture 3, of our Knee-bending Exercises).

B. Arm Exercises

Yogic tradition has not been particularly concerned about singling out the arms for special exercises. The main efforts have been directed at the torso and spine and at attaining a stable seated position in which the legs play a primary role. Except as needed for attaining and holding certain postures, the arms and hands have played largely a supporting role, and, when free, may serve to provide symbolic gestures.

However, we should recognize that the arms, like the legs, may bend in the middle, at the elbows, and may be twisted clockwise and counterclockwise. Since they can be swung around in a full circle from the shoulders, they have even greater possibilities than the legs so far as alternative forms are concerned. An arm, bent at the elbow to a right angle, may then be twisted more than 180 degrees with ease and has capacity for further twisting. The wrists have much greater pliability than the ankles and the fingers much more than the toes. Although yogins do also exercise their fingers, and develop amazing suppleness in them, these exercises apparently do not play a large role in postures as such. Classical Hindu dancers, however, make greater use of finger gestures than those of any other culture, doubtless.

Analogous kinds of movement may be noted in the arms, wrists and fingers, and in the legs, ankles and toes, and in the trunk and its appendages—and even, to an extent, in the neck and head. Each may bend forward and backward, and twist clockwise and counterclockwise, and both bend and twist at the same time. The arms, wrists, legs and ankles have similarities in being capable of turning symmetrically or asymmetrically, both in bending forward and backward and in twisting clockwise and counterclockwise, and in both bending and twisting. If one cares to, he may explore multitudes of posture possibilities. The traditional remark that there are eighty-four hundred thousand postures is quite believable after considering the alternatives calculable merely from the above-noted analogies.

Before turning to two not-yet-treated, traditionally recognized postures giving specific attention to the arms, we may recall that arms were also significantly involved in the Bound Lotus Posture, *Bandha-Padmasana,* and in the Upside-down Tortoise Posture, *Uttana-Kurmasana.* In the first, the arms were crossed behind the back while reaching downward to grasp the big toes. In the second, they were crossed behind the back while reaching upward to grasp the neck. Also, when the arms are placed behind the back, palms together, in a prayer position, as an optional form in some forward-bending postures such as *Yogasana,* they receive some twisting. However, we choose to mention two postures, one standing (*Garudasana,* the Eagle Posture) and one seated (the Cow-faced Posture, *Gomukhasana*) to illustrate attention to arms.

Garudasana, the Eagle Posture, consists in standing upright, trunk and head erect, on one leg, with the other leg "wound around" the first and with the arms "wound around" each other. The legs cross at about the middle of the thighs and the calf of the raised leg passes behind the knee of the straight leg and the instep of the raised leg rests on the back of the calf of the straight leg. Cross your arms just above your elbows and bend your elbows so that the forearms both point straight up in a vertical position. Then bring the palms of your two hands together in order to bring the palms closer to an even face-to-face position. Retain balance and an erect position. Repeat using the other leg and reversing the arm positions.

Gomukhasana, the Cow-faced Posture, is uniquely an arm-bending and twisting posture, but since it is also normally regarded as a seated posture, accounts of it usually begin by describing some favorite way of sitting. Actually the arm positions described here may be held with any of the seated postures (or standing postures, for that matter) in which the arms remain free. They may be combined, for example, with *Sukhasana,* the Easy Pose, *Samasana,* the Symmetrical Pose, *Siddhasana,* the Adept's Pose, *Muktasana,* the Free Pose, *Guptasana,* the Hidden Pose, *Svastikasana,* the Prosperous Pose, *Virasana,* the Hero Pose, or *Padmasana,* the Lotus Pose, all included as postures 1, 2 and 11 of our Leg-twisting Postures. Or they may be combined with *Vajrasana,* the Thunderbolt Posture, or any of its variations depicted as postures 1–5 of set E of our Knee-bending Postures. These variations include sitting on the ankles, soles up, soles out, soles in, sitting on the floor with ankles beside the hips, soles up, soles out, or soles in, sitting with both ankles crossed before sitting, or sitting on the floor with legs crossed at the thighs and feet at the sides. This lattter, called *Samkatasana* (the Contracted [or Dangerous] Posture), is favored; or it may be varied by sitting on one ankle with the other ankle beside its hip. The arm position, which surely everyone has tried at least once in his life, consists in dropping one hand behind his back from above and pushing the other up behind his back from below until both meet. One may merely lock his index fingers, or lock all four fingers of both hands or clasp his hands. With practice, one can increase the ease with which such locking or clasping occurs. Repeat, exchanging the positions of the two arms. Attend to making the spine and neck erect in a formal position.

C. Jaw and Tongue Exercises

We usually forget that the jaw is an appendage. We may not know that its muscles, too, become tense and stiff and that some relief from tension can come from extending them deliberately. Especially when, for any reason, we need to hold our jaws quiet or tight, we may benefit from stretching exercises. One who keeps a pipe, cigar or cigarette in his mouth much of the time or who does very little talking during the day may profit from regular mouth opening. The jaws move both down and up, backward and forward, and from side to side. One may open his mouth as wide as possible several times and hold it wide open for a while. Then he may move his jaw first to one side and then to the other as far as possible. A slow rotating motion, first clockwise and then counterclockwise, is easy. This can serve as a convenient little yoga at any time. Although one should avoid yawning in public, private yawning exercises can prove relaxing.

Likewise, the tongue is a muscular organ moved by muscles. It too may be held within a relatively small sphere of action and become tense, stiff and lifeless. Although not an appendage in the same sense as legs, fingers and jaws, which have bones in them, the tongue may be stuck out for some distance. Again, this is not a polite-society activity, but in privacy one may deliberately stretch his tongue out as far as it will go and move it up, down and sideways for exercise.

Both of these exercises have been combined significantly in one traditional posture called *Simhasana,* the Lion Posture, which consists in sitting on one's ankles in a Thunderbolt Posture and in stretching his jaw down and tongue out as far as possible. One will look more like a lion if he spreads his fingers out as wide as possible with the palms of his hands on his knees. The addition of eye exercises, which we will discuss next, may provide a quite hideous appearance. Presumably, the jaw and tongue benefits may be obtained also through other sitting, lying or standing positions.

D. Eye Exercises

Although eyes hardly rate as appendages, they too suffer from muscular fatigue and tension and can be relieved somewhat by deliberate attention to eye-muscle exercises. Like the appendages discussed above, eyes move up and down, from side to side, and may be rolled clockwise or counterclockwise. Not only can they be moved and rolled but they may also be "twisted" in the ways that occur when one looks cross-eyed and wall-eyed. When rolled, they may revolve both in the same direction or, with more difficulty, in opposite directions.

Although one should not overstrain eye muscles through stretching exercises, perhaps we need a reminder that a problem which faced us as children, or as parents of children—that of avoiding cross-eyed strain in the eyes of young children which have not yet been adequately coordinated and habituated—may have transformed itself into another problem. Oldsters, whose eye coordination has been not only perfected but hardened into fixed limited patterns, may need just the opposite kind of caution. It is well known that judicious massaging of eye muscles improves their tonus. Although one can easily overexaggerate claims for eye improvements through such exercises, not only as aids to relaxing tired eyes but also in actually improving eyesight, a bit of personal experimentation may be worth while. Persons with known eye diseases should, of course, use precaution and follow physicians' advice, but modest efforts to move eyes up, down, sideways or around should prove helpful to almost anyone.

In working out a routine for over-all stimulation and relaxation, one may do well to include just a bit of eye rolling. For example, when twisting your neck by moving your head from side to side, you may push your eyes farther in the direction in which your head turns. This obviously is an exercise which may be performed not only in the office but while driving or walking or in the thickest of company, for one normally turns his head somewhat anyway and this kind of stretching and limbering can be done without its appearing to be a relaxing exercise to anyone.

Yogic tradition not only recognizes the importance of eye muscles and their control but has some specific directions to recommend. Not only may one turn his eyes upward but also partly inward and hold them there for a while. Experience with this exercise will immediately reveal that one's attention becomes distracted from his other problems. This exercise or pose is described as gazing at the space between the eyebrows or *Bhrumadhya Dhrishti.* Or one may turn his eyes downward and partly inward. This may be described as nasal gazing, *Nasa Dhrishti,* or, better, as gazing at the tip of one's nose, *Nasikagra Dhrishti.* For relaxation purposes, movement both up and down may be better than either the one or the other alone.

Perhaps we should also mention navel gazing, which is more popular with onlookers and commentators than with practicing yogins. Although one may seek significance in the navel, as the center of the body, or in the space between the eyebrows, where the Brahman sacred symbolic mark is placed, as objects—the goal of yogic practice is subjective, not objective. The objects, as such, have little or no significance so far as physical exercise is concerned. They serve merely as means to guide efforts. One seeking limbering of his eye muscles, increased circulation of blood in such muscles and feelings of relief from fatigue will find that the exercises themselves, not the objects gazed at, are the goals to be sought.

We will not here review the ways in which eye exercises may be combined with other posture exercises. The role of eye movements has just been mentioned in discussing the Lion Pose, *Simhasana*. More detailed treatment of many traditional poses would include eye poses also. Specific abdominal massaging postures and some meditation postures traditionally include eye exercises. Sometimes the eyes remain open, sometimes they close entirely and sometimes they become half closed.

X. ABDOMEN-MASSAGING POSTURES

Massaging—whether of arm, neck, leg or spinal muscles or of internal organs—normally consists of putting external pressure on the body in such a way that the innermost parts receive their effects indirectly through other intervening tissues and organs. Yogic massaging, on the other hand, has internal sources: first, voluntary control, and then moving controlled muscles some of which are embedded deeply within the body. No external instruments play any role, except in the sense that one body organ is external to another. Hence yogic massaging functions primarily as a kind of self-massage, both in the sense that a person has full control over his own massaging activities and in the sense that the internal muscles massage themselves through the exercises in which deliberate attention is given to them. The yogic abdominal massage to be discussed here depends on no other person and use of no external force of fingers or hands or heel or knees, not even one's own.

Two distinguishable stages in practice which have become traditional should be noted. The first is easy. It consists in raising the diaphragm and drawing in the abdomen in certain specific ways. This is called *uddiyana.* The second is more difficult and, for persons with a thick layer of fat over their stomachs, may seem to be an impossibility. It consists in selective manipulation of the abdominal muscles. This is called *Nauli.* Both of these stages have been performed in either standing or floor-seated positions. However, they may also be performed in a kneeling position. I see no reason why one should not use them also while lying in bed at home, sitting in a chair in the office, or being transported in taxi or plane—or even, if one so chooses, while headstanding or shoulderstanding. Even if perfection in these stages cannot be obtained under such conditions, nevertheless some, even sufficient, benefit may be gained in them. Traditionally, they have been combined with breathing exercises and with the Lotus and Thunderbolt Postures and their variations, and may serve as an aid to preparing for full attainment of these postures.

Uddiyana, meaning "rising up," will be translated here simply as stomach exercise. The process and pose require something more than a mere drawing in of abdominal protrusion, of the kind commanded by drill sergeants: "Suck your guts in." Involved are both inward and upward movements, both diaphragm and ribs, both breathing and holding the breath, both tensing and releasing of some muscles while others remain tense, and use of arms and hands on knees or thighs. Begin by assuming either a seated or a standing position. If seated, in one of the standard poses such as the Adept's Pose, the Prosperous Pose or the Lotus Pose, put the palms of the hands on the knees for support. If standing, place the feet ten to fifteen inches apart, bend the legs slightly and clasp the hands on the thighs for support.

Beginners should practice abdominal breathing and complete breathing (discussed in Chapter III) a few times to accustom themselves to the functioning and limits of the breathing apparatus. First empty the lungs by exhaling forcibly and completely. In addition to quick expulsion of air in the larger branches of the lungs, continue a slower expiration of air from the smaller branches and sacs by further pressure. Then contract the abdomen, drawing its contents up into the expanded thoracic region by raising the ribs and diaphragm by means of a vacuum created in the thoracic area. In order to create and maintain such a vacuum, you must prevent air from entering the lungs. You may use one of the *bandha* considered in Chapter III, Section III, including *uddiyana bandha.* Since this posture remains incomplete until *uddiyana bandha* has been attained, it is more commonly named *uddiyana bandha* than merely *uddiyana.* Also, you may experience pressure upon the shoulders and arms created by the vacuum, so some effort by arm and shoulder muscles may be needed to help the rib muscles maintain it. This *bandha* or bound status serves as a fixed posture which one may hold for a very short while.

Next, try a vigorous mock inhalation by raising the ribs without permitting air to enter the lungs. At the same time, relax completely the front abdominal muscles, a simple task which may take some time for beginners to master. When you can no longer hold your breath with comfort, relax your neck, shoulders and ribs and inhale slowly. When the abdomen and chest have returned to their normal shape and you have inhaled sufficiently, one round has been completed. Beginners should stand up straight, if holding a standing position, or sit erect, when in a seated position, between rounds. You may raise and lower your diaphragm and lungs several times before inhaling, or during a single round of breathing. You may try three to five rounds, as seems needed for refreshing results. Bernard (*Hatha Yoga,* page 21) reports building up his ability until he reached 1,500 contractions (with as many as twenty contractions with each round of breathing) in a morning.

Let me caution not only against excessive abdominal exercise—especially by overzealous beginners—but also against persons indulging in this exercise who suffer from abdominal troubles or circulatory diseases, unless they have a physician's permission. Restraint by women during menstrual periods is also advised. Specific values include increased tonicity, improved digestion and elimination, invigorated circulation and slight reduction of abdomen size. The performer must judge for himself the total effect upon his general health and feelings of relaxed living. A few rounds may readily be included in one's daily posture routine as well as tried independently as an anti-fatigue measure during the day.

Nauli refers to abdominal muscle exercises presupposing ability to perform *uddiyana bandha*. Some slight acquaintance with abdominal muscular anatomy seems needed. Two sets of muscles, called "recti" ("rectus," singular), line the front of the abdomen, one spreading to the left of center and the other to the right, and both extending from the pubic bone at bottom to up under the ribs at the top. Other muscle tissues crisscross the front of the abdomen and line its sides. But *Nauli* exercises concentrate upon singling out for attention these two sets. Considerable experimentation with attempts at voluntary control of these muscles may be needed before ability can be attained. Persons with weakened recti, with thick layers of fat overlaying them, with huge stomach and intestinal structures, may be discouraged easily, since they will be unable to see results without tremendous efforts at reducing and remolding their torsos. They may, however, attain some of the benefits of *Nauli* exercises even without being able to see its effects in any dramatic way.

First, one needs to develop skill in drawing his abdominal contents in and up by creating a vacuum in his thorax as described above *(uddiyana bandha)*. When he has forced all air from his lungs, fixed his vacuum-held position, he may then experiment with relaxing and contracting the recti muscles at will. If he has not done this before, it will be a new experience for him. He should discover that he can attend to, and relax or contract, the muscles on one side—or the other side, or both sides together. He may need to play at such selective relaxing and contracting for some time before gaining satisfactory control over them. As control develops, he should be able to contract the muscles in such a way that they appear on the surface of the abdomen as a distinctly protruding tube or pair of tubes running from the pubic bone to under the ribs, if surface fat does not prevent such appearance. More clear isolation of the right rectus muscle *(Dakshina Nauli)* may be obtained by bending slightly forward on and toward the right knee, pressing the hand on the right thigh or knee harder than the hand on the left. Isolation of the left rectus muscle *(Vama Nauli)* may be obtained likewise by bending toward and pressing on the left thigh or knee. Concentrating and protruding both recti together may be referred to as central or middle *Nauli (Madhyama Nauli)*.

The next and final stage of the abdominal-massaging process is *Nauli* "rotation." If one can isolate both recti singly and together, then he is ready for contracting and relaxing them successively, and in a rhythmic pattern. After relaxing both, one may contract the right only, then the left only. This process may be repeated, starting with the right only, then both, then the left only. He thus creates the appearance of a repeated wave motion across his abdomen. He may then reverse the direction of the wave. Or, he may move them from right to left and then left to right, in a rolling or churning manner. The massaging qualities of *Nauli* rotation should be obvious and their effects, both beneficial and harmful, should be expected to be greater than those of *uddiyana* merely. One may observe that *uddiyana* effects come primarily from an up-and-down movement of the abdominal contents whereas *Nauli* effects result also from additional right-to-left and left-to-right motions.

XI. MEDITATION POSTURES

Except for surveying kinds of hand positions, only one new or additional posture will be considered in the present section. A few postures already discussed will be reviewed relative to their suitability for meditation. The purpose of the present section is threefold: (a) To summarize the nature and purpose of meditation, showing both why traditional goals may be expected not to interest business executives and professional people and how they may, nevertheless, prove useful to some of them; (b) To cite which postures serve best for meditation and to give reasons for such service; (c) To survey the thus-far neglected portion of traditional posturing, namely, the kinds of ways in which hands may be employed and the significance of these ways.

A. What Is Meditation?

Throughout this work we have followed the customary practice of referring to "meditation postures" as if the reader did, or could easily, understand what is meant by "meditation." However, the term meditation cannot convey very much insight into the nature and purpose of dharana, dhyana and samadhi, the last three stages, or "limbs," of raja yoga outlined by Patanjali, the classical formulator of yogic doctrine. No satisfactory English equivalents exist for these Sanskrit terms, and translation custom has come to rely upon the term meditation as perhaps least misleading.

The ultimate goal of yoga, union with the ultimate (see

my new edition of the *Yoga Sutras,* of Patanjali, *Yoga: Union with the Ultimate,* especially Book III, Sections 1–5, pages 117–126), is *kaivalya* (perfectly unattached freedom) or Nirvana (completely quiescent bliss), attained through a final act of liberating *(moksha* or *mukti)* pure soul from all, even the minutest and subtlest, disturbances. The first five of the eight stages of raja yoga, outlined in Chapter I, serve merely as preparatory. Concern for asanas (posture) and *pranayama* (breathing) constitute only the third and fourth of these preliminary attainments. The fifth stage, *pratyahara,* endeavors to shut out sensuous distractions and attain attentive stability. Some interpreters include this stage also under the broad and ambiguous term "meditation." But the last three stages, which may be gathered together under a mystical controlling process called *samyama,* seem more central to what is intended.

Of these three, the second, *dhyana* (Sanskrit) or *jhana* (Pali) or, derivatively *zen* (Japanese), has received most detailed attention. The process involved is one of attaining increased quiescence in mental activity–including cessation of desire, thought, imagination and feeling. The nature and significance of these details have been debated for centuries in Hindu, Jain and Buddhist philosophies. (See my *Philosophy of the Buddha,* especially Chapters 4–8.) But the nature of these processes has little to do with meditation which, in English, means "intending," "planning," "reflecting," "thinking," "especially closer or continued thought." Dhyana and meditation are alike in being subjective and mental and in being freed from aroused anxieties, bodily action and violent emotions; but the essential goal of raja yoga, complete elimination of all thought, imagination, desire and egoism, is not essential to the meaning of the English word meditation in its ordinary usage.

Hence, since the traditional purpose of those postures

selected as best for meditation can hardly be of use or interest to business executives or professional people, we might omit reference to them except for two reasons. The first is that anyone mildly interested in yogic breathing and posture techniques for purposes of relaxation should prefer not to be completely uninformed concerning postures held in highest esteem by yogic tradition. The second is that some may wish to explore meditation further since many Westerners who have done so report benefits beyond temporary relaxation. Both those disappointed with their initial efforts and those sufficiently satisfied with their successes through ensuppling exercises will have little further interest. But some say that yogic meditation is better than sleep. Many can discover for themselves that yogic exercises serve as aids to inducing sleep and curing insomnia. But one must go farther into yogic theory and practice than the suggestions outlined thus far in this volume to discover whether meditation is in fact more restful than sleep.

The task is enormous in the sense that one will have to reorient his outlook if he is to make much progress in this direction. But some distraught executives who have tried exercise, sex, liquor and the gamut of sedatives and tranquilizers, either in succession or in combination, and still remain harried, strained and fatigued, or sluggish and deadened, may find here another hope.

Speculation about how meditation is better than sleep should take into consideration the fact that a complexly disturbed and tensed nervous system tends to surrender itself to dreams, often more taxing than daytime efforts, soon after initial rest restores enough energy to reactivate it. Yogic meditation aims at deliberately retaining consciousness, or at least awareness, while at the same time eliminating desires, thoughts, memories and imaginings. By developing power and habits of controlling attention so completely that it cannot stray into energy-consuming nightmares, one may indeed retain and restore energy otherwise wasted in dream tensions. Thus, persons suffering from deep-seated omnistrain which cannot be relieved by easier methods may be led, finally, to explore for themselves the possibilities in yogic meditation which we cannot go into here. Nevertheless, we shall briefly sketch some pertinent facts about meditation postures.

B. Postures Best for Meditation

A zealous devotee may believe he must attain perfection in the Lotus Posture before he has any chance of further pursuits. In fact, he may read highly respected authors or hear from his guru that such is necessary. But the truth is that individual differences have been recognized by yogic instructors all along. Sivananda, for example, cites four asanas which are prescribed for meditation. "They are *Padma, Siddha, Svastika* and *Sukha*" (*Yoga Asanas,* page 28). Yet, in discussing the virtues of various other postures, he also remarks about their merits as aids to meditation. *Sama, gupta, mukta, vajra* and *pavanmukta* asanas may also be used.

It is true that, in surveying the amazing variety of postures and exercises, we have tended to emphasize their massaging, limbering, relaxing and health-giving aspects. Traditionally, most postures are recognized as serving in the process of developing complete voluntary self-control over even the involuntary musculature rather than as of direct use for meditation. Only a few postures prove suitable for meditation. But enough variety exists so that one does not need to wait for mastery of the Lotus Posture, a mastery which may never come, in order to begin pursuit of yogic meditation.

People trained in a chair-sitting culture will be interested to note an American development which consists of sitting erect with feet flat on the floor, knees together, eyes closed and hands in a relaxed, palms-upward, position on the lap, on a horizontal, straight, armless chair. This position is pictured in the November-December, 1955, *Self-Realization Magazine,* page 24, and entitled the "Self-Realization Fellowship Meditation Pose." A folded blanket lines the back and seat of the chair and extends under the feet on the floor. The poser is fully dressed in street clothes. Granted, this may be a makeshift and of temporary use for short periods of meditation. It may even be adapted to group techniques such as those used by the Self-Realization Fellowship. But the point is that the constant requirement that comfort remains essential to all yogic postures, whether for exercise or meditation, may lead individuals to experiment with seated postures other than those popularly considered essential.

However, the reasons for traditional postures should be known and the principles involved should be employed in personal revisions. A first requirement for a meditation posture is firmness and stability. Thus a seated rather than a standing posture is indicated. One needs to have as much of his body firmly planted on the floor as possible. At least three solid points, to maintain a triangular rigidity, should be sought. Four or more may be better, provided they do not involve opposing pressures which regularly force the body into a disequilibrium. Thus tradition requires a position in which the knees come into solid contact with the floor, if at all possible. Since one must breathe, each round of breathing entails a shifting of body weight. This fact may remain unnoticed in daily affairs, but, in the quiet of meditation practice, such shifting becomes noticeable, even when not a problem. If one sits too erect, he may tip over backward. If he leans too far forward, too much energy is needed to lift his weight during each breath. If he is unbalanced sideways, effort to compensate such imbalance will be needed. The problem of conscious attainment of an easy balance is such that standing on one leg and headstand exercises have been devised to help beginners. Development of automatic habits for readjusting weight without disturbance or strain is thus required so that dynamic movements needed in breathing occur without distracting from seemingly perfect stability.

Thus the seated posture must combine a fairly erect spine with relatively free movement of the abdominal muscles. Pressures upon the abdomen result both in less ease in respiratory movements and in tendencies which tip the body. The posture should be conducive to slow, steady breathing and to a slowing down of breathing patterns without disturbance or need for conscious readjustment. It should also permit easy performance of those movements needed for *kumbhaka,* or forced pauses in breathing, when these are used to induce deeper concentration. (See Chapter III, Section III.)

A second requirement is that a posture be such that it can be held for a long time without discomfort. The problems involved in attaining an experience of timelessly undisturbed awareness are time-consuming. One cannot enjoy even a "sip of eternity" so long as temporal intrusions of any sort interrupt.

A third requirement is retention of alert awareness. Novices naturally wonder why not lie down on the floor or in a bed or hammock or sit half-reclining in an easy chair. The first two requirements can be met by lying in *Savasana,* the Easiest Posture. But experience teaches that one who lies down soon either goes off to sleep, in which case his dreams take over and disturb his awareness with myriads of objects, interests and ambitions, or he drifts into daydreams, which do the same thing. In order to escape being a victim of one's subconscious tendencies, one must remain alertly conscious. But in order to eliminate consciousness of objects, ideas, images and memories which disquiet awareness, one must eventually become able to concentrate upon objectlessness. Hence staring at forehead, nosetip or navel may become an external part of a meditation posture. But one must retain an erect and alert, as well as stable and comfortable, posture in order to pursue yogic meditation very far.

Those interested in exploring yogic meditation may appreciate a few hints. The question of a rug or mat has already been dealt with. It should not be so hard that the legs or knees become numb from prolonged pressure or irritated by breathing movements. It should not be so soft that the body rolls back and forth upon it as it moves while breathing. People with fat legs or buttocks may have special problems to overcome, since their own flesh may serve as a rolling instrument which cannot be stilled. Early attempts to meditate, before one has attained comfort in a Lotus Posture, for example, may be aided by using a book or two to sit on so as to take some pressure off the bent, twisted legs. Use of a book, however, may introduce a host of problems. Books are hard. They may be too wide or not wide enough for persons with different hip spans. One may tend to roll off. The edges may dig into the flesh or bones. The height of the book must vary as one becomes more adjusted to his final meditation position. However, one may notice that a book prop enables him to get his knees down farther or easier and helps tighten his abdomen in initial phases of attaining stability. In any case, if one adopts for himself some variant mode of meditation posture, he should be sure to embody the above three requirements in it.

C. Significance of Hand Positions

First, let us glance at the possibilities regarding hand positions and, while we are at it, arm, hand and finger positions. Then let us observe some of the kinds of forms which have attained prominence in yogic tradition. Finally, let us notice how expression of symbolic meaning gives additional significance to meditative asanas through hand positions.

1. Possibilities

An amazing plethora of forms may be embodied in positions taken by our arms, hands and fingers. Most of us have never stopped to observe their quantity. Consider first your arms. They may be held straight or bent at the elbow in any of almost 180 degrees.

Notice the possibilities when one of your arms is held straight. Probably it can swing more than 180 degrees from front to back and more than 180 degrees up and down, and 360 degrees if swung in a complete circle. Thus one of your arms can occupy any of the radii of a hemisphere, relative to a fixed shoulder position. Not only does your other arm have the same possibilities, but your two arms together not merely double but multiply possibilities for, while one arm is occupying one radius of its hemisphere, the other may hold any of the positions in the radii of its hemisphere, and vice versa. Some find only the symmetrically related positions most interesting, though two different types of symmetry, or partial symmetry, may be noted: that type in which the arms hold a series of positions resulting, for example, from separating the arms from each other by equal additional units of distance; and that type in which they occupy a series of positions resulting from rotating them both clockwise, for example.

Consider, also, the possibilities occurring when one of your arms is bent at its elbow. Swing your forearm from a fully extended condition to a completely bent one so that your hand comes close to your shoulder. Then, holding it at a right angle to your upper arm, swing it as far up and back and as far forward and down as you can. If you can move it through 180 degrees, then your forearm, by itself, can occupy almost any of the radii of a hemisphere of its own, from any given elbow position. Compound this hemispheric set of possibilities with those of your other forearm, and then with those of your upper arms (even when your arm is completely bent, you may be able to swing it through this hemisphere), you cannot help but be astounded. Ignore, for the present, imagining compounding them also relative to positions of the body—whether standing, sitting, lying or upside down, and to leg positions—or you will get very dizzy.

Attend, next, to your hands. By bending them at the wrists, you may note that each has approximately a hemisphere of possibilities of its own, even when the fingers remain held straight and together. From any given symmetrical pair of arm positions, the numbers of possibilities suggested for straight arms and for bent forearms may be repeated. These two may be compounded with the previously mentioned possibilities. But let us turn now to your fingers. Each finger may bend through about ninety degrees at each knuckle. They may be held close together or separated. The thumb may be placed beside them or be opposed to them—to each one of them or to all four together. Thumb and a finger may form a circle, loose or tight, or a semicircle or a V shape and many other forms. Even the number of different ways in which two hands may be put together, by folding, clasping, with fingers interwoven in various ways, palms together, backs together, is greater than we realize before examining them. Yogic tradition has employed relatively few of these alternatives, or at least teaching processes have forced elimination of traditional mention of most of them. However, except for purposes of exercise and self-control, and ideally a yogin should attain control over every possibility, only a few arm, hand and finger combinations are needed for meditation purposes.

2. Kinds

Which kinds of hand-position forms have attained prominence? We will not review all the positions mentioned previously in describing the various asanas. In every posture and exercise, the hands must be somewhere: in the headstand they must be folded above the head; in some postures they are crossed or folded behind the back; in *Garudasana* they are twisted and forced together in front of the face; in *Garbhasana* they are thrust through the legs and then hold the ears; and in some breathing exercises they are used to close nostrils alternately. We limit consideration here to what one must, ought and may do with his hands while holding a meditation posture.

The hands must take some position. Either they touch the body somewhere or rest on the floor beside the body, for to hold them above the head or out from the shoulders will cause unnecessary strain. The fingers must be either open or closed. If open, the palms must be up or down or in some recognizable position. The positions of the two hands must be either symmetrical or asymmetrical. These simple musts seem obvious, though they merely state a problem rather than provide a solution.

One ought to do two things with his hands. First, he should prevent them from serving as distractions during meditation. In some conditions, they move or bind when the body weight shifts during breathing; they tickle or rub the skin; they press against or into the body; or they remain under strain or create a body imbalance which involves stress. Second, he should put them to maximum use, where benefit is possible. For, in addition to using them to get into a comfortable position, one ought, when possible, to employ them to promote the ends of meditation. What are some of these possibilities?

The hands may be merely dropped on the floor by one's sides, palms forward or up, in a most relaxed position. One who has not yet fully relaxed, may spread his fingers out on the floor with his palms down. In *Yogasana,* one may leave his hands on the floor palms backward and then up, as he bends forward to the floor. A most common position is to place the hands on the knees. Many alternatives exist, however. The palms may be turned down, and the fingers may be wrapped over the ends of the knees or hung loosely over the ends or held straight down over the ends. Or they may be turned upward and inward. The fingers may be held together, or spread out, and the thumb may be in line with the fingers or opposed to them. Their position may be with or without symbolic significance.

When symbolism is intended, then their position takes a form needed to express what is symbolized. The next, and perhaps most common, way of disposing of the hands is to let them drop into the lap, when a lap exists, as in *Padmasana.* Here the hands may drop separately, palms up, and remain apart. Or they may be folded around the feet. Or they may be put together, either by one nesting in the other, with both palms up, and with thumbs side by side or tip to tip, or by one hand clasping the other, with both palms toward the body and one thumb inside the other, or by interweaving the fingers. If one does not have specific directions in this matter from a teacher, he will experiment until he finds a most satisfactory condition. Christians, for example, may prefer to place their hands together in a prayer position, pointing them upward in front of the chest, if the meditation period is not long enough to produce tiring.

3. Symbolism

Strictly speaking, symbolism, involving one thing which means another, entails two things which are in some sense different from each other and thus a distinction of the very sort which yoga seeks ultimately to suppress. In Nirvana, no symbols exist because symbol and symbolized merge into a single unity. "Yoga" means "union," and ultimate union unites everything, including any differences or distinctions between a symbol and what it refers to. Nevertheless, one may wish to symbolize the ultimately nonsymbolical state which he seeks. So long as one has not yet reached the ultimate state, his present state is different from it and thus he may, without inconsistency, use symbols to mean that which is now different from his present state. To the extent that one's symbolizing faculties continue to function, he should put them to work symbolizing the ultimate. Since raja yoga aims at attaining perfect quiescence, awareness of and embodiment of a symbol of that perfect quiescence may induce an added dimension of quiescence into one's present condition. When this is so, the embodiment of a symbol of the goal in one's asana may, in effect, give that goal a symbolic embodiment and thus aid in occupying the self with the goal.

Concrete embodiment of such a goal-symbol may be accomplished in two ways during meditation periods. While exhaling, one may embody the omnisonal sacred symbol *om* in a single syllable enduring through a long period of exhalation. As in saying the Jewish-Christian "Amen," which doubtless originated from the same source as the Hindu *aum* or *om*, one pronounces the syllable with an attitude of assent, affirmation or acceptance which approaches perfection, and thus completion, or quiescence.

Likewise, one may embody in his hand positions some sacred symbol of ultimacy. Just as a Christian, when making the Sign of the Cross, intends to be embodying holiness within his gesture, so a yogin, when embodying the *Jnana Mudra* in his hands, intends to be embodying the attainment of holiness (yoga) in his asana. This symbol, called *Jnana Mudra* in Sanskrit and translated into English by various names, consists in holding three fingers straight and the index finger bent to meet the thumb. (See Plate 126.) Since it represents a feeling of attainment, it normally takes form after posture stability and some degree of mental tranquility has been achieved.

However, as with holding a crucifix, one may use a symbol also as an aid to such attainment. One may embody the symbol in his hands in any posture at any time while they remain free. When seated, one normally rests the side of his hand opposite the thumb upon his knee, straightens his hands completely, even stretching the fingers backward, if need be, to eliminate tension and tendency to grasp. Then, keeping three fingers stiffly straight, the index finger slowly bends to meet the thumb, tip to tip. Teachers may differ regarding details of placement of finger on thumb. After long practice, one assumes this hand position without effort or reflection. When one has held his hand in this position for a long time during a meditation period, his fingers may close somewhat. In any case, comfort should be maintained and embodiment of the symbol should be an aid to quiescence and not a distraction. Although one should seek perfection of form, whenever effort to maintain the form itself reduces quiescence, such effort should be abandoned.

Further study of symbolism must be foregone here. But we may mention that Hinduism, Buddhism and Jainism all have long histories of symbolic gestures which not only were embodied in living yogins, Buddhisattvas and Jainas but also have become enshrined in statues representing them. A study of the history of Oriental iconography can be most fascinating. But as statues of saints come to be shrines for worship, symbols tend to become instruments for teaching as well as signs of attained goals. Each hand forms itself into a different symbol, and multi-armed deities depict multiplicities of symbols. But here concern for multiplicity carries one away from the simplicity sought by the raja yogin. He symmetrically embodies the same symbol in both hands. Tradition regards a meditation posture as incomplete until a symbol of attainment is expressed, or until interest in symbolism has been surpassed by attainment of Nirvana itself. In fact, the Lotus Posture with *Jnana Mudra* has itself become the most famous symbol of the whole yogic tradition. A reader who cannot appreciate Hindu symbolism may adopt some attainment symbol of his own, or adapt one filled with significance from his own cultural tradition, as an aid to relaxation if he chooses.

XII. POSTURE ROUTINES

I refuse to recommend a single posture routine for all persons and times, not only because individuals differ so greatly in ability, need and circumstance but also because each individual changes from time to time in these ways. However, I will (a) suggest some principles regarding routines, (b) cite some references to advice on routines and (c) review one famous ancient routine called *Surya Namaskar* or "Sun Worship."

A. Principles

The first principle about routines is that you should have one. Neglecting to attain regular habits of practice accounts for more failures to achieve the benefits of yogic exercises than lack of ability to perform postures. Having some systematic way of continuing to persist in exercising is more important, generally speaking, than which particular routine you adopt.

A second principle, primarily for beginners though it holds as well for all at all times, may be stated as a warning: Do not attempt to do too much. Postures may be held too long. You may try too many at one practice period. The exercise period may be too protracted. You may try extreme postures before you are ready for them. Overdoing should be avoided, in yogic practice as in anything else.

A third principle, also one to which beginners should give special attention, though it applies generally, is that, if possible, a routine should contain a well-balanced program. Although, during an exploration period, a beginner will naturally emphasize one posture or exercise more than another, he should not be satisfied until he includes at least one back-stretching, one front-stretching, one side-stretching and one spine-twisting exercise in his pattern. Attention to legs, arms and neck, ankles and wrists, and fingers and toes should be included. An abdomen exercise and perhaps an upside-down posture, as well as breathing exercises, may be needed. As one persists and becomes more expert, he should be able to judge which exercises are most beneficial. One way of assuring balance is to prolong or repeat some exercises, e.g., front-stretching exercises, which may be more useful in counteracting continued back-stretching activities normal to a day's work.

A fourth principle has to do with rest and relaxation during a routine process. As Sivananda reminds us, "Relaxation of muscles is as important as contraction of muscles" (*Yogic Home Exercises,* page 77). Although perhaps no definite rule should be stated, one may try to spend as much time resting as exercising during each practice period. Persons differ relative to how much time should be devoted to such resting and exercising. Beginners who must strain themselves a bit to attain or maintain a posture may have to spend more time between attempts than others. After one becomes expert in attaining a posture, he does so with less effort, and he may be able to pause in a balanced state, even in a headstand, and deliberately relax many of his muscles during the posture. This principle, as well as others, holds for breathing exercises, since relaxing lung and rib muscles even momentarily may have a tremendous psychological effect.

A fifth principle pertains to integrating breathing with

posture exercises. Teachers differ regarding whether one should practice poses first or breathing first, and one will have to decide for himself which he will do. But wisdom seems to indicate interweaving both, especially by those concerned with health and mental relaxation in contrast to those training for yogic trances. I suggest considering a breathing exercise period both before beginning postures and during a supine relaxation pose at the end of a practice period, as well as during rest periods between postures, if a routine lasts very long. Relative to each particular posture, one may attend modestly to breathing efforts before entering the position and while holding the position—if it is held very long. Part of the purpose of some postures is to aid in promoting breathing exercises. In any case, develop some definite pattern for directing yourself into a continuing pattern interrelating breathing and posturing.

A sixth principle is the rather obvious one of setting aside some specific time or times each day for yogic efforts. Preplan both the time of day and the length of time for each period. Although life circumstances may determine whether a person can reserve more than one period a day, a person, when he is able, should distribute his efforts over several periods. It is probably better to have two, three or four shorter exercise periods throughout the day than to have a long period once a day. Morning and evening will be natural times for some, but may be impossible for others.

A seventh principle is to choose those exercises which your experience indicates give you the greatest relaxation and reinvigoration. Choose those which seem to reward you most. Do not demand of yourself attainment of a posture just because it happens to have received traditional recognition. Avoid those which yield constant or repeated frustration. To deliberately aim at repeating a frustrating experience merely adds to the day's problems and tensions rather than bringing relief from them. However, one should not be disappointed to find that the increased limbering gained from one day's exercise fails to carry over into the next day. If you bend down and fail to touch your toes, and then exercise until you can touch your toes, you may expect that tomorrow when you try this movement again you will again fail to touch your toes and that the same amount of, or even more, exercise may be needed all over again.

An eighth principle wisely directs you to select those exercises which carry over into your day's work, leaving more prolonged beneficial effects. For example, those breathing exercises which tend to generate in you a habit pattern of slow and steady breathing may yield a persisting result. Postures which tighten up the abdominal muscles may provide support for your posture pattern in a way which sets a tone for the day. No person is fit for his day's work until he has stood erect, pulled in his abdomen and breathed quietly for a few moments. One needs to brace up his posture, rest his mind and take stock of his confidence before plunging into duties and turmoil. Some do this with prayer, some through a posture routine, some by both.

A ninth principle concerns rigidity of routines. Some variability should be expected. Not only do individuals differ from each other, but each person changes in many ways during his lifetime and during his developing yogic habits. The items in a beginner's routine will be affected by his lack of skill and feelings of need for specific attainments. One who has developed enough, will design his routine for maximum effect in terms of skills already acquired. Age, illness, size, regularity of free periods, companions and variations in fatigue all function as factors in modifying routines. Different times of the year, which may be colder or hotter, different times of the week, when some days are busier than others, or different times of the day, such as morning, evening, noon or afternoon, make differences in what routines are possible. Finally, one needs to steer a course between too little and too much rigidity. One should seek sufficient regularity so that he will not have to worry about planning what to do each period. On the other hand, one should not become bored with a routine too long in operation. One may plan ahead for variations. He may use a different set of postures on different days, or have a basic unchanging pattern with one or two different daily variations throughout a week. Enough postures exist for almost endless variation, so one need never become bored.

B. References

Those who feel themselves unable to figure out a routine for themselves may wish some further suggestions. Following are some books, each of which makes recommendations. The suggestions differ somewhat, many pursuing their special interests further into related topics such as diet, irrigation, *kundalini,* meditation and prayer. For further details about these books, see the Bibliography.

Alain, *Yoga for Perfect Health,* pp. 101–106, has a Schedule of Exercises.

Déchanet, *Christian Yoga,* pp. 137–162, gives Practical Advice and Guidance for a Christian Yogi, including three training cycles and two patterns.

Devi, *Yoga for Americans,* devotes her whole book to six lessons for six weeks and may appeal especially to women.

Kuvalayananda, *Pranayama, Part I,* pp. 129–141, in a now-hard-to-get volume outlines three courses, A Full Course, A Short Course and An Easy Course.

Ramacharaka, *Hatha Yoga,* pp. 203–212, suggests Some Yogi Physical Exercises which include many well-known setting-up exercises.

Spring, *Yoga for Today,* p. 169, lists a Suggested Routine

consisting of twenty-three items requiring an estimated thirty-three minutes.

Vishnudevananda, *The Complete Illustrated Book of Yoga,* pp. 324–354, elaborates six Training Tables designed for differences in age, sickness, obesity and stiffness and outlining lessons for periods from two weeks to two years.

Yesudian, *Yoga and Health,* pp. 182–190, outlines twenty-one weeks of exercises.

Yogendra, *Yoga: Physical Education* and *Yoga Asanas Simplified,* pp. 165–166, offers a Guidetable with twenty-two exercises consuming about thirty minutes.

Yogendra Sitadevi, *Yoga: Physical Education,* Third Edition, p. 128, lists a Guidetable designed especially for women, with twenty-one postures taking thirty minutes.

C. Surya Namaskar

Surya Namaskar consists simply of a series of positions in which one begins by standing erect, then descends through precise stages to a prone position, then rises again to an erect standing position by repeating in reverse the same precise stages. *Surya* means "sun." *Namaskar* means variously "a bow of obedience," "a reverential salutation," "an exclamation of adoration" or "homage." Some translate *Surya Namaskar* as "Sun Prayers." I prefer the rendering "Sun Worship." Doubtless this series originated in an ancient sunrise ritual, performed facing the East or rising sun. It has become modified, adapted, and formalized somewhat to fit yogic practices, although it has also been adopted as a health measure by persons who have rejected, or who remain ignorant of, both yogic and ancient (orthodox yogins regard yoga as the original and most ancient truth) ideals and explanations.

Louise Morgan, London *News Chronicle* reporter, has edited a Fourth Edition of *The Ten-Point Way to Health,* a work attributed to Shrimant Balasahib Pandit Pratinidhi, the Rajah of Aundh. Her sceptical approach to the reasons for the extremely youthful appearance of the then seventy-year-old Rajah changed to approbation after personal experiences in regaining health through use of the series. This illustrated book gives an account of the Rajah's own modifications of the tradition which he learned. Other variations will be described below. But publication of this book illustrates how one particular routine not only retains some aspects reflecting a very ancient origin, but also exhibits both contemporary Indian ideals and practices and individual variations.

Although *Surya Namaskar* resembles, or is, a sunrise setting-up exercise, it emphasizes the back- and front-stretching exercises typical of yogic posture series, rather than the muscle-building tendencies of Western physical education programs. Beginners, however, may find the ideals expressed for many of its stages very strenuous. Those interested in pursuing and mastering this series may wisely adopt simplified modifications of some stages while trying to attain the benefits which come from the series as a whole. Let us turn now to a description of three versions of this series, the first a ten-stage series as depicted by Pratinidhi in the above-mentioned book, the second a twelve-stage series as depicted by Vishnudevananda in *The Complete Illustrated Book of Yoga,* pages 69–79, and the third a ten-stage series, combining features of the first two series, suggested by your author.

1. First Version

Pratinidhi recommends spreading a cloth on the floor. A cloth about two feet square appears to be about right. The purpose seems more to provide a line for marking positions for toes and palms than anything else. First, stand erect, with feet together and the two big toes barely touching the edge of the cloth. Place the palms of your hands together and raise them in front of the chest in a prayer position. Hold this position for a period while breathing deeply and drawing in your abdomen, raising and expanding your chest and throwing shoulders and head back. He then directs you to stiffen your body in a serial fashion, beginning with your feet and moving gradually toward the top of your head. This process seems much like that which we have described in Section IV on the Easiest Posture, except that there relaxation was emphasized whereas here a stiffening effort is stressed. You should concentrate your mind so as to shut out disturbing thoughts, displacing them with appreciation of the good you are enjoying by participating in this *Surya Namaskar*. Finally, inhale and hold your breath. This he calls breath 1.

The second stage consists in bending forward, dropping your hands on the floor, and exhaling completely, thereby terminating breath 1. The palms should be placed flat on the cloth, about a foot apart, in such a way that the back borders of your palms barely touch the edge of the cloth. Thus ideally the back borders of your two palms and the tips of your two big toes mark points on a straight line. The hands, once placed on the cloth, remain there throughout all of the positions until the last one. The feet, first one and then both, retake precisely the same position during the last three stages which they held at the beginning of the series. The position attained in this stage is very similar to those depicted as the fifth stages of our Prone-starting Hips-first and our Standing Bend-down series of our Back-stretching Postures, Section V, B, 1 and C, 1, and often called *Padahastasana*. The head should touch the knees.

The third stage begins with a deep inhalation, breath 2, causing pressure tending to separate head from knees. Lower your buttocks, bending both knees, but keeping one foot fixed while moving the other backward, placing its toes and and knee on the floor. On alternate rounds of this series, a

PICTOGRAPH CHART NO. 11

POSTURE ROUTINES
SURYA NAMASKAR

First Version

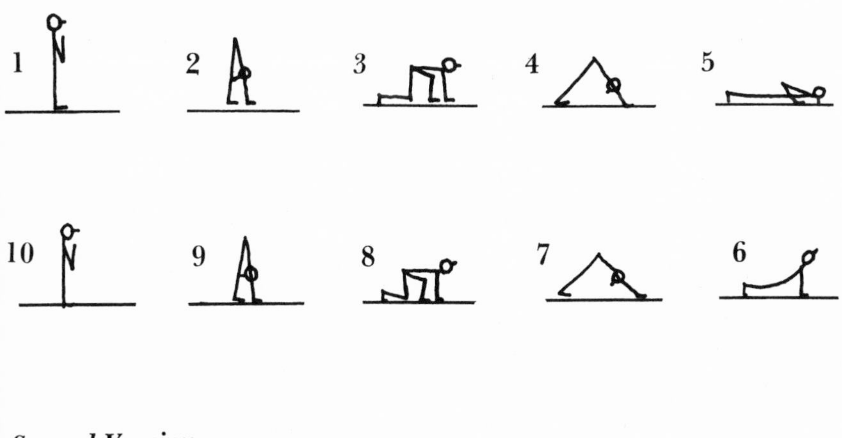

Second Version

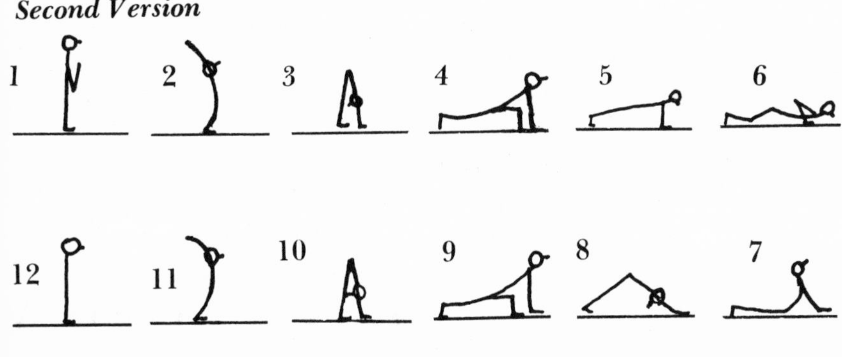

Third Version

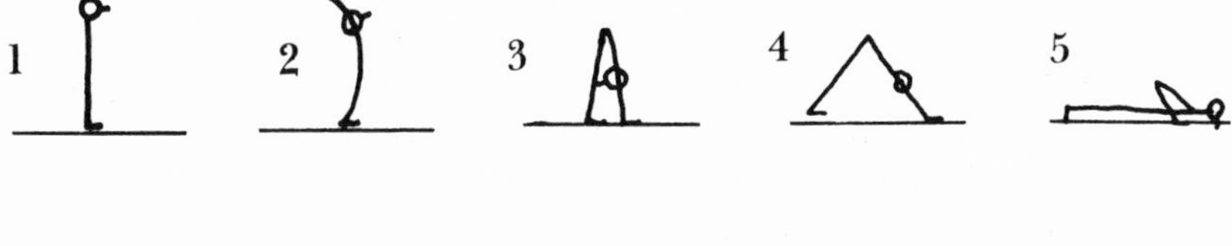

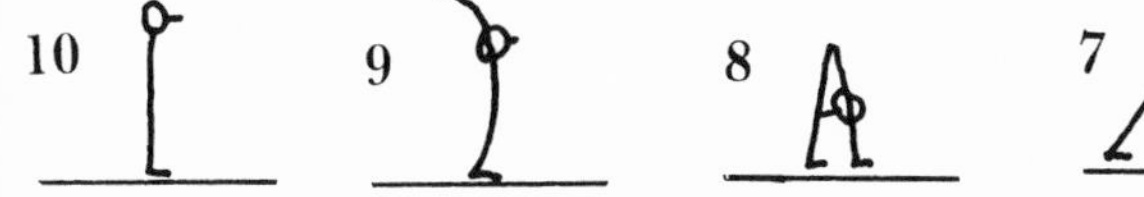

different leg is moved backward. The arms should be kept straight. The shoulders should remain vertical above the hands and the upper portion of the leg which has moved backward will be vertical, or parallel to the arms. The knee of the fixed foot should occupy a position between the arms. Finally, the head should be raised as high as possible and eyes directed upward. Breath 2 is held throughout this stage and the next and into the fifth.

The fourth stage consists in placing the fixed foot beside the moved foot and raising the buttocks high in the air. The arms remain straight, with palms still glued to the cloth, while the arms straighten and remain straight. The form of the body then appears like a pyramid, a position very similar to that depicted in stage 3 of our Prone-starting Hips-first Series (see Section V, B, 1). Although the lines of the pyramidal form should approximate a right angle, a sharper angle is easier to hold. A broader angle is harder to hold, both because more strain is placed upon the muscles of arms, legs and trunk and upon the heel tendons, since the heels should be kept on the floor. Pratinidhi advises bending the head in the direction of the knees in this position.

The fifth stage occurs simply by dropping to the floor, exhaling breath 2 and pulling in the abdomen. However, neither hands nor feet shift from their floor positions but the head and trunk move forward while the weight of the body rests mainly upon the bending arms. The legs remain straight while the bent torso straightens until the body approaches a prone position. Yet the hips and abdomen do not touch the floor but are kept away from it as far as possible. Although the forehead, nose and chest touch the floor, little weight is placed upon them. Keep chin in. Toes and knees remain on the floor but the weight of the body above the knees rests almost entirely on the hands.

The sixth stage embodies the Cobra Posture *(Bujangasana)*.

The bent arms should be straightened, thereby raising the shoulders up in the air while keeping the toes and knees on the floor, as in stage five. The head is bent back as far as it will go and eyes look upward as high as they can. During this process the chest is expanded and breath 3 is inhaled. Breath 3 is then held throughout stages 7 and 8 and exhaled during stage 9.

The seventh stage develops simply by retaking the position held in stage 4. Hands and feet remain in the same places on the floor kept throughout stages 4, 5 and 6. Raise the buttocks high in the air to re-embody a pyramidal form. The heels, which were raised from the floor while the feet rested on their toes during stages 5 and 6, return to the floor. The head, which was bent upward in stage 6, now bends downward.

The eighth stage repeats the position taken in stage 3, by dropping one knee to the floor and placing the foot of the other leg back in its original position with its big toe almost touching the cloth or line. Again one bends his head and eyes upward, keeping his arms straight, and still retaining his breath.

The ninth stage repeats *Padahastasana,* the posture assumed in stage 2, by bringing the other foot back to its original position and straightening the legs and raising the hips while keeping the arms straight. Exhale breath 3 during this process, completing exhalation as the head presses itself against the knees.

The tenth stage brings this series to a close by standing erect and again assuming a prayer position, with face straight forward. Inhale breath 4 as you rise and stand. If the series is repeated, breath 4 counts as breath 1 of the next series.

Pratinidhi, himself an expert, suggests that one complete series, or one single *Surya Namaskar,* can be done in twenty seconds. A beginner should proceed at his own pace and he may engage himself in considerable fumbling before getting a "feel" of the series of positions, even before integrating the restricted number of breaths recommended. Pratinidhi suggests that a beginner aim at fifteen *Namaskars* in five minutes, and should do about forty in ten minutes after six months of practice. He adds, "Do not be in a hurry."

2. Second Version

Vishnudevananda starts from the same position as does Pratinidhi but he inserts an additional second stage consisting in a backward bend. (See stage 2 of our second Half-circle Series, Section VI, B, 1.) The first inhalation occurs during this stage while the arms are raised and thrown backward. He then exhales while assuming his third stage which embodies *Padahastasana,* as in the second stage of our first version, except that he places his hands beside his feet, with thumbs touching the backs of his heels, instead of in front of his big toes. He uses no cloth or line. His stage 4 is like stage 3 of our first version except that he keeps the upper part of the extended leg in line with the trunk rather than in a vertical position. The knee and toes of this leg touch the floor but the upper portions of both legs oppose each other on a straight line rather than forming a right angle. Thus this position is harder to attain than that in our first version. Since the position of the extended foot is farther away from the position of the hands than in version 1, strain on the muscles required in some of the following stages is also greater.

Stage 5 differs greatly from stage 4 of version 1. The pyramidal form is replaced here by a form in which the body takes a straight line from heels to head, while propped up on straight vertical arms. This posture is attained by moving the foot from between the hands back beside the other and raising the other knee off the floor and straightening the body. A second breath is inhaled during this movement and held. It is exhaled as one moves into stage 6, which assumes a position like that of stage 5 of version 1 except that the nose is kept off the floor. One exhales as he enters this position.

Stage 7 embodies the Cobra Posture, but differently from that in stage 6 of version 1 by keeping the groin as well as knees and toes on the floor and by having the hands stay farther in front of the body—a consequence of placing the foot at a greater distance from the hands in stage 4. Inhalation takes place as the chest is raised from the floor. Stage 8 embodies a much more broadly based pyramidal form than that in stage 7, version 1, but Vishnudevananda sees no need for dipping his head downward in this posture. Exhalation occurs as one lifts his body from the floor.

Stage 9 repeats the posture in stage 4, with inhalation. Stage 10 repeats the posture in stage 3, with exhalation. Stage 11 repeats the backward bend, with arms thrust above the head, taken in stage 2, with inhalation. Stage 12 reassumes the posture in stage 1, except the arms drop by the sides (in a *Purna Padasana*) instead of returning to a prayer position, and one exhales and relaxes. Vishnudevananda advises us to repeat the series "twelve times daily," recalling that some yogins accompany each series by pronouncing one of the twelve names of "Lord Sun."

3. Third Version

Differences in the foregoing two versions suggest a somewhat more simplified series. The simplification consists in omitting stages 3 and 8 from the first version and stages 4 and 9 from the second version. This omission has both advantages and disadvantages, which will be explained below. By including stages 2 and 11 from the second version, our third version becomes a ten-stage series, as follows.

Its first stage is the same as the first stage of the first two versions. Its second stage is the same as the second stage of the second version. Its third stage is the same as the second stage of the first version and as the third stage of the second version. Its fourth stage is the same as the fourth stage of the first version. Its fifth stage is like the fifth and sixth stages of the first and second versions respectively. Its sixth stage is like that of the sixth and seventh stages of the first and second versions respectively. And its seventh, eight, ninth and tenth stages repeat, in reverse, its own fourth, third, second and first stages, respectively. Distance of placement of hands from feet in stage 4 becomes an optional matter; deliberate variation, gradually extending first and then diminishing the distance in successive cycles, is recommended. Inhalation accompanies stages 2, 4, 6 and 9; exhalation occurs during stages 3, 5, 8 and 10.

The advantage intended is a simplification in which both legs and feet are kept together at all times, thus eliminating the extending of one leg at a time and later retracting one leg at a time and any need for locating a precise position of foot in relation to hands. Although the first and second versions may be better for beginners, since one may go through initial trials more slowly, the third version has the advantage that one may whip through the whole series more quickly. There should be less strain involved in deliberately holding the breath, though this becomes a trivial matter as one becomes expert in any of the versions.

Disadvantages may, however, outweigh the advantages, especially if a person limits his exercise to repetitions of this series. The extending of one leg at a time produces a kind of stretching at the crotch as the muscles and ligaments of the two legs bend away from each other. By alternating the legs in successive series, a person gives both legs a beneficial limbering exercise. If he performs this function in other posture exercises, then no disadvantage occurs. If not, then either the first or second versions seems preferable.

No other versions will be discussed here. Harvey Day, in his *The Study and Practice of Yoga,* Plates 6 and 7, illustrates stages 5 and 6 of our first and third versions, keeping the body entirely away from the floor, resting all weight on toes and hands only. The arms are bent at right angles and the hands are placed closer to the feet in stage 5. Individual experimentation undoubtedly will result in still other versions.

CHAPTER V

Aids to Relaxation

The opening of a concluding chapter seems an appropriate place for restating the purpose of this volume. The widespread and increasing need for relief from nervous strain, the magnitude of which has come to be signified by the term omnistrain, may be met in part by techniques used by, or suggested by, hatha yoga—especially breathing, posture and attention techniques, developed in India throughout the centuries.

In general, the volume has a twofold significance. On the one hand, it may be taken as an example of deliberate promotion of intercultural cross-fertilization. As such, it illustrates how East-West influence functions as a two-way process. Western virtues centering about science and technology emphasize controlling conditions by means of instruments and gadgets external to the self. Hindu culture has excelled in developing ways of self-mastery without the aid or interference of instruments; its main concern has been with mental (including spiritual) and physical health; its approach is direct and its results can be intuitively apprehended. Orientals may be proud of their contribution to Western health. Westerners may appreciate receipt of help from an Oriental culture.

Also, this volume aims at helping individuals to relax.

Although persons in all walks of life may profit from it, it has been written with business executives and professional people specifically in mind. The survey of typical breathing and posture techniques in the two preceding chapters has aimed at remaining close to orthodox yogic tradition and many of the items considered go far beyond what a typical business executive can use.

In the present chapter, however, the author takes more liberty to offer his personal suggestions for relaxation. Most of these may seem to the reader as merely matters of common sense as, indeed, are most of the traditional yogic breathing and posture practices. Many readers will be acquainted already with much of what is said. But it may, nevertheless, serve as a reminder of techniques which they may have neglected, even forgotten—perhaps because they were not needed when learned, when the reader was younger, less burdened with anxieties and more vigorous. The purpose of this chapter is to offer suggestions which, although they fall short of traditional ideals of yogins engaging full time in quieting efforts, embody similar principles and may be used for immediate practical beneficial effects. Furthermore, these suggestions may be helpful to persons unfamiliar with yogic methods or even antagonistic to foreign ideas.

Persons who have tried to attain some of the postures outlined in the preceding chapter, who have been frustrated in repeated efforts to attain them, may have forgotten that this volume pertains primarily to relaxation. To confront new, baffling problems when seeking relief from new, baffling problems is to have failed in one's search. Unrealistic hope and overzealous effort to attain immediately what cannot be obtained immediately or even at all, can lead to tensions in trying to master yogic postures. But, just as one who goes for a boatride offshore in the ocean should not expect to reach the other side of the ocean, so one who stretches a muscle or two in yogic fashion should not expect to have mastered the astounding postures which full-time yogins finally achieve. A little boatride may be enjoyable in itself and a little muscle stretching may provide its own immediate rewards; but he who sets out to cross the ocean in a skiff creates for himself untold problems which the ocean, in itself, did not create. It is nice to know that the ocean is there and that opportunity for more persists; but he who is satisfied with his little ride is happier than he who remains forever on shore, struggling with efforts to get all the way across. This volume still aims at providing aids to relaxation, and the present chapter deals with methods which most readers should find easier to use, partly because they are adapted to everyday life in Western culture.

What, again, is relaxation? The nature of man or, indeed, the nature of the universe appears to entail a constant struggle between two natural polar tendencies. We cannot stop here to philosophize about generalizations concerning polar opposites. The sun rises and sets, creating day and night. We are born and we die. We desire to eat and then have our desires satisfied through eating. The naturalness and omnipresence of polar opposites has been depicted in ancient Chinese wisdom such as Tao, with its yang (initiative) and yin (completive) principles. (See my edition of *Tao Teh King* by Lao Tzu, especially pages 73–78.) The arousing of interest and attention and the withdrawal of interest and attention function as polar opposites. Like the successive waves of water, what is tensed needs to be followed by untensing. Man, as Lao Tzu warns us, tends to become artificial. That is, man tends to overdo or to remain tensed too long. Or, if he becomes completely untensed, he lapses into laziness. The problem of enjoying a most healthy balance between tension and untension remains perpetually. But for business executives, the problem is primarily one of reducing tension. Anxiety is natural. Relaxation is natural. But those who become too anxious or maintain their anxieties too long, suffer from destructive tendencies.

The proposals in this chapter reverse some aspects of traditionally yogic techniques while retaining others. Whereas most yogic posturing is done in private, many of the following suggestions pertain to ways of relaxing in public or in an office. Whereas yogins almost never use instruments, many of the following suggestions involve employment of common everyday instruments—beds, chairs, tables, desks and walls. Whereas yogic instruction and practice usually is individual, we shall note examples of deliberately sought "group therapy." The chapter is organized, somewhat arbitrarily, into sections on (1) little yogas, (2) easy stretching postures, (3) physical emphases, (4) attention techniques, (5) attitude techniques and (6) group therapy.

I. LITTLE YOGAS

I have deliberately coined the term "little yogas" to designate acts or positions which bring a little immediate relief from tension. "Big yogas," by contrast, are acts aimed, directly or indirectly, at ultimately perfect quiescence. Little yogas aim to quiet only a little. Their effect is temporary, except as they may have some cumulative effect when repeated constantly. They bring some momentary relief from anxiety, or reduce its overbearing effects in some small degree. One may choose to adopt his own terminology or prefer a single word, such as "yogettes" or "yogitas," if joining an ending derived from French or Spanish to a stem derived from Sanskrit does not disturb his linguistic sensibilities. (After all, English, French, Spanish and Sanskrit all originated in a common source and belong to the Indo-European family of languages.)

As must be expected, little yogas have comparatively little

value, judged from the standpoint of attaining a pervading calmness through traditional yogic methods. But they do have value and they are easily attainable. For those who cannot attain results through traditional ways and who do achieve results through little yogas, little yogas obviously have greater value. Although it may be true, as Yogendra says, that "the major yoga system cannot be easily grafted into our daily duties" (*Yoga Personal Hygiene,* Volume I, page 42), nevertheless many minor little yogas can be so "grafted," or rather found easily and enjoyed immediately.

Although anxiety and omnitension is experienced as an all-pervasive condition, we may approach reducing tension in the self as a whole by starting with some of its parts. The anxiety which spreads fatigue throughout the body begins in some part of the body; a self exists as an organic being in which whole and parts are interdependent. Any part may influence the whole; the whole in turn may influence any or all of the other parts. So, relaxing one part in such a way as to relax the whole even minutely may serve also to relax the other parts indirectly through the whole. At any rate, we propose to explore ways in which to relax some parts of the self, such as the hands, arms, legs, feet, torso and neck.

A. Hands

Like all tensed portions of the body, the hands tend to contract further as we become more anxious. When overwhelmed with fear, hatred or anxiety, we naturally contract our hands into a fist, and the more intense our emotions the tighter our fists clench. To relax, we must reverse this tendency. But more than a little bit. That is, releasing tension by changing from a tight to a loose fist is not enough. The hands need to be opened up completely, so that fingers and thumbs become spread out as far as possible. They should at least become straight. The first little yoga proposed here consists simply in straightening out curved, anxiety-ridden fingers. This may be done at any time and almost anywhere. However, some ways may be more effective than others.

The most obvious way is simply to stretch them, holding them straight deliberately. One may do this at his desk or while walking or talking. He may also do this in bed. Anyone who takes the trouble to observe that he has not gone to sleep as he had desired may notice that his hands remain closed, if not clenched, and that willful opening and stretching them may provide a little yoga. At his desk, committee table or typewriter, one may find it possible to spread his hands on the flat surface in front of him—even one at a time, if two at a time appear obtrusive. When he sits on a bench or a broad seat, as in a taxi or train, he may spread his fingers on the seat beside him and keep them there for a while.

One difficulty with hand-stretching efforts is that a person cannot keep them up for long. To counteract the protracted and intense pull of muscles in closing the hand, one should expect to have to succeed in producing an equally protracted and intense pull of muscles in keeping the hand open. But this would require its own energy, strain, muscle and nervous tension, and fatigue. Hence, if possible, one should seek a way to prop his hands open and then keep them open without effort. If he simply drops them in his lap, on the table, by his side or on his bed, he will notice that his fingers gradually close up again. Thus, on these occasions, he should look for ways to keep his fingers spread. While in bed, for example, one may lie on his hands after straightening them, or let his hand hang over the side and flatten itself on the floor with a slight pressure from his body weight, or flatten his hand upon the headboard or the wall at the head of his bed.

Hands may be stretched not only all at once but one finger at a time. You may find opportunity on most any occasion to place a finger on your desk, knee, book or any object and bend the finger back just a bit farther than usual. If you notice the relaxing effect, you will then proceed with the others in turn. Earlier I described with amazement the suppleness of Swami Chidananda's fingers as he counted off some serial items on them. Thus right before us in a public audience he was stretching his fingers one at a time while proceeding with his lecture. Any business executive can find ways of doing this if he bothers to take the trouble.

B. Arms

The arms, too, tend to bend and their muscles contract as we become increasingly nervous. How can you voluntarily extend them? In your office chair, you can drop them and let them hang loosely at your sides. Unfortunately, business executives normally acquire office chairs with armrests which naturally keep their arms bent. They purchase armless chairs for their secretaries, and part of the reason given for secretarial chairs is that one becomes less fatigued when sitting in them for long periods. Why not trade chairs with your secretary, as I have done, and gain the fatigue-reducing advantages for yourself? Now I feel sorry for my secretary but, since she works only part-time, I have not yet been moved to do anything about it.

While driving or riding in a taxi, plane or train, if the seat next to you is vacant and it is possible to extend your arm along its top, you may attain some straight-arm relaxation while traveling. Although one-armed driving cannot be recommended, the natural need for curling fingers around the steering wheel and bending the arms to turn it or hold it steady aggravates the tensions already present from other causes. If a person can hold one arm straight with fingers stretched out and bent back as far as they can go for a while, he may experience a significantly observable amount of relief.

I cannot refrain from reporting here my admiration for the way in which Tom Popejoy, President of the University of New Mexico, manages his handshaking duties at each annual Commencement exercise. Earlier, when only a hundred or so graduates passed on the platform before him, he seemed to do what was natural. He not only tensed his hand and arm for a first handshake, but kept them tensed in preparation for the next and the next and the next which were to follow in rapid succession. The engineering of a smooth public-platform handshake with each of a long series of nervous graduates, each with a slightly different hand size and shape and power of grip, required a constant sensitivity to myriads of alternatives and thus a perpetual and anxious alertness, to say nothing of the other problems facing him as a presiding officer. Reports of sore hands, stiff arm muscles and special hot bathing remedies signify the magnitude of this annual chore.

However, even though the number of graduates has grown enormously, President Popejoy now appears to manage the task with little trouble and no ill effects. Somewhere he learned to practice what I am calling a little yoga. As soon as a handclasp is finished, he relaxes both his hand and arm muscles and lets his arm hand limply at his side. Then as the next graduate approaches, he executes a well-timed raising of his arm to accomplish a smooth result. He takes a slight initiative so as to guide both pressure and length of time for the handclasp. Although he must adjust his maneuvers to the speed at which the announcer sends graduates to him, I have observed that the periods during which his hand hangs limp at his side exceed in total duration the periods during which it is in action. During the action period, his hand does not become tensed until immediately before the clasp, and it relaxes immediately afterward, even though the arm must remain in some tension until limp at his side. Few if any persons in his audience realize that his smooth, cordial handshakes are made possible by an unobtrusive use of a little yoga.

Before leaving our consideration of ways of stretching hands and arms, I must comment also upon Oriental versus Western ways of manifesting greetings. The handshake has become so firmly established in Western tradition that Westerners have difficulty in realizing that most Orientals never do it. Contrasts between East and West come out clearly here. The Westerner demands active physical contact and mutual shaking; the more cordially he wishes to express himself, the more vigorous his hand pumping, the firmer his grip, the more prolonged his gyrations. All this requires tension, exercise and effort. The Oriental more typically expresses his greetings peacefully, and hence passively, quiescently, gently. Each person places his own hands before his chest with palms together, fingers matching each other perfectly, with his fingers thus stretched out, rather than curved as required by a handshake, and oftentimes his arms are bent at their wrists. Since Hindus idealize quiescence, the more reverently one esteems the person he greets, the more peaceful and quiet his greeting. The more prolonged the moment of silence, the more cordially one has been greeted—a situation which completely baffles the Westerner, who naturally demands action and tension rather than a pause and relaxation in his greetings. If he could but stop to think for a minute, he could realize that he still uses the Oriental gesture of peace when he approaches God in prayer. The prayer position of the hands, which has come to be interpreted as pointing upward toward God, is really an Oriental handshake, a peaceful one which embodies in itself a bit of holiness. For the Oriental, the peace is present, not just up yonder, as it is also for the Westerners who enjoy peacefully a "sweet hour of prayer."

In case the reader is not clear how holding his hands in a prayer position can constitute a concrete symbol of holiness, perhaps some explanation is needed. A symbol is something, in this case the physical hands with palms together held in front of the chest, which refers to something else. Western theists tend to think of holiness as something existing perfectly in God who is above and as descending from above in diminished degrees. Hands in prayer position may, indeed, be symbols, but they are thought of as signs which refer, by pointing, to something else which is primarily elsewhere—above.

Hindus tend to think of holiness in terms of wholeness or unity. ("Holiness" and "wholeness" derive from the same stem and have essentially the same meaning.) Now the unity of the universe is believed to exist within rather than outside the person. Awareness of such unity or holiness has its source primarily inside a self, not outside or above. One's own willingness to be pacific, which must result in embodiment of such pacificity in one's body and behavior if it is to be realized at all, is the source of peace and holiness. Now, when one pacifies his hands, by bringing them both to inactivity and to a relaxed position in which the fingers and wrists are stretched, he embodies peace within them. Hands in the prayer position are concrete physical things. They are symbolic in referring to something else, not above, but to the spiritual peace which, although in some respects different from the physical hands, is embodied within them. Hindus seem less interested in the symbolical character than in the peace or holiness embodied.

Further ideas may be of interest relative to hand positions in greetings. The Westerner seems more concerned about peaceful relations between two persons on meeting, but less attentive to their inner spirits and whether they remain anxious, tense or in inner turmoil. The Oriental seems typically more interested in knowing that each is at peace with himself. "Peace be with you" is not merely an afterthought like a "good-luck wish." It is also a preparatory and precautionary concern, for peace between men is more likely to prevail when each is at peace with himself. A person who cannot manifest his pacific nature and intentions in a peace pause as a greeting cannot be trusted to deal peacefully with another.

Thus, for the Oriental, the seemingly aggressive Western approach which thrusts out a vigorous hand naturally creates distrust, until he also becomes accustomed to the perpetually active, unpacific, hence unholy, nature of the Westerner. Of course, not every Oriental is aware of the spiritual significance of his mode of greeting any more than every Westerner realizes the origin and significance of a vigorous handshake. Although a business executive cannot wish to reduce the spirit of cordiality naturally expressed through a handshake greeting, he may give thought to the ways of reducing anxiety in a nervous client or colleague by finding ways to utilize little yogas in his manner of greeting.

C. Legs

As anxiety increases, leg muscles tend to contract and legs to bend more. If one sits in a chair, he finds his legs drawn up under it as far as they can go. If the chair has rungs, his feet will prop themselves upon them, in front or on the sides. If the chair has a pedestal, his legs tend to wind themselves around it. If he cannot move his legs backward, he tends to cross them at the ankles or knees. Crossing the legs usually can be taken as a sign of nervousness. The obvious little yoga indicated here is to unwind or uncross the legs and get the feet back on the floor.

But bending legs back to a ninety-degree angle from a sharper angle is not enough as long as one can do more. He may, keeping his feet flat on the floor, move them forward from the chair a bit farther. Another obvious move is to prop the feet up on a desk. Since this is both improper and inconvenient for paperwork and tends to create forward bending in chest, shoulders and neck, it is hardly available to most business executives except in very informal sessions. But, if one tries, he may find ways of straightening his legs more often. Standing up whenever possible, going for short walks, even pacing up and down the room (itself a sign of anxiety), may provide inconspicuous little yogas for the nervous businessman.

One of the easiest places to make use of leg-stretching little yogas is in bed. When a person takes his anxieties to bed with him, he tends to contract his legs, as well as arms, hands and neck. When he becomes aware of his condition, he can then deliberately straighten them. Lying in *Savasana,* the Most Relaxed Posture, is indicated. But, as anxieties continue, he will find that his tendencies to contract his muscles express themselves as a discomfort leading him to roll over. But if he will notice that, as he rolls over, his legs, arms and fingers all bend again, he will have to straighten them out again. Then *Advasana,* the Prone Posture, or *Dradhasana,* the Firm (Side) Posture, may be sought deliberately, if one cannot force himself to maintain *Savasana.* Breathing exercises, especially Archiyoga, combined with the series of voluntary single-muscle relaxation efforts, help to maintain the Most Relaxed Posture and gain the advantages of leg stretching entailed therein.

D. Feet

Stretching the feet may, on the one hand, seem more difficult, especially when they are encased in shoes. Yet, if one tries, he can wiggle his toes, vigorously and continuously and yet quite unobtrusively, since they remain hidden in the shoes. He may bend his feet at the ankles, both up, down and sideways, with noticeable effect; and he may do this repeatedly, even continuously, without distracting the attention of others or even without taking his mind completely off his work. Although going barefoot—which can aid in discharging static electricity accumulating in the body, aggravated by anxieties—may be out of the question, most professional people fail to make use of the little yogas available to them in their offices and conference rooms through twisting their feet and ankles.

E. Torso

Attention to straightening the trunk and drawing in a protruding abdomen may provide most rewarding little yogas. Anxiety causes the trunk to bend forward. When sitting at a desk, one tends to crouch over it. When sitting back in a chair, one tends to sink into a slouchy position. The obvious counter-movement consists in sitting erect. As one slouches, his belly protrudes a bit more and his chest sags, diminishing the air space in the lungs. The more nervous a person becomes, the more his muscle contractions tend to roll him into a ball. Little yogas can be sought through reversing these tendencies by tightening the abdominal muscles. Although not all back ailments and slipped disks are due to slouching, many of them result in part from conditions which follow from slouching tendencies. One need merely notice the disproportionate amount of body size and weight in front of the spine in persons with bigger bellies. The larger your abdomen becomes, the more your spine and back muscles must endure strains involved in carrying a lopsided load. When forces due to nervous contractions of muscles become added to this load, the resulting persisting strain should be expected to have deleterious effects.

Except for the fact that one finds it difficult to counteract his habits, he may discover that common advice to sit erect is not only the easiest way to reduce nervousness but also one constantly available to him in his office or conference room. No one should complain about his anxiety and lack of health so long as he fails to employ this simplest of all methods.

Of course, one may deliberately bend backward and sideward occasionally while seated in a chair. He may also bend down to the floor, especially whenever something has been dropped. We usually regard picking up an article dropped by someone else as an act of courtesy. But, also, the person who bends over gains an additional stretch in the process and should regard the occasion as a healthy opportunity rather than as an etiquettical duty.

F. Neck

Urgency forces your head forward and down. Neck muscles tighten and strain. Often, under continued stress, the bearing of your head become stiff, rigid. Little yogas may be obtained by deliberately reversing all this. Not only should the head be held erect, and deliberately so, again and again and again as it droops repeatedly during a day's work, but occasionally it should be pushed backward. Take a look at the ceiling every once in a while. You can stretch your neck muscles not only by tipping your head from side to side but also by twisting your head by turning it around backward. Here is a little yoga which may be used repeatedly during office hours and committee sessions—and no one will notice. Each occasion for turning your head to look at, listen to or address another person may be an opportunity for twisting your neck muscles a little farther. Continued practice ensures surprising agility and suppleness in head turning.

Also, while driving your automobile, you often have occasion to turn your head to look out for cross-traffic at intersections, street signs and cars approaching from the side or rear. When tired, you may develop a tendency to keep your head stiff and to look only straight ahead. But when you realize that head twisting can provide some small degree of relief, you may deliberately twist your head farther on every opportunity. Although at high speeds you cannot safely take your eyes off the road ahead, whenever you slow down or stop at a traffic signal you may find safe opportunities. You might even develop a habit of correlating the extent of your neck twist with slowness of speed, and give it a fuller twist whenever you pull out of a parking space into a traffic lane.

Once attention has been drawn to the values of stretching muscles, a person can notice additional ways for achieving these values. He may roll his eyes, rotate his jaw, wiggle his ears, contract his scalp, nose and cheek muscles, and even twist and squeeze his tongue. A yawn always helps—when it can be managed in privacy and when it signifies relief rather than fatigue or boredom. One may exercise his anal sphincter, and the other internal muscles mentioned in our section on abdominal massage, while seated at work.

The point of listing all these items is not to present a catalogue of possibilities so much as to make the reader aware of multitudes of opportunities for employing little yogas. Even though each one alone may have only a minute effect, not only repetitions of each but also successive or even simultaneous uses of many of them may combine to contribute a noticeable amount of mental relaxation. The business executive, professional person or office worker of any sort, who pities himself because he is tied down to anxiety-producing duties which prevent him from refreshing himself at sports, really has immediately at hand resources for relaxation which he fails to use so long as he neglects to exploit the multitudes of little yogas available to him.

G. Deceleration

Another very subtle aspect of anxiety is its tendency to accelerate your movements, such acceleration in turn contributing to increasing anxiety. Here is another always-reliable technique which may not only be used inconspicuously, but which may also influence others in the direction of quietude. Both anxiety and sedateness are "catching." The person who speaks and moves more slowly exhibits an air of confidence, assurance, serenity. Deliberate reintroduction of slower paces into situations where public anxiety prevails may well pay off in reduced fatigue and irritability.

Slackening of pace may be introduced into almost any kind of activity. A most obvious form is slowed speech, more clear and full-rounded enunciation, lengthened pauses and a tone of deliberation. Deceleration of breathing rhythms promotes deeper, more relaxed breathing. Slower body movements—from moving the hand when giving or getting a paper to rhythm rate of steps when walking—provide a psychological effect of ease. While eating a meal, one may pause before each bite, chew more slowly, even retard his rate of swallowing. It is not merely a slow rate of activity but the noticeable feeling experienced, especially during the decelerating change of pace, which needs to be sought. Integrating a decelerating temperament with erect posture, deep breathing and habits of making use of opportunities for stretching should result in beneficial consequences for those needing relaxation at work.

II. EASY STRETCHING POSTURES

We turn now from little yogas, easy exercises which can be performed inconspicuously in public, to exercises which approximate some traditional yogic postures in amount of muscle stretching and physical benefit and yet which may seem easier because they are adapted to ways of behaving which are common and natural in Western culture. Whereas yogic postures normally employ no instruments, here frank and unabashed use of instruments—such as beds, chairs and walls—is presupposed. Our treatment will be limited to six varieties, all of which may be performed on a bed, though some other opportunities will also be noted. For the sake of brevity, these will be called by partially descriptive terms: Leg Backward, Leg Frontward, Wall Spread, Wall Walk, Edge Hang and Floor Roll.

A. Leg Backward

Lie on your back on a bed. Move near the side of the bed so that the line of your body is parallel to the side of the bed. First, let the leg nearest to the side drop over the edge until its heel touches the floor, keeping both legs straight. Proceed slowly, comfortably, restfully. Secondly, bend the leg which is touching the floor so that the top of its foot comes to rest on the floor and its knee also rests on the floor, if the bed is low enough. A third stage in this backward bending of a leg is reached when the upper leg attains a vertical position, while its knee and top of foot remain on the floor. Springiness of mattress and distance of top of bed from the floor may require some readjustments. This is about as far as one should expect to go in backward bending but one may, if he wishes, distinguish a fourth stage in which the angle of the bent leg to the one remaining straight on top of the bed is greater than a right angle. Feelings of comfort and relaxation should guide the distance through which the leg is bent, not some specific angle. Repeat the whole process, using the other leg.

B. Leg Frontward

Lie on your front on a bed. Move near the side of the bed, keeping your body parallel to this side. First, allow the leg

PICTOGRAPH CHART NO. 12

EASY STRETCHING POSTURES

A. Leg Backward

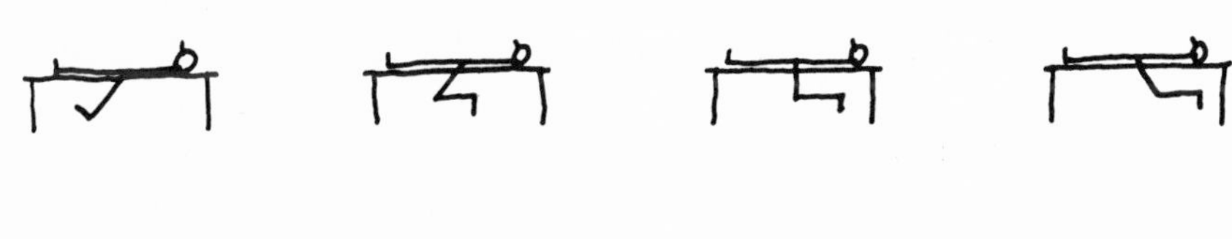

B. Leg Forward

C. Wall Spread

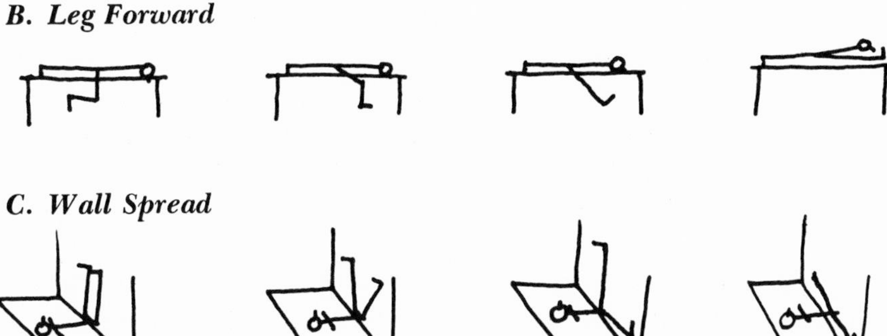

D. Wall Walk

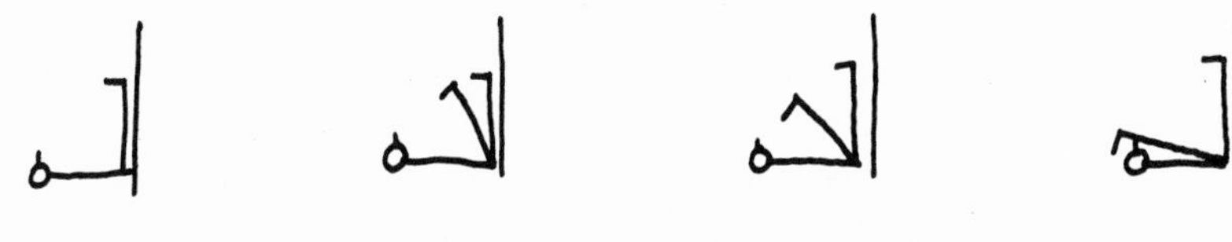

E. Edge Hang

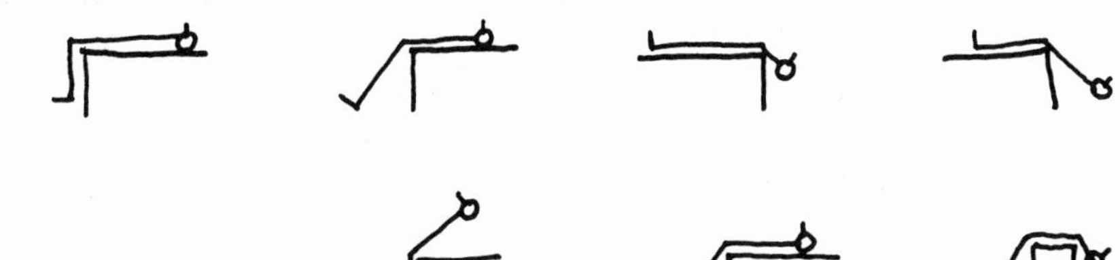

closest to this side to slide over the edge until its knee touches the floor and the top of its foot or toes lie on the floor. If the height and springiness of the bed permit, the upper leg will tend to take a vertical position. Secondly, move this bent leg forward so that its foot moves along the floor until the foot is flat on the floor. This may be a slow process requiring weeks of practice to attain a position in which the foot is flat on the floor and the lower leg is in a vertical position. This is about as far as anyone should expect to go with this exercise, but we mark out two additional stages for those who want something more to aim at. A third stage is reached when the bent leg is straightened. This will involve moving the foot still farther forward along the floor; caution about rushing into this stage should be heeded. A fourth stage is included only for extremists and those trying to prepare themselves for perfecting the various one-leg bending series previously outlined. This stage is reached when the stretched leg is placed upon the head of your bed, with your two legs approximating a straight line but pointing in opposite directions. Try this "leg frontward" exercise over again with the other leg.

C. Wall Spread

Prerequisite to our next kind of exercise is either a bed next to a wall or a bit of floor space next to a wall. The wall must be vacant for about five or six feet. Lie on your back, on the bed or floor. Then move your buttocks to the wall so that you appear to be sitting on the wall while lying on your back. Put both legs up the wall and keep them straight. This position gives many of the advantages of those yogic postures in which the head is held down and the feet up, causing blood pressure to increase in the head and decrease in the feet. Beginners should hold this position only a short time, especially if they notice any discomfort. After one has discovered what dangers or benefits accrue to himself in this position, he will avoid or prolong it, as the case may be.

A second exercise consists in retaining this position except for separating the legs, at first slightly, then a little more, allowing the feet to slide gradually along the wall. Dirty feet or shoes should, of course, be avoided. Keep the legs straight and buttocks close to the wall during this process. Stretching of muscles and ligaments in the crotch occurs. As tension develops in the cords and muscles on the inside of the legs, one should stop and reverse his leg movements until he feels relaxed and completely comfortable. Do not hold this position longer than you can do so with ease.

A third goal to aim at is the stretching of the legs spread on the wall until they form at least a right angle to each other. Many will be unable to attain this position. One possible method consists in keeping one leg in a vertical position on the wall while sliding the other along the wall toward the floor. By alternating legs, a person may find that he makes some progress this way more easily than by moving both legs at the same time. If his seat separates itself from the wall as his legs move, he should adjust his back position so that he touches the wall again.

A fourth posture, which is beyond all except those who can do "the splits," is to allow both legs to slide down the wall until both touch the floor in opposite directions. One who remembers that the goal is the exercise, stretching and relaxation that comes from it, and not the feet touching the floor, will keep himself from feeling frustrated.

D. Wall Walk

The same initial conditions must be attained for this as for the previous kind of exercise. Lie on your back on a bed or floor next to a wall. Keep your buttocks close to the wall while extending both legs straight up in the air flat against the wall. After a period of relaxing in this position, move one foot directly away from the wall a short distance, then move the other. Alternating these movements simulates walking—not walking on the wall but away from it. Here is an exercise which almost any person can profit from and perform with convenience and relative ease. He can continue to take longer and longer steps away from the wall until, perhaps, he can touch his head with his leg. Legs should be kept straight for maximum benefit and the seat should remain against the wall. If one becomes sufficiently limber, he may walk, or rather jump, both legs away from the wall at once. He may even dispense with the wall and "walk in the air." Although most convenient as a home exercise, and one handy for inducing sleep, this and the previous exercise may be adapted to office use, when a person is so inclined, has privacy and can find sufficient spare wall and floor space.

E. Edge Hang

A most effective way to reverse the perpetual forward crouch of the body is to bend over backward with the aid of a piece of furniture such as a bed, chair, table, stand or even a hassock, box or trunk. The simplest, and least effective, is to lie on your back on a bed with your feet hanging over the edge. Since you bend your knees while sitting, the gain comes merely from bending your trunk backward so that it is straight with your upper legs.

But this simple way may be a natural preliminary to a second way, which consists in straightening your legs and sliding your body progressively toward your feet. You may stop at any point and prolong the stretch; but you may notice that stopping so that the edge of the bed comes either just below the buttocks, in the middle of the buttocks or just above them has some different effects. If the posture attained seems sufficiently comfortable, one may hold it for a long time. Too many postures can be maintained for only a moment or a very few minutes.

You may also stretch the top part of your body by letting it hang over the edge. A first way is to let your head hang down over the side of the bed as you lie on your back. Your arms may remain on the bed or fall off, as you like. Your head may rest in this neck-stretching position for quite a while. Further stretching comes naturally from sliding your body gradually off the bed in the direction of your declining head. You may stop, with slightly differing effects, at various places along the way, until your hips reach the edge of the bed. Use of hands and arms in such movement is advisable for beginners, and caution about haste and about moving too far off the bed so that you cannot recover your starting position safely may be needed.

In order to stretch both top and bottom of your body at the same time, you will need to be very tall and have a narrow bed or transfer your operations to a chair or hassock. Bruises may be avoided by becoming concerned in advance about the softness of edges which may be improved with pillows; but pillows have a disadvantage in slipping as you move. The chair should be both solid and stable, for a tip-over might be disastrous. The height of the chair from the floor is a matter to consider, especially by shorter and fatter people. A beginner should start with a very low chair or hassock and change to higher chairs as his ability to adjust to, and profit by, them improves. This exercise may be performed with your clothes on and may be adapted to daytime use if you have office privacy.

Some offices possess only armchairs, so one may wish to be reminded that he can bend backward also with the aid of a desk or table. The table must not only stand firmly but not move when you lean against it. It should be cleared of papers, pens, etc., to avoid the dangers of slipping or rolling off.

Stand with your back to the table and lean backward, slightly at first, then more and more, without using your hands to brace yourself as you move. Care should be taken not to let your feet slip suddenly from under you, for you may fall either backward onto the table or down on the floor. As you bend back farther and farther, you will tend to lie down on the table; one advantage of lying down is that you may be able to rest for a while in this position. Another is that you can then adjust the position of the edge of the table relative to your spine, buttocks and legs, changing positions so as to obtain the maximum ways of stretching. Do not get up too quickly, especially from a tall table or if your legs do not touch the floor, since you may fall on the floor on your face. The sharpness of the edge of the table or desk will pose a problem for some, but an essential precaution consists in becoming assured that the table will not tip over as you move your weight about on it.

Finally, we come to a suggestion which will go beyond what most persons can make use of. In order to stretch backward farther than you can on a chair, a higher piece of furniture, such as a narrow stand or stool, may be sought. Previous precautions need to be magnified since the higher the stand and the narrower its base, the greater the danger of tipping over and falling.

Since one needs to stretch sideways as well as backward to obtain fuller relaxation, one may experiment with bending sideways also as he hangs over the edge of his bed or chair. But I hesitate to make recommendations or even detailed suggestions here, because the risks of injury may multiply as more movements become involved. Personal experimentation here, as elsewhere, seems indicated.

F. Floor Roll

Finally, as should be obvious to almost everyone, rolling along the floor, first in the direction of one side and then of the other, brings many muscles into play. This is a different posture and exercise from what you are accustomed to in your daily work. The lessons taught you as a child, to get up and stay up off the floor, may now have to be unlearned for the sake of health and relaxation. Although you may roll along on your bed, and roll along its edge with part of your body hanging off, with good effect, the solidity of a floor may provide additional massaging benefits and involve less danger of falling off. This is one, too, which may serve as an office relaxation technique for anyone interested.

III. BE PHYSICAL

Man is a psychophysical organism whose mental and physical functions are interdependent, interacting intimately. Physical exertion which exhausts energy supply diminishes mental work capacity. Mental concentration which drains physical energy from the body results in both mental and physical fatigue. The problem facing the responsible business administrator and professional specialist overwhelmed with omnistrain becomes that of how to relax, physically and mentally, in the midst of duties which cannot be unloaded except for short periods. Imbalance of devotion to mental activities, with resulting anxieties, brings a need for balancing emphases upon physical activities. All this is well known to most business and professional people, but the way to accomplishing this balancing seems to escape them.

The purpose of the present section is to offer reminders of ways—most of which are already known to the reader but have been forgotten or at least neglected—which may be exploited for "being physical." When younger, one had sufficient reserve so that he did not need to bother with these ways. Untapped physical strength could be mobilized for energetic sports—such as basketball, tennis, squash, handball, once or twice a week—which provided rejuvenation that lasted for a few days. But aging processes tend to make these sports, as well as golf or hiking, unavailable to many. Reserves of strength built up by morning setting-up exercises may help but the older one gets, the more he feels he cannot spare the energy needed for them, and their effects do not last throughout the day. More little ways of being physical become needed. What are some of them?

In addition to breathing and posture exercises outlined in Chapters III and IV and the little yogas and easy-stretching postures sketched in the two preceding sections, all of which can be used as aids to being physical, the following may be recalled for the reader's consideration. If he is interested enough in his own nervous fatigue to read this volume, he may now find himself in an appropriate psychological mood to resolve to make actual use of neglected items of information which he already knows. These will be merely listed and not discussed in any detail.

A most obvious relaxing technique to take a shower or tub bath—hot or cold or both. A well-equipped office building has facilities. Or a nearby club, hotel or recreational building may serve. Steam baths, Turkish or Russian or Swedish style, may be available in some districts. Although a merely warm shower can help, an increasingly hot or cold shower or bath tends to produce a deeper revitalization and a fuller withdrawal of attention from business matters. What, precisely, are the physical and physiological mechanisms and processes involved, I cannot say, but some transference of accumulated static electricity from body to water occurs; in any case, anyone may notice for himself, if he takes the trouble to observe, that some feeling of relief from nervous tension normally accompanies taking a bath. This knowledge should be exploited oftener during the day by those who have facilities and opportunity. Even a person with severely restricted opportunities may wash his face and hands slowly in hot or cold water, each trip to the restroom, for psycho-physical as well as for sanitary purposes.

Nudity may have virtues for those enjoying a private dressing room. Removal of clothes often results in changes in skin temperature, with an accompanying need for some physiological readjustment. Deliberately seeking a cooler or warmer breeze of air upon the skin may both increase a feeling of being physical and shift attention from business to bodily objects. Simple self-observation tends to have an effect, of the kind already noted in explaining the attentive series in treating the Most Relaxed Posture, which emphasizes physical aspects of the various portions of one's body merely by attending to them. Just looking at your own body may produce a mild form of emphasis upon the physical and thus a little relief from being overwhelmed by the mental.

Some change in the electrostatic conditions of the body in relation to long-worn clothes occurs as one takes off his clothes. Fresh clothes may provide a new set of electrostatic conditions. Attention to the fabrics one wears may offer some clue to rate of nervous fatigue. With rubber soles and heels, rubber-padded chairs, carpeted floors, one's body becomes more insulated from conductors which draw off electrical excesses that may accumulate from prolonged nervous activity. One may find some mental relief from just taking off shoes and socks, even if he cannot attain complete nudity. Contact of feet with a cool floor, or with a metal conductor, can hardly bring us back to childhood enjoyment of barefoot walking, but if moments of relief may be obtained thereby, why should not a business executive exploit this simple technique?

Few can enjoy the convenience of a daily sunbath unless they live in a sunny climate, as I do in Albuquerque, but sunbathing is a well-known device for promoting relaxation. Perspiration, massage and deep breathing, however produced, tend to relax. Drinking, whether hot or cold liquids, has some effect, unless the drinks are gulped so fast as to nullify possible benefits. Coffee breaks have demonstrated their psychophysical values; but the tendency to indulge in stimulants and to shift attention to alternative nervous irritants often partly negates such values. Substitution of yoga breaks for coffee breaks is hardly likely to become popular. But an individual who becomes aware of his own anxiety problems may figure out some way to increase his being physical if he tries.

One such method derived from yogic tradition may be called "water sniffing." This consists simply in sniffing water up the nose. Its effectiveness, for those who have not tried it, may be inferred from recollections about having water in the nose while swimming or bathing. One may experiment by sniffing just a little. The whole inside of his head feels involved. Although one may prefer to use a paper cup, most will hold just a bit of water in the palm of the hand, easily obtainable from a restroom water tap or even a drinking fountain. Hold the cup or palm to the nose and sniff. As one discovers both the effects of different amounts of water and ways for disposing of excesses, he can adjust the amount of water intake. This is a device which can be used many times a day, whether in an office or while traveling about.

Although I refrain from commenting on the roles of diet and laxatives in promoting physical and mental health, and from recommending the virtues of another Hindu practice, namely, fasting, I must recall one current Indian practice which may be worth attention: tea in bed before arising. I was introduced to a custom for improving the daily routine, apparently British in origin, while attending an annual meeting of the Indian Congress of Philosophy at Nagpur University recently. I was awakened, rudely, I thought, by a knock at my door and a bustle and clatter in the hallway of the dormitory where Congress guests were housed. A servant brought in some tea. A friendly gesture, no doubt, but why so early in the morning? Why not let a person get all he can of badly needed sleep? The reason, I found out later, is that serving tea in bed starts one's digestive system working so he can empty his bowels on arising and get a smelly chore out of the way before he bathes and eats his breakfast.

Persons who get up and dash off to work before eliminating excreta commonly find themselves in need of interrupting their work by a trip to the toilet. Or, if work concentration prevents this, poisons accumulate and may be reabsorbed into the system, increasing tendencies toward irritability, nervousness and fatigue. Constipation, headaches and ripening conditions for digestive and circulatory diseases may result.

Although Americans may offer the excuse that such a custom is unfeasible because we lack inexpensive servants, on the other hand we do have plenty of automatic gadgets, to turn on an electric teapot and to awaken us, all without the problems of personal involvement with servants. After tea we can turn over in bed and nap, or go back to sleep, and have a second alarm arouse us for scheduled duties. The sleep we get just before rising in the morning is said to be less restful than what we get earlier in the night anyway. And, starting off the day with a cleansed and replenished digestive system conduces to both physical and mental buoyancy. If one cannot go back to sleep after initial waking, he may either begin mild yogic exercises or think over the day's projects under conditions of morning calm and freshness which may provide a more objective perspective than is possible during the day's practical pressures. Tea in bed may, indeed, prove to be a potent aid to relaxation. Coffee, of course, or wine, fruit juices or carbonated beverages may produce the same kind of result. But the principle of early stimulation of the digestive system remains the same regardless of one's favorite, or most effective, morning stimulant.

IV. ATTENTION TECHNIQUES

An organic relation exists between object and subject, or between the problems which worry us and our worrying about them. The more complex, challenging and serious the problem, the more disturbed, tense and anxious our minds become. The more restless, fatigued, distraught our mental condition, the more problems irritate us. Thus, there exist two ways of approaching problems of anxiety. One is to remove disturbing objects or remove our awareness of them and attention to them. The other is to modify and pacify our mental attitude so that we can manage objective disturbances with greater equanimity. The present section will concern itself with techniques for replacing more disturbing by less disturbing objects. The next section will focus upon methods for replacing more anxious attitudes by less anxious attitudes.

During our normal waking hours, we can hardly escape awareness of objects, except, perhaps, for moments at a time. Attention involves *objects* of attention. But we may deliberately shift our attention from tension-producing objects to mind-quieting objects, at least during those periods when we seek relief from mental strain. The reader may not have realized that most of the exercises and postures treated thus far in the present volume have been activities requiring attention to physical, subjective and relatively quiescent objects. The benefits derivable from such activities are not wholly mental, for each person is a psychophysical being, but they are basically mental as well as physical. In the previous section we emphasized being physical. But one can be physical only by *attending* to being physical. The present and following sections stress mental or subjective approaches to relaxation, not by avoiding the physical, but by intentional effort exerted to turning away from disturbing objects and to presenting an undisturbed mental attitude toward objects.

From myriads of possibilities, we arbitrarily select three pairs of topics around which to organize our remarks: sounds and silence, symbols and nonsymbolic objects, attention to body rhythms and to nonrhythmic status.

A. Sounds

One may shift attention from sounds which communicate ideas to sounds which seem either meaningless or convey meanings so familiar as to be quiescent or even boring. One may, if he wishes, select and attend to some continuing sound, such as the hum of a motor or fan. He may switch on a buzzer and persist in listening to it. He may vocalize continuously a monotone. He may pronounce *om* or *aum,* the Hindu omnisonal sacred symbol. He may turn from a single sound to series, such as a pattern of non-sense symbols. Familiar jingles, or poems or standardized prayers, reiterated again and again, may provide a steadying effect. Chanting or *japa* (continuous repetition of a holy word or prayer or verse) normally has a quieting effect. Persistent listening to sounds which in any way suggest snoring may reduce tension.

"Music hath charms." The restful effects of background music, provided it is soothing and not exciting, have been amply demonstrated. An individual selecting background music for himself should choose familiar, stabilizing tunes rather than new, interesting varieties which arouse a challenge to become acquainted with them—if his motive is entirely that of seeking peace. Some persons may have a music-listening room where they can turn up the volume so loud that their whole being becomes overwhelmed by and carried along with the music. Such a technique almost forcefully eliminates attention to disturbing objects. Some may whistle, hum or sing to themselves. Whatever method is used, while attention is focused upon restful sounds and series of sounds, it is withdrawn from disturbing objects. Such withdrawal provides at least momentary relief from tensions.

B. Silence

For the nervous executive, silence seems outside the range of possibility. Yet deliberate effort to remain silent for a few minutes every hour may have telling effects. Try it. Even where sounds cannot all be shut out, directing attention to silence may have some effect. The person who has a soundproofed music room sufficient for loud music may use the same room for a period of silence. The purpose of this suggestion is not freedom from sounds so that the mind will wander off in imaginative daydreams but so that silence, vacancy, voidness will become the objects of attention. Persons accustomed to idealizing activity may find this little trick too difficult.

C. Symbols

The use of symbols is not in itself conducive to quietude, but if one can employ effective symbols of quietude or symbolic objects which have a quieting effect, he certainly should. General advice here is out of the question, since one man's pacifier may be another man's antagonizer. But when one already appreciates certain symbols as rest-producing, whether they be personal, political, historical, religious or whatnot, he may deliberately keep them around as instruments to produce restfulness. Some find feelings of repose when confronted with a crucifix, a yin-yang symbol, or a national flag. Sometimes a picture of a sedate ancestor, a political hero, an innocent child, a calendar girl, a familiar landscape or a favorite animal creates a mood of stability in a world of bustle. Framed diplomas, certificates, awards and honors may provide an air of stability in the midst of effervescent troubles. Some post notices to themselves, such as THINK; but a blunt QUIET or some more subtle sedative idea might be posted, not for others but for oneself to heed.

D. Nonsymbols

Whereas symbols point, indicate or direct attention—even when at or toward quietude—nonsymbolic objects tend to retain attention in themselves. Thus those who seek the greatest degree of relief from troublesome objects will turn from symbolic to nonsymbolic things. Part of the indescribable ecstasy of a vacation ramble in a meadow often comes from lying on your back and gazing up at a perfectly blue sky. Clouds provide shapes which stimulate imagination. But a completely cloudless sky overwhelms us with its peaceful expanse. A blank wall is a poor substitute but, especially if it happens to be painted with a favorite restful color, it may serve to provide a few moments of rest. A nonobjective painting, provided it is really nonobjective in the sense that it arouses no feelings of controversy or apologetic explanation to unappreciative visitors, may serve this purpose. A bit of statuary which can hold your attention without directing your thoughts may serve the same purpose. If either symbolic or nonsymbolic objects serve to regularize your breathing and straighten your posture as well as to quiet your mind, they will do double or triple duty.

E. Body Rhythms

Those who can remember when rocking chairs and lawn swings produced a soothing effect upon rambunctious spirits may feel inclined to try to recapture their virtues. Are rocking chairs entirely out of place in contemporary offices? Some desk chairs not only swivel but also rock. If this technique works, many office personnel already have their instrument at hand. One may, if he can prop the legs of his chair with a book until his feet no longer reach the floor, swing his lower legs under the desk unobtrusively. One can, if he has a table or desk or stool tall enough, sit on it with a leg hanging down pendulously. One may, while seated, sway his body very slightly from side to side, slowly, ponderously, rhythmically. The point of all these rhythms is that they can serve as foci of your attention when you wish to keep it from pursuing troublesome trains of thought. Recall our earlier mention of Taoist yoga which consists simply in listening to your breathing, with its regular rhythmic movements, until it is heard no more. While listening attentively, your attention is kept away from disturbing thoughts.

F. Attention to Being

Although some will find their distraught minds soothed in some degree by attention to rhythmic motions, unmoved being has a still more quiet nature than moving being. Those who can direct their minds toward being itself should feel themselves coming to a fuller stop than those who find some rest in swaying movement. The ultimate goal of yogic endeavors is to attain *sat-chit-ananda,* blissful awareness of being and nothing else. To have your awareness *(chit)* fully occupied with pure being *(sat)* is believed to be the ultimate in the way of bliss *(ananda).* Without either understanding or seeking the ultimate goal of yogins, one may nevertheless experiment for himself to find whether, and how much, relief from tension may be obtained by focusing and retaining his attention upon being, just being. Care not for the morrow, nor even the next moment. Can you say or think to yourself: "I am"? Not "I am this or that or the other or not this or not that and not that other," but merely "I am"? Practice presence. Some will prefer to "Practice the presence of God," and this will work so long as God is conceived as an unmoved, timeless stability—but not so well if God appears as a perpetually disturbing conscience. Think not "I will," which demands more nervous effort, but "I am," which signifies completion and promotes subsidence of anxiety. Have you tried this one?

We must forego discussion of other suggestions, such as burning incense to provide a pervasive atmosphere of satisfying saturation—for those who might be affected by this—or chewing gum, tasting tobacco, sniffing snuff, half closing the eyelids or crossing one's eyes in nasal or forehead gazing. Once the nature of the problem and varieties of solutions have been opened up for consideration, the intelligent reader will look for devices and methods suited to his own personal needs and circumstances.

V. ATTITUDE TECHNIQUES

Our final suggestions pertain to ways of relaxing while working. In addition to rebuilding energy away from office and work and in addition to preserving and temporarily restoring energy by short periods of resting on the job, there are ways of relaxing not only on the job but while at work. Most of this volume has dealt with methods for re-creating mental and physical pliability in private, some of which may be adapted to office work. The previous section outlined a few ways to withhold attention from troublesome objects by turning it to pacifying objects. Now we turn to the possibilities for relaxing while dealing attentively with troublesome objects.

How may one come to grips with important, complex, perplexing demanding problems for long periods without becoming nervous, fatigued, anxious? Work without worry, responsibility without anxiety, prolonged mental effort without fatigue—this is what every weary business and professional person seeks. Although worry, anxiety and fatigue cannot be eliminated entirely, they may be reduced surprisingly. The way is both easy and hard. It is easy in the sense that all that is required is a change in attitude; it is hard because few can bring about this change of attitude in themselves and maintain it for long periods of time.

In general, this way consists in attaining and retaining the attitude that both the problems you face and the solutions actually attained are just what you want. It requires adoption of an outlook upon life which sees both the annoyances, perplexities and predicaments and the frustrations, defeats and disappointments as your lot, as what life has in store for you, and as constituting what is really best for you. Since you naturally want more than you are going to get and naturally become disappointed when you do not get this, you can accept this way only by becoming aware of a paradox—that you want to be disappointed as much as you are going to be disappointed—and accepting this paradox which you would prefer to believe is not so. Thus, you can adopt this attitude only by overcoming certain natural inclinations. They can be overcome, however, but only by penetrating more deeply into the philosophical foundations of life than most ambitious executives and professional people are willing to do.

Less generally, this way has been depicted differently in the historically developed perspectives now indigenous to various cultural traditions. Four of these will be mentioned. (1) Orthodox Hindus and Buddhists subscribe to a Law of Karma which justly determines their lot in life and their predicaments each day. To want their life and its daily provocations to be different from the way they are is to demand injustice and create further misery for themselves. (2) Chinese Taoists and Confucianists see Tao, the Way of Life, as naturally good and as made evil by man's willful intervention in the natural course of Nature's way. "Those too eager for activity soon become fatigued. Such impatience is against Nature. What is against Nature dies young" (*Tao Teh King* by Lao Tzu, my edition, page 87). (3) Ancient Greek ideals endowed Western civilization with the idea of "Fate," which contributed to the development of mechanism and determinism. One who believes that both his business circumstances and his ability and will to deal with them are fated or determined may keep in awareness a realization that greater anxiety about one's lot is foolish when it merely creates discomfort for himself. (4) Theists, including many Jews, Christians and Moslems, conceive the world and life as determined by an omnipotent, omnibenevolent will of God, whether arbitrary or necessary. The way to acceptance of the paradox of wanting what you are going to get even when you seem not to want it is to surrender your will completely to the will of God.

This way, sketched above first very generally and then as depicted generally in four cultural traditions, may be illustrated in somewhat more specific ways. The completeness with which a person has arranged his preconceptions in accordance with his native culture will determine, to a large extent, his ability to accept a specific explanation of how to assent to this way and its paradoxes. We arbitrarily limit our treatment to four examples: religion, prayer, Zen and humor.

A. Religion

Being religious consists in maintaining an attitude of "yea-saying," of saying "yes" to one's lot. Theists conceive yea-saying as saying yes to the "Will of God." Yogins, Vedantists and many Buddhists interpret yea-saying as surrender ("extinction") of desire for illusory objects and values. Taoists depict yea-saying as "Let Nature (Tao) take its course." Confucianists add to yea-saying a willingness to conform to the principle of reciprocity. (See my edition of *Tao Teh King,* pages 107–114.) Mechanistic determinists and fatalists may say yes by quoting Omar Khayyam, "Take the Cash and let the Credit go" for "The Wordly Hope men set their Hearts upon Turns Ashes—or it Prospers; and . . . lighting a little hour or two—is gone."

However conceived, the task is the same: wanting what you are going to get or, better, enjoying what you have as what you now want. Whether inspired by the words of Jesus ("Care not for the morrow") or Lao Tzu ("The way to succeed is this: having achieved your goal be satisfied not to go further" [*ibid.*, page 87]) or Buddha ("Destruction of craving is Nirvana" [see my *Philosophy of the Buddha*, page 59]), one must somehow realize that his own desirousness is the main source of his anxiety and that relief from anxiety can be attained only by reducing the intensity of the zeal, ambition and insistence with which he wants to remake the world and "mold it closer to his own desires."

The religious task is difficult because the world is complex and one's desires arise spontaneously. How can one ever want precisely what he is going to get or exactly what he has when the very nature of wanting is to desire something which is lacking? An executive is committed to wanting to solve problems which, when they present themselves, are not yet solved. The very nature of his task is to want what he does not yet have. He cannot escape such wanting unless he abandons his responsibilities, and this he cannot do and remain an executive.

But the religious task is not the naïvely apparent solution of abandoning business, but the more subtle one of retaining a pervasive realization of wanting the worries which business entails so long as one wants to remain in business. So long as retention of awareness of a feeling of satisfaction about being in business and being responsible predominates one's mentality, then a particular trouble may be attended to with minimal anxiety. But when one concentrates his whole attention upon the frustrating aspects of a specific predicament, his anxiety may overwhelm him and fatigue him. The attitude technique suggested here consists in "seeing life steadily and seeing it whole." When you want neither more nor less of anxiety than you are going to get, then "wherever you go, you shall go in comfort" (*ibid.*, page 17). (For further suggestions about relaxing religiously, see my *The World's Living Religions,* Dell Publishing Co., Inc., New York, 1964.)

B. Prayer

Turning from religion generally to prayer as a more specific religious technique, we must notice, first, that many different kinds of prayer exist and that we limit our consideration to two: those prayers in which we express our desire to have things other than as they are and those in which we express our willingness to accept our lot of satisfactions and frustrations for what they are. A person who uses prayer as an occasion for becoming aware that what he really wants is what he deserves, and neither less nor more than he deserves, thereby puts himself in a frame of mind which helps him to realize that he is already getting what he wants. He who learns how to "pray without ceasing," in this latter sense, finds himself quite relaxed while doing business. Most of us cannot attend to too many things at the same time, so specific time deliberately devoted to pursuing acts of attention for realizing that we already have what we want, at least in a large measure, may serve as specific relaxing periods. Prayer, in this sense, functions as an aid to relaxation.

Prayer, and prayer periods, may have other uses in promoting peaceful, confident living. The lazy may use it for arousing resolve for action. The dying may use it to sustain hope. But when the fatigued use it to whip their consciences into goading themselves further, or to agonize over deficiencies, or to aggravate fears about guilt or depravity, or to suffer morbid dismay about failure to overdo their abilities, surely they misuse it. To pray anxiously serves to aggravate anxiety. To pray for peace peacefully itself aids in bringing peace on earth. Unfortunately, those who interpret The Lord's Prayer "Give us this day . . ." in such a way as to emphasize the "gimme" more than we would otherwise have coming, rather than "this day" in which we should "care not for the morrow," are ill prepared to use such a prayer to reduce anxiety. One had better simply repeat again and again the "Amen" or *aum,* or the above-noted "I am," to emphasize feelings of sufficiency and satisfaction, or of already *being* rather than awaiting more becoming, than dream about what things more he might yet be given or may yet get, when what he most needs given him is relief from anxiety.

C. Zen

We introduce Zen in a volume on yoga not as a substitute but as a supplement. The demonstrable values of yogic breathing and posture exercises, both for physical and mental health, as outlined in Chapter II, are in no way diminished by indicating that some additional values may be found in Zen by those seeking aid for relaxation. Although Zen has historical roots in Hindu yoga, Zen developed an emphasis upon relaxing while acting instead of relaxing by refraining from action. Yogic exercises may be used to restore energy which buoys up vitality during work; Zen attitudes may be used to refrain from using energy wastefully during work. The yogin seeks to rest by withdrawal from tension; to be in Zen is to be finding rest within tension. The yogin tries to withdraw his attention from disturbing mental activities; when in Zen, one may attend to vigorous mental activities constantly without feelings of disturbance.

Zen, or *Satori,* once you are in it, consists of an alert, sensitive, appreciative attitude in which you completely accept each presented challenge, or lack of it, as just what you now want. Concern for the future or past as such is missing. No regrets about the past, no fears about the future, no dissatisfaction with the present disturb the spontaneous and instant assent to dealing positively (appreciatively) with whatever appears for attention. I cannot take time to explain how Zen occurs, why one may only with great difficulty, if ever, get into it, or what preconceptions must be overcome in order to begin to grasp its nature. (See section on Zen in Chapter IX of *The World's Living Religions.*) But I do hope to whet curiosity somewhat so that those who do have additional capacity to deal with another paradoxical Oriental way to relaxation may look farther. Those who dislike paradoxes, however, should avoid wasting their time with Zen.

At first glance, Zen, like yoga, seems antagonistic to business and professional endeavor. But deeper penetration reverses the picture and one may discover that both, or at least the principles embodied in both, are essential to successful business practice and satisfactory living. When in Zen, one does not try to impose his will upon life but he wills to enjoy it as it is. One does not plan his future. But business executives must plan and, indeed, often serve as full-time planners. Zen, used by Samurai warriors and Kamikaze pilots, is relevant everywhere. But, paradoxically and dialectically, in Zen, when one is confronted with plans and need for business planning, he accepts them appreciatively as just what he wanted to be confronted with at the moment. He thus adopts an unplanned attitude toward planning; and he plans and plans without planning either to plan or not to plan. When you can do this, you can enjoy a kind or degree of relaxation, while working vigorously, which cannot be obtained in any other way. One may use Zen in business provided he subordinates Zen to business and not business entirely to Zen.

D. Humor

Nothing is more relaxing than a genuine, good-hearted, deep-seated laugh. A person who has been lucky enough to have acquired a ready sense of humor enjoys his work and suffers less from working fatigue and anxiety than those whose funnybone has atrophied or whose susceptibilities to humor must be stimulated by others before they can function. We refer here not to artificial intrusion of stale jokes into valuable business conversation, but to one's attitude of willingness to enjoy life as a great joke even when it is a joke on him. Lin Yutang has expressed as well as anyone the urbane spirit pervading Chinese culture which embodies in its mature citizens a characteristic called "mellowness." (See his *The Importance of Living* and *My Country and My People.*)

The executive cannot easily laugh at a serious mistake. But he can laugh at the fact that his failure to laugh makes him an all-the-more pitiful creature. You can hardly entertain a sense of humor without standing back, so to speak, and taking a more distant and objective view of what you are laughing at. This psychical backward step automatically broadens your perspective in such a way that you will see your momentary troubles as less than the whole world. It places them in a truer perspective, and permits you to reduce your tension and anxiety over them in some degree, as well as massaging your muscles and inner organs when the laugh is hearty enough. Business is serious. But business without humor is too serious.

In concluding this section on Attitude Techniques, I must remark that which "attitude methods" may be used, and the extent to which they can be used by individuals, will depend somewhat upon the philosophical preconceptions conditioning their outlooks. Surely all philosophies, religions and business psychologies must deal effectively with the problem of how to relax, if they are to be wholly adequate. The writer has refrained from explicit introduction of his own philosophy, Organicism, into this work. For those who are curious, preliminary sketches of it are in his *Philosophy, An Introduc-*

tion, Chapter 20 and page 439, and his *Types of Intuition.* A technical tidbit presented popularly distinguishes between "Aesthetic Experience and Moral Experience." (See *The Journal of Philosophy,* Sept. 25, 1958, pages 37–846.) And a provocative challenge appears as "The New Philosophy Names Its Enemies" (*New Mexico Quarterly,* Summer, 1959).

VI. GROUP THERAPY

Most readers of this volume should be relatively self-sufficient, self-directing and practical people who can figure out and apply ideas which they may put to work by themselves. But since many have been conditioned to seek solutions to anxiety problems socially or have exhausted their ingenuity elsewhere, some further suggestions may be welcomed. One can, of course, seek instruction in how to practice *asanas* and breathing exercises. Yogic tradition warns that a person cannot learn to perform these properly by himself. Hence, he is advised to seek a guru or teacher. Competent instructors in yogic asanas are available in major cities in the United States and Canada, but they remain few and scattered. No standards as yet exist for yogic instruction, so each American yogin is free to offer his services as he pleases. Some limit themselves to instruction in meditation entirely without practicing asanas, so will refuse to provide assistance here. Some hold the more ultimate goal of yogic endeavors so firmly in mind that they may refuse to instruct persons who have only a lower end in view. Some will insist that *kundalini* and the arousing of mystical powers are more important than the merely preparatory asanas. But a discriminating person may still be able to obtain assistance. Also, reliable instruction in yogic postures may be obtained from teachers who are not yogins.

Classes in yoga are offered in many places. One remarkable

institution, the Self-Realization Fellowship of America, with headquarters in Los Angeles and branches in several states and countries, not only offers posture instruction but conducts weekly group meetings in which energizing techniques are taught and practiced by groups. The leaders of this Fellowship have been adept at adopting and adapting yogic ideas to needs of Americans. Their use of chair-seated meditation postures in place of floor-seated postures has been mentioned previously. Their "double-breathing" exercise can be used by individuals at work as well as in groups. Group endeavors may be organized by local clubs, churches or YMCAs and group support of competent yogic instruction may be arranged. Group action, however, remains a means to an end. For your anxieties are your own, and your own will and willingness play the most important role in your success in attaining and retaining relaxation.

BIBLIOGRAPHY

Books consulted during the preparation of this volume include the following:

Alain, *Yoga for Perfect Health,* Thorsons Publishers Ltd., London, 1957, 1959.

Bahm, Archie J., *Yoga: Union with the Ultimate,* Frederick Ungar Publishing Co., New York, 1961.

Behanan, Kovoor T., *Yoga: A Scientific Evaluation,* The Macmillan Co., New York, 1937.

Bernard, Theos, *Hatha Yoga,* Columbia University Press, New York, 1944.

Bharati, Yogi Suddhananda, *Yoga for the Modern World,* Ganesh and Co., Ltd., Madras, 1955.

Bragdon, Claude, *Yoga for You,* Alfred A. Knopf, New York, 1943, 1959.

Carlson, Anton J., and Victor Johnson, *The Machinery of the Body,* Fourth Edition, University of Chicago Press, 1937, 1953.

Chidananda, Swami, *Forest Academy Lectures on Yoga,* the Yoga-Vedanta Forest Academy, Rishikesh, Himalayas, 1960.

Danielou, Alain, *Yoga: The Method of Reintegration,* University Books, Book Publishers, New York, 1949, 1955.

Day, Harvey, *The Study and Practice of Yoga,* Thorsons Publishers Ltd., London, 1933, 1959.

Déchanet, J. M., O.S.B., *Christian Yoga,* Harper and Brothers, Publishers, New York, 1956, 1960.

Devi, Indra, *Forever Young, Forever Healthy,* Prentice-Hall, Inc., Englewood Cliffs, New Jersey, 1953.

Devi, Indra, *Yoga for Americans,* Prentice-Hall, Inc., Englewood Cliffs, New Jersey, 1959.

Gunaji, N. V., *Scientific and Efficient Breathing,* Nagesh Vasudev Gunajii, Bombay, 1948.

Kuvalayananda, Swami, *Pranayama,* Parts I and II, Swami Kuvalayananda, Lonavla, Bombay, 1931, 1950, 1958.

Marshall, Clyde, and Edgar L. Lazier, *An Introduction to Human Anatomy,* Fourth Edition, W. B. Saunders Co., Philadelphia, 1935, 1955.

Morehouse, Laurence E., and August T. Miller, *Physiology of Exercise,* Third Edition, C. V. Mosby Co., St. Louis, 1948, 1959.

Narayananda, Swami, *The Secrets of Prana, Pranayama and Yoga-Asanas,* N. K. Prasad and Co., Rishikesh, 1959.

Pratinidhi, Shrimant Balasahib Pandit, *The Ten-Point Way to Health,* J. M. Dent and Sons Ltd., London, 1938, 1956.

Ramacharaka, Yogi, *Hatha Yoga,* The Yogi Publication Society, and L. N. Fowler and Co. Ltd., London, no date given.

Ramacharaka, Yogi, *The Hindu-Yogi Science of Breath,* The Yogi Publication Society, Chicago, 1903, and L. N. Fowler and Co. Ltd., London, no date given.

Rele, V. G., *Yoga Asanas for Health and Vigour,* D. B. Taraporevala Sons and Co. Private Ltd., Bombay, 1960.

Shastri, Hari Prasad, *Yoga,* W. and G. Foyle Ltd., London, 1957.

Sivananda, Swami, *Yoga Asanas,* Revised Tenth Edition, P. K. Vinayagam and Co., Madras, 1934, 1955.

Sivananda, Swami, *Yogic Home Exercises,* D. B. Taraporevala Sons and Co. Private Ltd., Bombay, 1944, 1959.

Sivananda, Swami, *Yogic Therapy,* Swami Bijnanananda Saraswati, Kamakhya, Assam, 1950, 1957,

Spring, Clara, and Madeleine Goss, *Yoga for Today,* Henry Holt and Co., New York, 1959.

Vishnudevananda, Swami, *The Complete Illustrated Book of Yoga,* Julian Press, Inc., New York, 1960.

Wood, Ernest, *Yoga,* Penguin Books Ltd., Harmondsworth, 1959.

Woodroffe, John, *The Serpent Power,* Sixth Edition, Ganesh and Co. Private Ltd., Madras, 1918, 1958.

Yesudian, Selvarajan, and Elisabeth Haich, *Yoga and Health,* Harper and Brothers, New York, 1953.

Yogendra, Shri, *Yoga: Personal Hygiene,* Vols. I and II, The Yoga Institute, Santa Cruz, Bombay, 1931, 1958.

Yogendra, Shri, *Yoga: Physical Education* (paperback reprint entitled: *Yoga: Asanas Simplified*), The Yoga Institute, Bombay, 1928, 1956.

Yogendra, Shrimati Sitadevi, *Yoga: Physical Education* (for women), The Yoga Institute, Bombay, 1934, 1947.

ACKNOWLEDGMENTS

Three kinds of acknowledgments are needed, namely, to certain men for ideas, to several publishers for quotations, and to those who assisted in producing the photographic plates.

For ideas, I am most indebted to three men, Swami Sivananda, Swami Kuvalayananda and Swami Vishnudevananda, in that order. Swami Sivananda (His Holiness Sri Swami Sivananda Saraswati, of Ananda Kutir, Rishikesh, Himalayas), a lifelong yogin and guru, teacher of many hatha yogins, is author of *Yoga Asanas,* among other works. I have used mainly his Revised Tenth Edition, published by P. K. Vinayagam and Co., Madras, 1955. Swami Kuvalayananda, whose *Pranayama, Parts I and II,* first appeared in 1853, presided over an Ashram which later, in 1932, established a Yogic Health Center in Bombay. I have profited by the 1950 and 1958 editions published by Kuvalyadhama, Lonavla, Bombay, especially regarding breathing exercises. Swami Vishnudevananda, student of Sivananda, Director of the Sivananda Yoga Vedanta Center, Montreal, has taught hatha yoga in many places in the United States and Canada, notably at the Sivananda Yoga Vedanta Center, Cornish Arms Hotel, New York City, for many years. His *Complete Illustrated Book of Yoga,* published by Julian Press, Inc., New York, 1960, having 146 photographs of poses, has been cited several times in the present volume.

I have profited also from illustrations and descriptions by C. Bernard, B. Tesniere, M.D., and Brahmachari Leland appearing almost monthly from 1952 to 1962 in the *Self-Realization Magazine,* published by the Self-Realization Fellowship, Los Angeles.

For quotations and other references, I am indebted to many publishers. Specific acknowledgment is due Harper and Brothers, New York, and Burnes and Oates Ltd., London, for permission to quote passages from J. M. Déchanet's *Christian Yoga,* published by them in 1960 as a translation from the original French edition, *La Voie du Silence,* published by Desclée de Brouwer, 1956.

For photographic plates, I am indebted to Glenn Wills, KNME-TV cameraman, for poses; to William M. Shimer, KNME-TV Director of Public Relations, for photography; and to Claude Hempen, Manager of KNME-TV, for use of a studio. The pictures do not represent poses of a professional yogin but of a self-taught amateur with very little practice, illustrating how easily an untaught American can approximate traditional standard yogic postures. All of the pictures were taken during one evening and the next morning. There would have been more headstand pictures, but Mr. Wills suffered from a sunburned head.

LIST OF ASANAS (Sanskrit-English)

Adva-ardha-padmasana, Prone Half-Lotus Posture
Adva-matsyasana, Prone Fish Posture
Advasana, Prone Posture
Anjaneyasana, Leg-split Posture
Ardha-bandha-padmasana, Modified Bound Lotus Posture
Ardha-bhujangasana, Half-cobra Posture
Ardha-chakrasana, Half-circle Posture
Ardha-chandrasana, Half-moon Posture
Ardha-halasana, Half-plough Posture
Ardha-kurmasana, Half-tortoise Posture
Ardha-matsyendrasana, Half-spinal-twist Posture
Ardha-padmasana, Half-lotus Posture
Ardha-salabhasana, Half-locust Posture
Ardha-savasana, Semi-supine Posture
Ardha-urdhva-padmasana, Half-aloft Lotus Posture
Bakasana, Crane, or Heron, Posture
Baddha Padmasana (*see* Bandha Padmasana)
Bandha Padmasana, Bound Lotus Posture
Bhadrasana, Gentle, or Auspicious, Posture
Bhujangasana, Cobra, or Snake or Serpent, Posture
Chakrasana, Circle, or Wheel, Posture
Dhanurasana, Bow Posture
Dradhasana, Firm (side) Posture
Eka-padasana, One-foot Posture
Garbhasana, Foetus Posture
Garudasana, Eagle Posture
Gomukhasana, Cowface Posture
Gorakshasana, Cowherd, or Goatherd, Posture
Guptasana, Hidden Posture
Halasana, Plough, or Plow, Posture

Hamasana (*see* Mayurasana)
Hastapadangustasana, Hand-foot-stretching Posture
Jalandhara Bandha, Chin Lock
Kakasana, Crow Posture
Karnapitasana, Ear-covering Posture
Khandapitasana, Crippled, or Clubfoot, Posture
Kukkutasana, Cock Posture
Kurmasana, Tortoise Posture
Lolasana, Swinging Posture
Makarasana, Crocodile, or Dolphin, Posture
Mandukasana, Frog Posture
Matsyasana, Fish Posture
Matsyendrasana, Spinal-twist Posture, or Matsyendra's Posture
Mayurasana, Peacock Posture
Mayura-padamasana, Peacock Lotus Posture
Mrtasana (*see* Savasana)
Muktasana, Free, or Freed, Posture
Natarajasana, Nataraja's Posture
Nauli, Stomach, or Abdominal, Exercise
Navasana, Boat Posture
Padahastasana, Feet-and-Hands Posture
Padangushtanasana, Balancing Posture
Padasana, Foot Posture
Padmasana, Lotus Posture
Parvatasana, Mountain Posture
Paschimottanasana, Back-stretching Posture
Pasini Mudra, Noose Posture
Pavanmuktasana, Wind-freeing Posture
Prarthanasana, Prayer Posture
Purna Chakrasana, Full-circle Posture
Purna Halasana, Full-plough Posture
Purna Padasana, Erect-standing Posture
Salabhasana, Locust Posture
Samasana, Symmetrical, or Equal, Posture
Samkatasana, Contracted, or Dangerous, Posture
Sarvanga-ardha-padmasana, Shoulderstand Half-lotus Posture
Sarvangasana, Shoulderstand, or All-members, Posture

Sarvanga-padmasana, Shoulderstand Lotus Posture
Sarvanga-vajrasana, Shoulderstand Thunderbolt Posture
Savasana, Most Relaxed, or Supine, or Corpse, Posture
Siddhasana, Adept's, or Perfect, or Perfected, Posture
Simhasana, Lion Posture
Shirshasana (*see* Sirshasana)
Sirsha-ardha-padamasana, Headstand Half-lotus Posture
Sirsha-padmasana, Headstand Lotus Posture
Sirshasana, Headstand, or Topsy-turvy, Posture
Sirsha-vajrasana, Headstand Thunderbolt Posture
Sthasana, Stable Posture
Sthitasana, Standing Upright Posture
Sthita-paschimottasana, Standing Back-stretching Posture
Sukhasana, Easy Posture
Supta-ardha-padmasana, Supine Half-lotus Posture
Supta-padmasana, Supine Lotus Posture
Supta-vajrasana, Supine, or Sleeping, Thunderbolt Posture
Surya Namaskar, Sun-worship Posture Series
Svastikasana, Prosperous, or Auspicious, Posture
Swastikasana (*see* Svastikasana)
Tolangulasana, Balance Posture
Trikonasana, Triangle Posture
Tulasana (*see* Tolangulasana)
Tulitasana (*see* Tolangulasana)
Uddiyana, Abdominal Posture
Uddiyana Bandha, Bound Abdominal Posture
Urdhva-padmasana, Aloft, or Elevated, Lotus Posture
Ustrasana, Camel Posture
Utkatasana, Difficult, or Hazardous, Posture
Uttana Kurmasana, Upside-down Tortoise Posture
Uttana Padasana, Raised-feet Posture
Utthita Kurmasana, Raised Tortoise Posture
Utthita Padmasana, Elevated Lotus Posture
Vajrasana, Thunderbolt Posture
Vakrasana, Twisting Posture
Vatyasana, Banyan Tree Posture
Virasana, Hero Posture

LIST OF POSTURES (English-Sanskrit)

The Abdominal Posture, Nauli
The Abdominal Posture, Uddiyana
The Adamantine Posture (*see* Thunderbolt Posture)
The Adept's Posture, Siddhasana
The All-members Posture, Sarvangasana
The Aloft Lotus Posture, Urdhva-padmasana
The Auspicious Posture, Bhadrasana
The Auspicious Posture, Svastikasana
The Back-stretching Posture, Paschimottanasana
The Balance Posture, Tolangulasana, etc.
The Balancing Posture, Padangushtanasana
The Banyan Tree Posture, Vatyasana
The Boat Posture, Navasana
The Bound Abdominal Posture, Uddiyana Bandha
The Bound Lotus Posture, Bandha Padmasana
The Bow Posture, Dhanurasana
The Camel Posture, Ustrasana
The Candle Posture (*see* Shoulderstand Posture)
The Chin Lock, Jalandhara Bandha
The Circle Posture, Chakrasana
The Clubfoot Posture, Khandapitasana
The Cobra Posture, Bhujangasana
The Cock Posture, Kukkutasana
The Contracted Posture, Samkatasana
The Corpse Posture, Savasana
The Cowface Posture, Gomukhasana
The Cowherd Posture, Gorakshasana
The Crane Posture, Bakasana
The Crippled Posture, Khandapitasana
The Crocodile Posture, Makarasana

The Crow Posture, Kakasana
The Dangerous Posture, Samkatasana
The Difficult Posture, Utkatasana
The Dolphin Posture, Makarasana
The Eagle Posture, Garudasana
The Ear-covering Posture, Karnapitasana
The Easy Posture, Sukhasana
The Elevated Lotus Posture, Utthita Padmasana
The Equal Posture, Samasana
The Erect-standing Posture, Purna Padasana
The Feet-and-Hands Posture, Padahastasana
The Firm (Side) Posture, Dradhasana
The Fish Posture, Matsyasana
The Foetus Posture, Garbhasana
The Foot Posture, Padasana
The Free (Freed) Posture, Muktasana
The Frog Posture, Mandukasana
The Full-circle Posture, Purna Chakrasana
The Full-plough Posture, Purna Halasana
The Gentle Posture, Bhadrasana
The Goatherd Posture, Gorakshasana
The Half-aloft Lotus Posture, Ardha-urdhva-padmasana
The Half-circle Posture, Ardha-chakrasana
The Half-cobra Posture, Ardha-bhujangasana
The Half-locust Posture, Ardha-salabhasana
The Half-lotus Posture, Ardha-padmasana
The Half-moon Posture, Ardha-chandrasana
The Half-plough Posture, Ardha-halasana
The Half-spinal-twist Posture, Ardha-Matsyendrasana
The Half-tortoise Posture, Ardha-kurmasana
The Hand-foot-stretching Posture, Hastapadangustasana
The Hazardous Posture, Utkatasana
The Headstand Half-lotus Posture, Sirsha-ardha-padmasana
The Headstand Lotus Posture, Sirsha-padmasana
The Headstand Posture, Sirshasana
The Headstand Thunderbolt Posture, Sirsha-vajrasana
The Hero Posture, Virasana

The Hidden Posture, Guptasana
The Leg-split Posture, Anjaneyasana
The Lion Posture, Simhasana
The Locust Posture, Salabhasana
The Lotus Posture, Padmasana
Matsyendra's Posture, Matsyendrasana
The Modified Bound Lotus Posture, Ardha-bandha-padmasana
The Most Relaxed Posture, Savasana
The Mountain Posture, Parvatasana
Nataraja's Posture, Natarajasana
The Noose Posture, Pasini Mudra
The One-foot Posture, Eka-padasana
The Peacock Posture, Mayurasana
The Peacock Lotus Posture, Mayura-padmasana
The Perfect (Perfected) Posture, Siddhasana
The Plough Posture, Halasana
The Pole Posture (*see* Headstand Posture)
The Prayer Posture, Prarthanasana
The Prone Posture, Advasana
The Prone Fish Posture, Adva-matsyasana
The Prone Half-lotus Posture, Adva-ardha-padmasana
The Prosperous Posture, Svastikasana
The Raised-feet Posture, Uttana Padasana
The Raised-tortoise Posture, Utthita-kurmasana
The Scorpion Posture, Vrichikasana
The Semi-supine Posture, Adhva-savasana
The Serpent Posture, Bhujangasana
The Shoulderstand Posture, Sarvangasana
The Shoulderstand Half-lotus Posture, Sarvanga-ardha-padmasana
The Shoulderstand Lotus Posture, Sarvanga-padmasana
The Shoulderstand Thunderbolt Posture, Sarvanga-vajrasana
The Side Pose (*see* Firm Pose)
The Sleeping Thunderbolt Posture, Supta-vajrasana
The Snake Posture, Bhujangasana
The Spinal-twist Posture, Matsyendrasana
The Stable Posture, Sthasana
The Standing Back-stretching Posture, Sthita-paschimottanasana

The Standing Upright Posture, Sthitasana
The Stick Posture, Yastikasana
The Stomach Exercise, Nauli
The Sun Worship Series, Surya Namaskar
The Supine Posture, Savasana
The Supine Half-lotus Posture, Supta-ardha-padmasana
The Supine Lotus Posture, Supta-padmasana
The Supine Thunderbolt Posture, Supta-vajrasana
The Swinging Posture, Lolasana
The Symmetrical Posture, Samasana
The Thunderbolt Posture, Vajrasana
The Topsy-turvy Posture, Sirshasana
The Tortoise Posture, Kurmasana
The Tree Posture, Vrikshasana
The Triangle Posture, Trikonasana
The Twisting Posture, Vakrasana
The Upside-down Tortoise Posture, Uttana-kurmasana
The Wheel Posture, Chakrasana
The Whole-body Posture, Sarvangasana
The Wind-relieving Posture, Pavanmuktasana
The Yoga Posture, Yogasana, Yoga Mudra

Index